Lesser Forefoot Surgery

Edited by

Joshua Gerbert, DPM, FACFAS

Professor and Former Chair, Department of Podiatric Surgery, California School of Podiatric Medicine at Samuel Merritt University, Oakland, CA;

Chief of Podiatric Surgery Department, St. Mary's Medical Center, San Francisco, CA;

Fellow, American College of Foot and Ankle Surgeons;

Board certified in foot and ankle surgery, American Board of Podiatric Surgery;

Private practice in San Francisco, CA

Published by
Data Trace Publishing Company
P.O. Box 1239
Brooklandville, Maryland 21022-9978
410-494-4994   Fax: 410-494-0515
www.datatrace.com/medical

Copyright 2009, Data Trace Publishing Company
All rights reserved, First Edition
Printed in the United States of America

ISBN: 978-1-57400-126-6

Care has been taken to confirm the accuracy of the information presented and to describe generally accepted practices. However, the authors, editor, and publisher are not responsible for errors or omissions or for any consequences from application of the information in this book and make no warranty, expressed or implied, with respect to the currency, completeness, or accuracy of the contents of the publication. Application of this information in a particular situation remains the professional responsibility of the practitioner.

The authors, editor, and publisher have exerted every effort to ensure that drug selection and dosage set forth in this text are in accordance with current recommendations and practice at the time of publication. However, in view of ongoing research, changes in government regulations, and the constant flow of information relating to drug therapy and drug reactions, the reader is urged to check the package insert for each drug for any change in indications and dosage and for added warnings and precautions. This is particularly important when the recommended agent is a new or infrequently employed drug.

The authors and editor have endeavored to locate the copyright owners and to request permission for the use of all copyrighted material reprinted in this book; except for those references deemed to be fair use under the Copyright Act.

Library of Congress Cataloging-in-Publication Data

Lesser forefoot surgery / edited by Joshua Gerbert. — 1st ed.

   p. ; cm.

  ISBN 978-1-57400-126-6

  1. Foot—Surgery—Textbooks.   I. Gerbert, Joshua. [DNLM: 1. Forefoot, Human—pathology. 2. Forefoot, Human—surgery. 3. Foot Diseases—surgery. WE 880 L638 2008]
  RD563.L375 2008
  617.5'85059—dc22

                                                                      2008053663

Contributors

Albert E. Burns, DPM, FACFAS
Past Dean for Academic Affairs and Professor and Former Chair, Department of Podiatric Surgery, California School of Podiatric Medicine at Samuel Merritt University, Oakland, CA.
Fellow, American College of Foot and Ankle Surgeons.
Board certified in foot and ankle surgery, American Board of Podiatric Surgery.
Private practice in Pacifica, CA.

Joel R. Clark, DPM, FACFAS
Professor, Department of Podiatric Surgery, California School of Podiatric Medicine at Samuel Merritt University, Oakland, CA.
Fellow, American College of Foot and Ankle Surgeons.
Board certified in foot and ankle surgery, American Board of Podiatric Surgery.
Private practice in San Francisco, CA.

William M. Jenkin, DPM, FACFAS
Professor and Chair, Department of Podiatric Surgery, California School of Podiatric Medicine at Samuel Merritt University, Oakland, CA.
Fellow, American College of Foot and Ankle Surgeons.
Board certified in foot and ankle surgery, American Board of Podiatric Surgery.
Private practice in San Francisco, CA.

Joshua Gerbert, DPM, FACFAS
Professor and Former Chair, Department of Podiatric Surgery, California School of Podiatric Medicine at Samuel Merritt University, Oakland, CA.
Chief of Podiatric Surgery Department, St. Mary's Medical Center, San Francisco, CA.
Fellow, American College of Foot and Ankle Surgeons.
Board certified in foot and ankle surgery, American Board of Podiatric Surgery.
Private practice in San Francisco, CA.

Preface

The surgery department at the California School of Podiatric Medicine at Samuel Merritt University has believed for some time that there were no textbooks which adequately cover surgical correction of pathology involving lesser forefoot pathology. While there are a few textbooks that cover certain aspects of this subject, none provided an in-depth perspective.

This text will present the pathomechanics of the most common lesser forefoot pathologies which can not be found in any current published textbook. It will also present in a "cookbook" format the indications and contraindications for the common surgical procedures utilized to correct lesser forefoot pathology along with a detailed description of the surgical techniques. Each chapter involving the surgical procedures will also discuss the recommended postoperative management and the inherent complications associated with the procedure. This textbook is a compilation of 30 years of experiences by the members of the surgery department at the California School of Podiatric Medicine in evaluating and determining the most effective surgical therapies for the more common problems of the lesser forefoot.

This textbook is intended for the podiatric student, the podiatric and orthopedic resident and the practicing podiatrists and for those orthopedists who treat forefoot conditions. It is my hope that this text will serve to assist in better understanding, better evaluation, more effective surgical management and proper postoperative management for the more common lesser forefoot pathologies encountered in practice.

I would like to thank my wife Barbara for allowing me the time to once again undertake a medical textbook project and my colleagues in the Department of Podiatric Surgery at the California School of Podiatric Medicine who were willing to share their years of clinical and academic experiences by agreeing to write specific chapters in this text.

Joshua Gerbert, DPM, FACFAS

Lesser Forefoot Surgery

Joshua Gerbert, DPM, FACFAS, Editor

Table of Contents

Pathophysiology of Metatarsalgia and Digital Deformities

1

William M. Jenkin, DPM, FACFAS

Introduction:

Metatarsalgia is a non-specific term referring to pain located within the forefoot. The term *forefoot* represents the dorsal and plantar aspects of the distal metatarsal shafts, metatarsal heads and corresponding phalanges (toes). Inclusive with the above osseous structures are the soft tissue interface (skin, fat, tendon/sheath, nerve); the metatarsal phalangeal joint (MTPJ); interphalangeal joint (IPJ) (cartilage, synovium, ligaments, capsule); the intermetatarsal; and the submetatarsal space. The "ball" of the foot refers to the MTPJs and the area plantar to the metatarsal heads.

Pain localized to metatarsal 2, 3, and 4 is referred to as central metatarsalgia, pain localized to the first ray is referred to as medial metatarsalgia and pain localized to the fifth ray is referred to as lateral metatarsalgia. If first ray load bearing is compromised for whatever reason, ground reactive stress is transferred to the central metatarsals, primarily the second or the second and third. If the transfer of stress results in forefoot pain, it is referred to as transfer metatarsalgia.

The etiology of metatarsalgia is multi-factorial. It may occur as an isolated entity or as a composite of mixed disorders which may be clinically difficult to differentiate from each other. It can be secondary to a systemic disease such as rheumatoid arthritis or be entirely related to structural or mechanical etiologies.

Aside from possessing knowledge of which systemic diseases affect the foot, the surgeon needs to possess an appreciation of the normal anatomy and biomechanics of the forefoot. This knowledge is essential in understanding the pathomechanics behind each cause of metatarsalgia, allowing for thorough evaluation and individualized problem-specific non-surgical and surgical management.

Functional Forefoot Anatomy:

Functional anatomy includes the osseous, fibrous connective tissue, and myotendinous structures forming and controlling the metatarsophalangeal and interphalangeal joints.

Osseous Structures

Metatarsals and Phalanges:

The osseous structure of the forefoot consists of the five metatarsals connected by a ligamentous framework along with the corresponding phalanges of the toes. The term *central metatarsals* refers to metatarsals 2, 3, and 4; the term *lesser metatarsals* refers to metatarsals 2, 3, 4, and 5.

Medial and Lateral Columns:

The five metatarsals with their tarsal bones combine with the phalanges to form a ray and contribute to the formation of the medial and lateral columns of the foot. The medial column of the foot involves metatarsals I, II, and III, along with the phalanges, cuneiforms, navicular, and talus. It is flexible and is involved mostly with shock absorption and adaptation to the supporting surface while enabling the first ray to bear proper load prior to propulsion. It is dependent upon proper functioning of the windlass mechanism especially to the first ray. Metatarsals IV and V along with the phalanges, cuboid and calcaneus combine to form the lateral column of the foot. The lateral column of the foot is essentially rigid and functions mostly as a lever for propulsion. Its function is primarily dependent upon the ability of the calcaneo-cuboid joint to stabilize or "lock" when the midtarsal joint itself is maximally pronated (Fig. 1-1 A, B, C).

Phalanges:

Each toe provides transverse plane stability to juxtaposed neighbors by acting as a buttress. The head of the proximal phalanx of a given digit rests against the proximal phalangeal neck of its medial neighbor. This spatial relationship provides for stability in the transverse plane. Although each phalanx is of a different size as the overall length of the toes decreases, it is the intermediate phalanx which demonstrates the greatest decrease in both absolute and proportionate length while the proximal phalanx remains relatively constant in length. This provides for a proximal phalangeal parabola established by the different proximal phalangeal length patterns which increases from the fifth to the second toes. During gait, as each digit bears load it serves as a lever arm for the plantar fascia and connective tissue frame work of the ball of the forefoot which attach to the plantar aspect of the base of the proximal phalanx. Due to the longer combined metatarsal and phalangeal lengths, the longer lever arm of the medial column toes provides for a better "windlass effect" upon the plantar aponeurosis. When the stable toe is dorsiflexed, the plantar aponeurosis will help to tense the skin of the ball of the foot. Tensing the skin of the ball of the foot allows for the shear forces to be transferred to the skeleton by restricting passive movements of the skin.

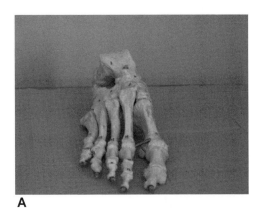

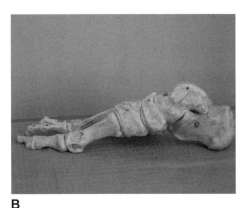

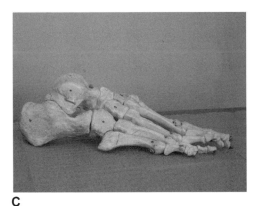

Figure 1-1: A: Photograph of frontal plane view of osseous medial and lateral column. **B:** Photograph of sagittal plane view of osseous medial column. **C:** Photograph of sagittal plane view of osseous lateral column.

Metatarsal Length Pattern:

The five metatarsals are of different lengths. In most metatarsal length pattern formulas the second metatarsal is the longest (2>1>3>4>5 or 2>1=3>4>5). Because of the greatest length of the second metatarsal, there is no common axis for the five MTPJs. There is, however, a transverse axis consisting of the first and second MTPJs and an oblique axis consisting of the second through fifth MTPJs (Fig. 1-2).

The metatarsals are curved longitudinally forming a longitudinal arch with the central metatarsals extending the farthest distally. This configuration allows for a proximal transverse metatarsal arch high medially and low laterally with the apex at the second metatarsal base corresponding with the arch of the cuneiforms while distally the metatarsals are on one plane (Fig. 1-3 A, B).

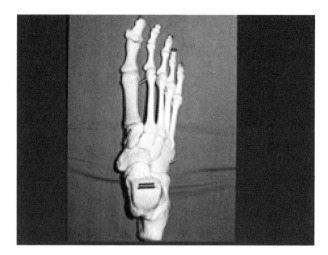

Figure 1-2: Photograph of dorsal view of foot skeleton demonstrating a transverse MTPJ axis consisting of the first and second MTPJs and an oblique MTPJ axis consisting of the second through fifth MTPJs.

As long as the entire foot is weight bearing, the metatarsals share a common load. The ratio of weight distribution, however, is 2:1:1:1:1 with the first metatarsal carrying a double load. Because of the different metatarsal lengths, the common sharing of the load between metatarsal heads comes to an end as soon as the heel leaves the ground.

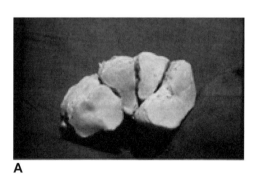

A

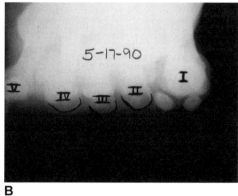

B

Figure 1-3: A: Photograph of frontal plane view of foot skeleton demonstrating a proximal transverse arch consisting of the cuneiforms and cuboid bone. **B:** Frontal plane plantar axial X-ray view demonstrating that distally all of the metatarsal heads rest on one plane.

Together with the different length phalanges, they provide a sequence of resistance arms of increasing lengths which aid in the transfer of the center of pressure under the foot during forward motion from the heel to the lateral part of the ball of the foot and onto the middle portion of the great toe. In normal gait, as the heel leaves the ground the weight is transferred onto the metatarsals, utilizing the oblique MTPJ axis starting with the shortest metatarsal and ending with the longest while off loading the fifth MTPJ, fourth MTPJ, third MTPJ and continuing on to the transverse MTPJ axis passing through metatarsal heads I and II and eventually through the tip of the hallux. It is the body's forward momentum, not muscular contraction, which causes the ultimate push-off.

When primarily utilizing the transverse MTPJ axis, metatarsal heads V, IV, and III are relieved of weight in that order: when the oblique MTPJ axis is used, the first metatarsal is the first to be relieved of weight bearing. If the patient has pain in the first MTPJ such as with hallux limitus or rigidus and has sufficient internal rotation of the leg available, she/he will often adduct the foot in order to utilize the oblique MTPJ axis rather than the transverse axis during the propulsive phase of gait. If, on the other hand, the patient experiences pain within the lesser MTPJs, often the patient will externally rotate the leg and abduct the foot thus utilizing mostly the transverse MTPJ axis.

The second or third MTPJs are the joints which are most often involved when there is an arthrosis of a MTPJ. This is explained by anatomic structural and biomechanical relationships. The second MTPJ is common to both axes. Therefore, it bears ground-reactive stress regardless of which axis is being used. Additionally, the second and the third metatarsals are firmly anchored at their bases with strong plantar metatarsal tarsal ligaments such that they cannot dorsiflex or move up when ground reactive force is applied. Furthermore, the first and fifth rays have separate ranges of motion from the central metatarsals. They are able to independently move above and below the central metatarsals. Consequently, any ground reactive stress which is going to be transferred to the central metatarsals secondary to a biomechanical fault of the first and or the fifth is going to be fully borne by the central MTPJs — primarily, the second and third MTPJs. The fourth metatarsal is less firmly anchored at its base and is often able to dorsiflex with ground reactive forces, thereby avoiding the abnormal stress.

Structurally, if the first metatarsal is short or the second and/or third metatarsal are excessively long, this creates the problem of abnormal weight transfer as a greater ground reactive force is applied to the longer metatarsal and MTPJ and for a longer time.

Prolapsed Metatarsals:

It should be noted that the central metatarsals, even though they are not capable of being dorsiflexed, can be individually plantarflexed at their respective metatarsal tarsal joints. Therefore, the metatarsal can become "prolapsed" or plantarly prominent. This occurs as a result of a digital deformity: the digit no longer bears proper load and instead causes a retrograde plantarly-directed force upon the metatarsal head so that the metatarsal functions in a plantarflexed position (Fig. 1-4 A, B). This position can

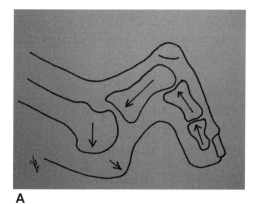
A

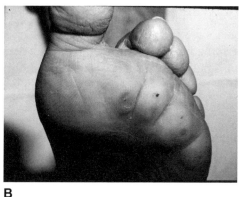
B

Figure 1-4: A: Sagittal plane diagram demonstrating hammertoe deformity causing retrograde plantarflexory force upon metatarsal. **B:** Clinical photograph of plantar foot demonstrating prolapsed metatarsals.

become fixed over time resulting in a structurally plantarflexed metatarsal. This is often referred to as a "fallen anterior arch." The plantarly prominent metatarsal head results in a pressure point which causes a mechanically induced hyperkeratosis. Any enlargement or hypertrophy of the plantar condyle will compound the problem.

Osteochondral Shape of MTPJ:

The shape of both the metatarsal head and corresponding proximal phalangeal base creates the vertical as well as the horizontal axis of each individual joint. The head is quadrilateral and convex. It is covered with articular cartilage which extends further proximally plantarly than dorsally. The plantar articular component consists of two condyles separated by a concave surface. The lateral condyle usually extends further plantarly than the medial condyle. The proper shape also provides sufficient volume to satisfy the internal cubic content of the joint to allow for proper function. Osteochondral adaptation or change in the shape may occur with chronic stress, trauma, erosive arthritis or osteonecrosis (Freiberg's Infraction) (Fig. 1-5). Once the shape has changed the quality and quantity of joint motion will be compromised resulting in a painful arthrosis.

Connective Tissue Framework:

MTPJ Capsule and Intra - articular Ligaments:

The capsule varies in thickness from a thin membrane to a strong fibrous band. The thickened, fibrocartilaginous plantar capsule reinforced by various ligamentous

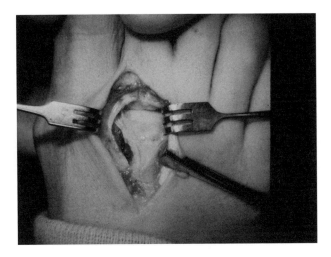

Figure 1-5: Clinical photograph demonstrating abnormally shaped metatarsal head associated with Freiberg's Infraction.

aponeurotic insertions become the flexor (plantar) plate. Within the joint capsule the collateral and the suspensory ligaments are found. They are strong, inelastic structures which guide and align the joint throughout flexion and extension and serve as checkreins for the ends of motion. The ligaments are stronger and thicker on the lateral side. The ligaments originate from the epicondyle on each side of the metatarsal head. The suspensory ligaments fan out plantarly inserting into the flexor plate while the collateral ligaments insert into the plantar sides of the proximal phalanx (Fig. 1-6 A, B, C).

Flexor (Plantar) Plate:

The plantar plate is the most significant factor in stabilizing the MTPJ due to its central location and multiple important attachments. The length of the plate varies from 17.0 mm in the fourth and fifth toes up to 20 mm in the second and third toes. Its thickness is 2 mm being thickest at its mid portion distal to its metatarsal insertion and proximal to the phalangeal insertion. The width corresponds to the width of the proximal phalanx base. The plate consists of Type I collagen fibrocartilage similar to the meniscus of the knee. The strongest attachment of the plate is into the proximal phalanx directly adjacent to the articular cartilage creating a socket for the metatarsal head. Proximally also is a strong attachment to the plantar fascia longitudinal band which is the most significant attachment of the plantar fascia distally. As it nears the plate, the longitudinal band divides in two and passes on either side of the flexor tendons. The bands insert directly onto the medial and lateral sides of the plate at its proximal aspect.

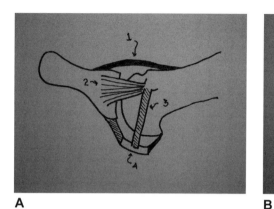

A

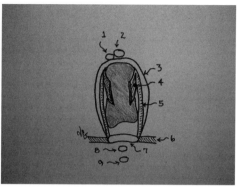

B

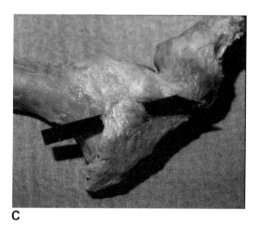

C

Figure 1-6: A: Diagram demonstrating MTPJ intra-articular ligaments in the sagittal plane: 1. Dorsal MTPJ capsule, 2. Collateral ligament, 3. Suspensory ligament, 4. Flexor plate. **B:** Diagram demonstrating MTPJ intra – articular ligaments in the frontal plane: 1. Extensor digitorum brevis, 2. Extensor digitorum longus, 3. MTPJ capsule, 4. Collateral ligament, 5. Suspensory ligament, 6. Deep transverse metatarsal ligament, 7. Flexor plate, 8. Flexor digitorum brevis, 9. Flexor digitorum longus. **C:** Clinical photograph demonstrating MTPJ collateral and suspensory ligament attaching to metatarsal epicondyle.

Through the flexor plates, the plantar aponeurosis is attached firmly to the bases of the proximal phalanges. Proximally, the flexor plate is connected loosely to the metatarsals just proximal to the articular surface by a thin (0.4 mm) capsule with synovial folds. The flexor plate moves with the proximal phalanx and this configuration allows the flexor plate to glide unrestricted forward and backwards, as the proximal phalanx is dorsi- or plantar-flexed (Fig. 1-7 A, B, C). The flexor plate serves as a checkrein to prevent hyperextension and works with the plantar condyles to maintain joint congruity and function. Sectioning of the plantar plate creates an unstable joint. The most commonly reported area of rupture is just adjacent to the phalangeal rim of the base of the proximal phalanx.

Deep Transverse Intermetatarsal Ligament:

The deep transverse metatarsal ligament runs as a continuous ligament below the metatarsal heads from the first to the fifth. Below each metatarsophalangeal joint, it

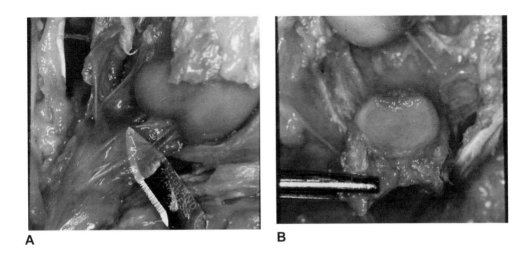

A   B

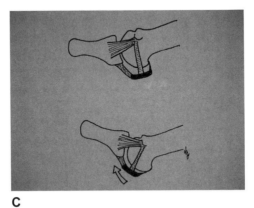

C

Figure 1-7: **A:** Clinical photograph demonstrating thin, loose attachment of plantar capsule proximally to under surface of metatarsal. **B:** Clinical photograph demonstrating firm attachment of flexor plate to plantar base of proximal phalanx. **C:** Sagittal plane diagram demonstrating how flexor plate moves forward and backward freely with the proximal phalanx.

incorporates the lower third of the flexor plate (plantar ligament) and becomes firmly attached to the proximal phalanx. Through the suspensory ligaments inserting into the epicondyle on the lateral fifth metatarsal head and into the flexor plate below the fifth metatarsal, and the flexor plate's connection with the intermetatarsal ligament, the deep transverse metatarsal ligament is literally attached from the lateral side of the head of the fifth to the medial side of the head of the first metatarsal.

The transverse fibers of the intermetatarsal ligament continue distally into the toes as transverse lamellae called plantar interdigital ligaments, which are attached to the sides of the flexor sheaths found in the toes and extend from the medial to lateral margin of the foot.

The plantar interdigital ligaments end in a round mooring ligament which arches from one phalanx to the next, securing the transverse stability of the toes while at the same time allowing individual extension of a toe. It is important to note that the common digital nerve passes plantar to the intermetatarsal ligament and dorsal to the mooring ligament as it continues into the toes. With MTPJ instability and digital deformity this configuration contributes to a torque force being placed upon the nerve.

It is through the above framework that each of the MTPJs and digits are capable of functioning independently yet are bound to each other. Since all of the MTPJs and digits are directly or indirectly connected, what affects one affects all to some degree. This concept has to be considered in the evaluation process as well as in treatment. The MTPJs of the medial column appear to be the most significant as far as forefoot stability is concerned, with their importance decreasing from medial to lateral.

Plantar Aponeurosis:

The plantar aponeurosis (plantar fascia) and flexor plate are critical to forefoot function and stability of the MTPJ. The central slip of the plantar aponeurosis originates from the medial tubercle of the calcaneus and proceeds into the forefoot dividing into a superficial and a deep system. The superficial fibers insert into the ball of the forefoot while the deep fibers insert into the flexor plate (Fig. 1-8 A, B). The deep fibers of the plantar aponeurosis form two marginal and eight intermediate sagittal septa, which pass along the sides of the flexor tendons separating them from the lumbricales, nerves and vessels to the sides of the fibrous flexor sheath. The longitudinal fibers now join with the plantar capsule in forming the dorsal two-thirds of the flexor plate and, through them, insert into the base of the proximal phalanx.

Immediately anterior to the septa insertion to the flexor plate and below each metatarsal head, vertical fibers form a connective tissue cushion of encapsulated fat. The vertical fibers come from the sides of the flexor tendon sheath, the flexor plate and the plantar ligaments and insert into the superficial portion of the plantar aponeurosis and, through them, into the skin.

The tension within the plantar fascial slip to the digit is critical. If the fascial slip is on a slack such as when the metatarsal is short, the toe does not purchase the ground. This is demonstrated clinically when someone has a congenitally short metatarsal (brachymetatarsia) and the toe is found to be in a dorsal position with no ground

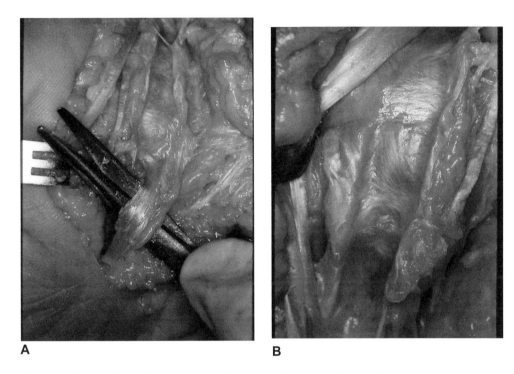

A   **B**

Figure 1-8: A: Clinical photograph demonstrating insertion of plantar aponeurosis slip into flexor plate. **B:** Clinical photograph demonstrating plantar aspect of flexor plate while flexor tendon is retracted.

purchase. If the metatarsal is lengthened, the toe is pulled down by the plantar aponeurosis slip and assumes ground purchase (Fig. 1-9). For this reason, it is recommended that when a metatarsal is shortened as when performing a Weil osteotomy, a flexor tendon transfer and/or PIPJ arthrodesis is performed as an adjunctive procedure to stabilize the MTPJ in order to help prevent a post-operative floating toe deformity.

Windlass Mechanism:

It is by way of the above attachments that the skin of the ball of the foot is tensed, the medial column articulations are "tightened" or stabilized and the arch of the foot is raised and shortened. Dorsiflexion of the toes at the MTPJ exerts a pull of the plantar aponeurosis: plantar-flexing the forefoot on the rearfoot, "raising" the arch at the tarsus and inverting the heel. This motion is called the "windlass action" of the plantar aponeurosis which when engaged creates supination of the foot resulting in external rotation of the leg (Fig. 1-10 A, B, C). The flexion of the forefoot on the rearfoot occurs at the cuneonavicular and metatarsocuneiform joints of the medial column.

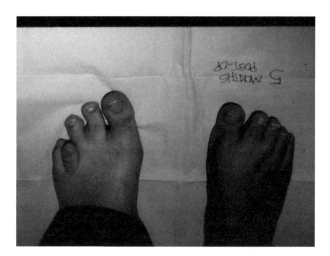

Figure 1-9: Clinical photograph demonstrating a congenital brachymetatarsia with dorsally located fourth digit on the left foot and a fourth toe which purchases the ground on the right foot status post fourth metatarsal lengthening procedure.

The windlass mechanism working through the "metatarsal–phalangeal capsuloligamentous complex" is passive and depends entirely on normal bony alignment, ligamentous and flexor plate integrity and the ability of proximal joints to stabilize for its function. It has its most effect upon function in the medial column, especially the first ray, and progressively less functional effect as one proceeds laterally across the foot.

The larger size of the first metatarsal head as well as inclusion of the sesamoids allows the plantar aponeurosis to have a greater effect upon the windlass mechanism of the first ray. The first ray flexes an average of 10 degrees when the plantar aponeurosis is tensed where the central rays flex about five degrees. This contributes to the first ray bearing twice the load as the central metatarsals during forefoot ground contact.

Myotendinous Structures:

Extensor Tendons:

Tendons crossing the MTPJ and inserting into the digit are divided into those which originate in the leg (extrinsic) and those whose origins are in the foot (intrinsic).

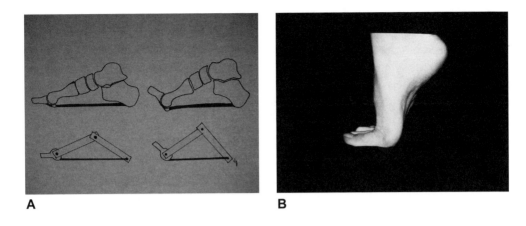

A   B

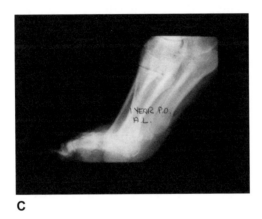

C

Figure 1-10: A: Diagram demonstrating the Windlass mechanism unengaged and engaged. **B:** Clinical photograph demonstrating a weight bearing foot with the windlass mechanism engaged. **C:** Lateral X-ray of forefoot demonstrating windlass mechanism engaged.

The action of the tendons passing the MTPJ is related to their location to and distance from the joint axis. Tendons passing above the joint axis create extension; those below create flexion, etc. The closer the tendon is to the joint axis, the more it functions to stabilize the joint and the less to create motion. The combined action of the tendons creates the dynamic stabilization of the MTPJ as well as movement of the joint within the restraints of the ligaments and flexor plate. The intrinsic muscles primarily stabilize the MTPJ, so that the extrinsic muscles may create motion by eccentric and concentric contraction.

The extensor digitorum longus (EDL) tendon runs dorsal to the MTPJ and onto the digit where it trifurcates proximal to the proximal interphalangeal joint. The medial and lateral slip of the trifurcation pass to the sides of the PIPJ only to become one tendon over the DIPJ and then inserts on the terminal phalanx. The central slip inserts on the dorsal aspect of the base of the intermediate phalanx. This arrangement allows for a restrained but greater plantar flexion of the PIPJ than if the tendon was in one piece, while at the same time limiting flexion of the DIPJ. At the level of the MTPJ on toes two to four, the EDL is joined laterally by the extensor digitorum brevis (EDB) tendon. The EDB either inserts onto the EDL tendon laterally or forms the entire lateral slip of the trifurcation.

Extensor Expansion:

The extensor system is held in a central location to the MTPJ by the extensor expansion. This fibroaponeurotic band extends from the MTPJ to the proximal interphalangeal joint (Fig. 1-11). The proximal segment of this extensor expansion has transversely oriented fibers originating from the lateral medial borders of the flat aponeurotic tunnel surrounding the corresponding extensor tendon. The fibers extend around the capsule of the MTPJ and blend on the plantar side with the flexor plate, the deep transverse metatarsal ligament, the flexor tendon sheath and the base of the proximal phalanx.

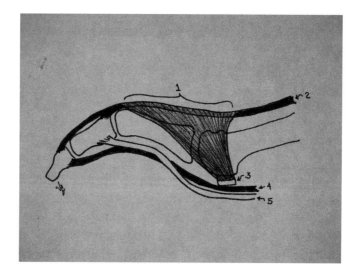

Figure 1-11: Diagram demonstrating sagittal view of extensor expansion: 1. Extensor expansion, 2. Extensor digitorum longus tendon, 3. Flexor plate, 4. Flexor digitorum longus tendon, 5. Flexor digitorum brevis tendon.

This sling like structure (extensor sling) firmly anchors the EDL to the plantar aspect of the MTPJ and proximal phalanx. The EDL actually has no dorsal attachment to the proximal phalanx. Consequently, when the muscle contracts it lifts the metatarsal phalangeal apparatus which is suspended from the EDL by the extensor sling.

The distal segment of the extensor expansion on each side of the toe is composed of the obliquely oriented fibers of the extensor wing or hood. This distal arrangement unites the intrinsic muscles with the trifurcation of the EDL. It enables the tendons of the lumbricales, dorsal and plantar interossei to pass plantar to the axis of motion at the MTPJ and dorsal to the axis of motion at the proximal and distal interphalangeal joints. When contraction of these muscles occurs, it results in flexion at the MTPJ and extension at the PIPJ and DIPJ.

Intrinsic Tendons:

The lumbricale tendon terminates medially into the extensor wing and essentially comprises the medial portion of the wing. After passing below the intermetatarsal ligament, it flexes the MTPJ by pulling on the extensor wing in a plantar direction at the same time as it extends the interphalangeal joint. The lumbricale also exerts an adductory force on the digit. The dorsal and plantar interossei are weak extensors of these joints (PIPJ and DIPJ), but strong flexor-pressors of the MTPJ. They have a firm attachment to the flexor plate and proximal phalanx. Also, the dorsal interossei adduct and the plantar interossei abduct the central toes.

Flexor Tendons:

At the level of the plantar plate, both tendons enter a fibroosseous tunnel. The flexor digitorum brevis (FDB) is still more plantar to the flexor digitorum longus (FDL). The FDB divides into two slips at the level of the base of the proximal phalanx. The tendon of the FDL passes through the bifurcation and continues its distal course now located more plantar to the tendon of the brevis. The FDB inserts into the plantar sides of the intermediate phalanx while the FDL continues distally to insert into the terminal phalanx. Within the fibroosseous tunnel, the flexor tendons are independently surrounded by synovial sheaths extending from the metatarsal heads to the base of the distal phalanx (Fig. 1-12). The FDLs act from their distal insertion. During 30 to 55 percent of the gait cycle while the MTPJs are extending, the FDLs are in concentric contraction and act as stabilizers of the toes, invertors of the hind foot and plantar-flexors of the ankle.

First Ray Dysfunction:

The first ray and especially the first MTPJ is critical as far as forefoot stability is concerned. Once the integrity of the first MTP joint is compromised, the entire forefoot is affected. The integrity of the first MTPJ can be compromised by disease (rheumatoid arthritis, gout), biomechanical faults, or structural insufficiencies. Each

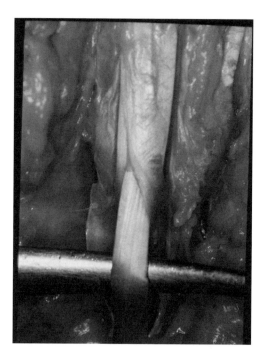

Figure 1-12: Clinical photograph of plantar forefoot demonstrating flexor tendon and its synovially lined sheath.

of these compromises the effect of the windlass mechanism on the first ray's ability to bear its metatarsal load share.

Structural Dysfunction:

Structural first ray dysfunction can be congenital or acquired as a result of trauma or as a side effect or complication of certain surgical procedures. Whatever the cause, there is an inability to bear the proper load beneath the first MTPJ-sesamoid apparatus. This causes a transfer of forces to the fixed central metatarsals, placing a ground reactive stress upon the MTPJ. A short first metatarsal may not purchase the ground, transferring stress to the central metatarsals (Fig. 1-13). In this case, the windlass mechanism can engage but is not effective. A long first metatarsal will not allow the windlass mechanism to engage and essentially functions like an elevated metatarsal causing limited first MTPJ motion (Fig. 1-14). An elevated first metatarsal which is fixed in position is not capable of moving in the sagittal plane and does not allow the windlass mechanism to engage (Fig. 1-15).

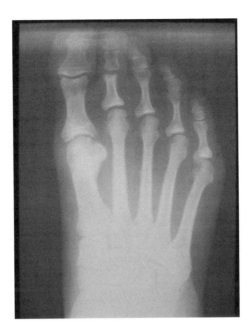

Figure 1-13: AP X-ray view demonstrating a short first metatarsal (Morton's Foot).

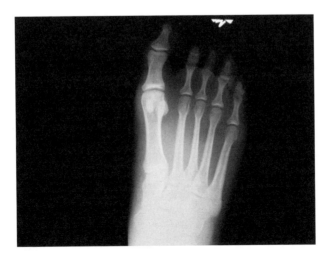

Figure 1-14: AP X-ray view demonstrating a long first metatarsal.

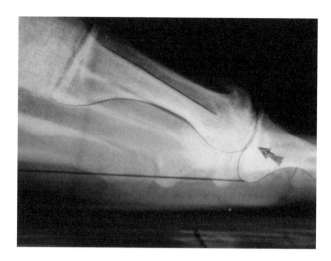

Figure 1-15: Lateral X-ray view demonstrating an elevated first metatarsal.

Post surgical load transfer is found as a side effect after Keller arthroplasty, first MTPJ implant arthroplasty, or any procedure or complication which causes excessive shortening (AVN) or elevation of the first metatarsal. It is epitomized by amputation of the hallux or first ray.

Biomechanical Dysfunction:

Biomechanical dysfunction of the first ray occurs as a result of instability of the first MTPJ alone or in combination with one or more of the proximal first ray joints (first metatarsal cuneiform joint, cuneiform navicular, talonavicular and intercuneiform joint). It is referred to as contiguous instability or hypermobility of the first ray.

The unstable first ray maximally elevates upon weight bearing, resulting in either a metatarsus elevatus with limited first MTPJ motion (functional hallux limitus) or an increase metatarsus primus adductus with a hallux abductus deformity. If the metatarsus elevatus becomes structurally fixed, the first MTPJ becomes arthritic and rigid (hallux rigidus). With limited first MTPJ motion, the windlass mechanism does not engage and the first ray does not bear load.

If present the consequences of the first ray no longer bearing proper load must be factored into surgical planning for treatment of central metatarsalgia. The ability to restore function to the first ray either with orthotic control or through various surgical procedures will improve the prognosis.

Central MTPJ Instability and Digital Deformity:

Central MTPJ instability is a multifactorial problem. In essence it occurs when the proximal phalanx can no longer be stabilized in its neutral position upon the metatarsal head. This instability ultimately results in some degree of forefoot deformity, often causing pain and pressure reactions such as mechanically induced hyperkeratosis, thickened nails and ulcerations. The source of the pain varies. It can be secondary to an inflammatory process such as an adventitious bursitis, tendinitis, or synovitis, or from sources such as nerve entrapments (neuromata), or degenerative joint disease.

The pathophysiology of instability of the MTPJ essentially involves the loss of integrity of the capsuloligamentous complex of the joint. It is insidious, occurring in stages unless secondary to an acute traumatic rupture of the flexor plate or ligaments.

Sagittal Plane Instability:

Sagittal plane stability of the metatarsophalangeal joint is provided by the insertion of the slips of the plantar aponeurosis into the flexor plate as well as the intrinsic muscles which pass below the horizontal axis of the MTPJ and insert into the digits. These create MTP joint stability and plantar-flexion of the proximal phalanx upon the metatarsal head (pressor effect).

When the intrinsic muscles fail to stabilize the proximal phalanx onto the metatarsal head, a hammertoe or claw toe deformity develops (Fig. 1-16). The FDB produces flexion of the proximal interphalangeal joint, resulting in a retrograde force of the intermediate phalanx against the proximal phalanx, creating hyperextension of the MTPJ. The long flexor strongly contributes to this action by acting on the terminal

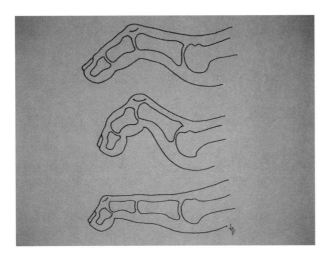

Figure 1-16: Sagittal plane diagram demonstrating a hammertoe, claw toe, and mallet toe deformity.

phalanx plantar-flexing the interphalangeal joints. The relationship between the intrinsic musculature, which normally places a plantar-flexory stabilizing force on the proximal phalanx, and the toe extensors is disrupted as the extensors contract with the result of reinforcing the abnormal proximal phalangeal dorsiflexion by the long and short extensor tendon. As the proximal phalanx dorsi-flexes, its retrograde force plantar-flexes the respective metatarsal. The metatarsal head becomes more susceptible to ground reactive stress. An excessively elongated digit primarily involving a long intermediate phalanx often results in a mallet toe deformity especially if there is contracture of the FDL tendons. This digital deformity only involves the DIPJ (Fig. 1-16).

Transverse Plane Instability:

In the transverse plane the centralization of the long extensor tendons relative to the vertical axis passing through the metatarsal head is of prime importance. If the tendon shifts lateral to this axis, it will act as an abductor. If the tendon shifts medially, it will act primarily as an adductor. With failure of a collateral ligament the toe initially deviates in an abductory or adductory direction at the MTPJ, creating a space between the adjacent digits. This results in a digital adductus/abductus deformity or a crossover toe deformity (Fig. 1-17).

Additionally, the fifth, fourth, and sometimes third toes in the foot with intrinsic instability as a result of abnormal pronation will tend to assume an adductovarus deformity because of the more medially-directed pull of the flexor digitorum longus tendon (Fig. 1-18 A, B).

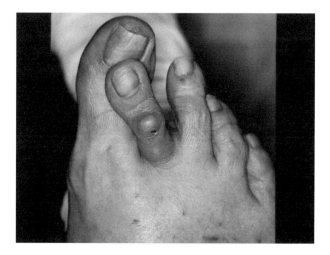

Figure 1-17: Clinical photograph demonstrating digital adductus and an overlapping second toe deformity in the transverse plane.

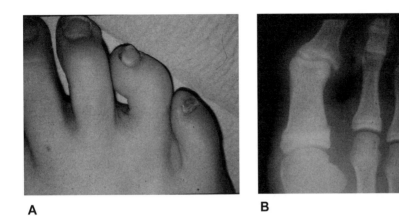

A   B

Figure 1-18: **A:** Clinical photograph demonstrating an adductovarus deformity of the fourth and fifth toe. **B:** AP X-ray view demonstrating an adductovarus deformity of the fourth and fifth toe.

Accompanying this process, the suspensory ligament also fails, allowing the plantar structures including capsule, the flexor plate along with its insertions and the flexor tendons to move in the direction of the proximal phalanx. These structures eventually become relocated on the side of the MTPJ and, along with the capsule, contract. Instead of providing a stabilizing plantar-flexory force upon the proximal phalanx at the MTPJ, they now exert a deforming adductory or abductory force. With time, secondary to ground reactive forces and dorsiflexory forces of the extensor tendons, the proximal phalanx hyperextends upon the metatarsal head, causing the toe to deviate dorsally at the MTPJ, buckle or curl at the IPJs, causing subluxation or dislocation at the MTPJ. This allows a retrograde plantar-flexory force to occur upon the metatarsal, resulting in a prominent plantar metatarsal head. Additionally, a retrograde abductory or adductory force is placed upon the corresponding metatarsal head from the proximal phalanx, occasionally resulting in a narrowing of the intermetatarsal angle between this and the adjacent metatarsal, which further aids in the adduction or abduction of the toe.

The plantar structures continue to follow the proximal phalanx, leading to more anterior as well as dorsal subluxation or dislocation. This allows capsulodesis of the plantar capsule to the undersurface of the metatarsal head, making the deformity non-reducible.

The dorsal structures including extensor tendons, extensor expansion and capsule are secondary players in this process. Nevertheless, they do help to cause and maintain the deformity. With no plantar-flexing stabilizing force upon the proximal phalanx, the extensor tendons secondarily contract as the toe moves dorsally.

Additionally, since the dorsal structures also follow the proximal phalanx, the extensor apparatus of the toe becomes relocated to the side of the contraction, resulting in an adductory or abductory force to the toe.

Mechanically Induced Hyperkeratosis (MIH):

Mechanically induced hyperkeratosis (MIH) is the generic name given to the acquired, hyperkeratotic skin reaction occurring over or under pressure points. Although given different names based upon location and moisture content, the pathological process for any MIH is essentially the same. This process occurs as a physical response and is not a result of imperfect keratinization. The initial phase is merely an inflammatory reaction which is easily reversible with rest. If the abnormal physical stress continues and becomes chronic, a hyperkeratotic phase or callus (tyloma) formation occurs. Eventually, while the skin continues to thicken, it too is pushed deeper, disrupting the lower layers of the skin as a keratin "core" or "nucleus" is formed over the areas of maximum pressure. This process often results in an epidermal inclusion cyst at its deepest part (Fig. 1-19).

On the dorsal aspect of the toes, the MIH is referred to as the heloma durum (HD) or hard corn. On the end of the toe it is referred to as a distal heloma durum (DHD). If the lesion is in the web space between the toes, it is referred to as a heloma molle (HM) and is often soft due to absorption of interdigital perspiration. If the MIH occurs on the plantar aspect beneath metatarsal heads, it is referred to as a plantar tyloma. If it has a clear keratin deep seated core (nucleated) within the tyloma, it is referred to as the intractable plantar keratoma (IPK). The IPK is more painful with direct pressure than pressure from side to side, which distinguishes it from a porokeratosis plantaris discreta (keratin plugged eccrine sweat gland duct) or plantar verrucae.

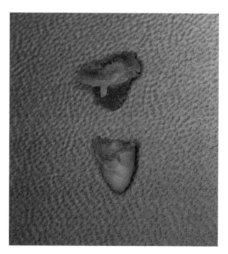

Figure 1-19:   Clinical photograph demonstrating an epidermal inclusion cyst enucleated from the core of an IPK.

MTPJ Stress Syndrome:

Metatarsal phalangeal joint (MTPJ) stress syndrome is a specific mechanically-induced synovitis found mostly in the second MTPJ; it can involve other central MTP joints as well. It is due to mechanical overload of the MTPJ such that the flexor tendons can no longer overpower the ground-reactive forces with resultant joint, ligament, flexor tendon and flexor plate strain or attenuation. It is a progressive functional disorder. Eventually, the stabilizing structures lose their integrity, resulting in instability of the MTPJ. Ultimately, this leads to ligament and flexor plate rupture ending in MTPJ dislocation. It presents as a pre-dislocation phase or a dislocation phase. The symptoms and signs are dependent upon the structures involved and the phase at presentation.

Pre-dislocation Phase:

The patient presents with forefoot pain located at the second and/or third MTPJ area with weight-bearing. The patient will often say the pain is worse when not wearing shoes. The pain is often referred to as a burning sensation which does not radiate. It can also be described as a dull ache within the joint. The signs are few and subtle. A dactylitis of the base of the toe may be noted. There may be a mild to moderate separation of the second and third toe as the second toe begins to overlap the hallux in the transverse plane, rotate into varus in the frontal plane and begins to form a hammertoe deformity in the sagittal plane (Fig 1-20 A, B, C). The physical examination confirms the diagnosis when there is pain to palpation along the flexor tendon into the toe as well as when the joint is palpated dorsally or when the joint is stressed. The MTPJ luxation or Modified Lachman Test as described in the Clinical Evaluation section below is positive for pain and in later stages for pain and subluxation/dislocation. The symptom complex is secondary to joint instability, reactive synovitis, joint effusion and flexor tendinitis or tenosynovitis. The presence of a common digital nerve entrapment must be considered and appropriately ruled out.

Radiographic evaluation may reveal little information or contribute to the diagnosis if not surgical planning. Subluxation of the second MTPJ may be present along with an elongated second metatarsal (Fig. 1-21). A digital deformity may or may not be present.

Dislocation Phase:

In this phase the patient typically presents with complaints referable to the effects of chronic lesser MTPJ dislocation in addition to MTPJ pain. The source of pain is primarily associated with digital deformity and pressure reactions (mechanically-induced hyperkeratosis, bursitis, ulceration, etc.), and shoe fitting concerns. The involved digit is dislocated out of the MTPJ, often forming a hammertoe or claw toe deformity which can override the hallux or just contract dorsally upon the second metatarsal head.

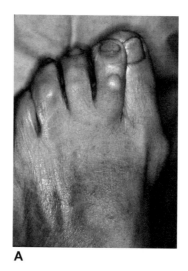

A

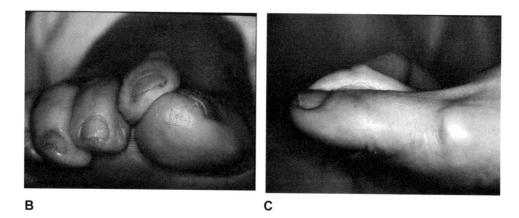

B   C

Figure 1-20: A: Transverse plane clinical photograph of foot in the pre-dislocation phase of an MTPJ stress syndrome demonstrating digital splaying and the beginning of an overlapping second toe deformity. **B:** Clinical photograph of frontal plane view of pre-dislocation phase demonstrating second toe varus. **C:** Clinical photograph of sagittal plane view of pre-dislocation phase demonstrating beginning of a second toe hammertoe deformity.

Radiographic evaluation will reveal a dislocated MTPJ with or without an elongated second metatarsal. The second digit often adducts towards the hallux and the intermetatarsal angle between metatarsal 2 and 3, or 2, 3 and 4 is diminished. Erosive changes or shape changes of the metatarsal head may be present (Fig. 1-22 A, B).

Magnetic resonance imaging (MRI) may be helpful in identifying an attenuated or ruptured flexor plate (Fig. 1-23 A, B).

An acute hyperextension force on the MTPJ can result in a traumatic rupture of the flexor plate. This results in a dislocation of the MTPJ without a pre-dislocation phase.

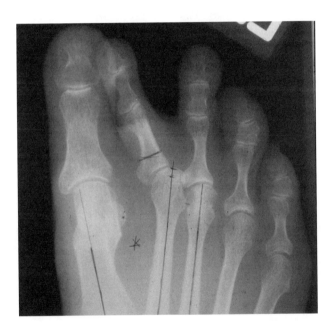

Figure 1-21: AP X-ray view demonstrating a subluxed MTPJ associate with a long second metatarsal in the end stage of a pre-dislocation phase.

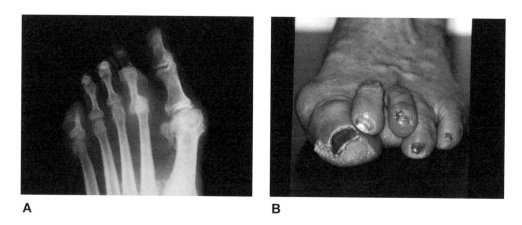

A   B

Figure 1-22: A: AP X-ray view demonstrating second MTPJ dislocation. **B:** Frontal plane clinical photograph demonstrating dislocated second and third MTPJs and lack of toe purchase associated with the dislocation phase of the MTPJ stress syndrome.

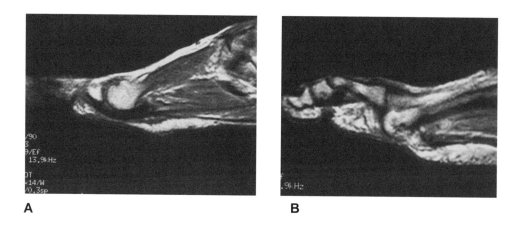

A   B

Figure 1-23: A: Sagittal plane MR image of normal MTPJ and flexor plate. **B:** Sagittal plane MR image of ruptured flexor plate with dorsally dislocated MTPJ.

Metatarsalgia Evaluation (Exhibit I)

Non – Weight Bearing Portion:

Observation:

The examination begins with non-weight bearing observation for signs of asymmetry: normal, symmetric or prominent tendon visibility due to tendon contracture, or non-visible tendons due to dorsal edema or rupture; gross digital deformity (hammer toe, claw toe, mallet toe, adductus/abductus); increase in toe girth; edema (dactylitis); dorsal skin contractures; plantar digital skin contracture; and plantar skin bulk at base of digit. Irritation areas defined by swelling, redness, increased warmth and mechanically-induced hyperkeratosis are noted.

Location of Pain:

The location of pain is determined from the history, observation of the patient's response to the palpating hand and results of diagnostic procedures. **If the source of pain is primarily associated with digital deformity and pressure reactions (mechanically-induced hyperkeratosis, bursitis, ulceration, etc), the examination should proceed directly to digital evaluation.** If, however, the source of discomfort is at the level of the MTPJs, then metatarsalgia work up proceeds to attempt to determine if the source of pain is intra-articular, peri-articular, or extra-articular and to determine if the pain is in the intermetatarsal space below IML, in the intermetatarsal space above IML, in the submetatarsal space, or osseous in origin.

Palpation Pain:

Palpation for areas of forefoot tenderness involves palpation of the distal metatarsal shafts, distal metatarsal interspaces, the plantar aspect of the metatarsal head or flexor plate, and along the flexor tendons into the toes, dorsal to the MTPJ, and along the extensor tendons.

- **Direct palpation of metatarsal interspace:**

    Pain with direct dorsal-plantar palpation of the distal metatarsal interspace could be indicative of an intermetatarsal bursitis, neuritis, or neuroma (Fig. 1-24 A).

    Pain with direct plantar palpation of the distal metatarsal interspace could be indicative of a neuritis or neuroma (Fig. 1-24 B).

- **Lateral-Medial Squeeze Test:** (Fig. 1-25). Pain produced within the involved interspace by squeezing the lateral and medial aspects of the forefoot is indicative of intermetatarsal bursitis, MTP joint effusion, or arthritis. This maneuver in no way evaluates for a neuroma, since the involved common digital nerve lies beneath the transverse metatarsal ligament below the metatarsal head. Therefore, the common digital nerve cannot be compressed between the metatarsal heads when they are squeezed together.

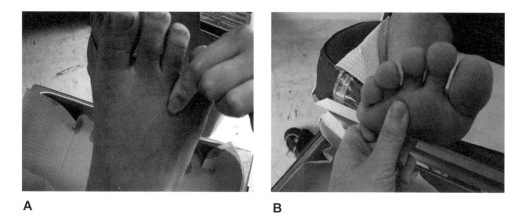

A   B

Figure 1-24: A: Clinical photograph demonstrating dorsal-plantar palpation of the distal metatarsal interspace between thumb and index finger. **B:** Clinical photograph demonstrating plantar palpation of distal metatarsal interspace with the examiner's thumb.

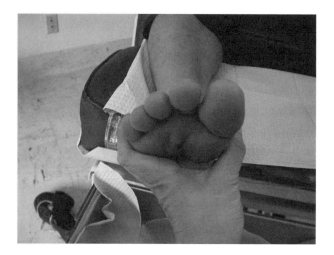

Figure 1-25: Clinical photograph demonstrating the Medial to Lateral Squeeze Test by compressing the metatarsal heads together.

- **Mulder's Click:** (Fig. 1-26 A, B). Mulder's click or maneuver evaluates for the presence of a neuroma. It is performed by applying pressure to the involved distal interspace at the level just proximal to the metatarsal ligament. Dorsal pressure is applied with the index finger and plantarly with the thumb while at the same time with the opposite hand squeezing the foot from medial to lateral. The plantarly placed thumb is then dragged distally. If pain and a clicking sensation occur, this is referred to as a positive Mulder's click or sign. It is indicative of a neuroma or other space-occupying lesion involving the nerve. The clicking sensation is due to bringing the enlarged portion of the nerve (neuroma) over the distal aspect of the transverse metatarsal ligament.

Neurological Evaluation:

Sensation to the digits is established by testing the ends of the toes and each side of the web for hypesthesia, hyperesthesia, or anesthesia. Proximal nerve involvement can be sought by palpating the tarsal tunnel for nerve tenderness, enlargements, or by percussing the nerve to elicit a Tinnel's sign.

Range of Motion:

Range of motion (ROM) along with various stress manipulation studies are performed to further evaluate the MTPJ for painful synovitis, instability, lack of

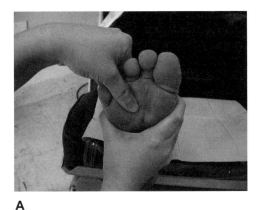 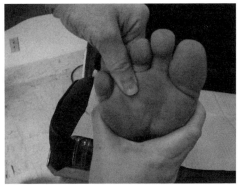

A   **B**

Figure 1-26: A, B: Clinical photograph demonstrating an attempt at eliciting a Mulder's click to evaluate for a neuroma of the common digital nerve at the level of the intermetatarsal ligament.

motion especially in flexion, excessive motion and arthritis. Pain emanating from the tendon or its sheath is noted during passive ROM, active ROM and resistive ROM.

Passive ROM Pain at End Range and Joint Distraction Pain:

Pain from synovitis is suspected when there is edema (joint effusion), hyperemia and range of motion pain only at the ends of the range when the synovium is "pinched" between the metatarsal head and phalangeal base, or when the capsule and ligament are placed on stretch when the joint is distracted distally. If the synovitis is advanced, pain from the lateral squeeze test will be present.

- **Passive ROM Pain and Crepitus:**

     Pain from synovitis as well as erosive arthritis is suspected if joint motion pain is present throughout the entire range and crepitus or grinding sensation is felt.

- **Retrograde ROM Pain:**

     The presence of erosive arthritis is confirmed by noting a painful response obtained with retrograde compression of the proximal phalanx upon the metatarsal head while also taking the joint through its range of motion.

- **Active ROM Pain:**

     Pain from synovitis and erosive arthritis occurs with this motion as a retrograde force is created by the pull of the tendons. It is also present with tenosynovitis as the tendon glides within the tendon sheath.

- **Resistive ROM Pain:**

     Pain from tendinitis is more pronounced if while having the patient perform a movement requiring tendon contracture, a resistive force is applied in the opposite direction placing more tension within the tendon.

- **MTPJ Luxation Test (Modified Lachman Test):**

     Pain alone or pain accompanied with luxation of the MTPJ joint is positive for intra-articular pathology. It is indicative of the MTPJ Stress Syndrome. The test evaluates sagittal plane instability by attempting to dislocate the proximal phalangeal base dorsally out of the MTPJ. It has been referred to as the modified Lachman Test, but it is best called the MTPJ Luxation Test as this terminology describes what it is attempting to accomplish. The test is performed by stabilizing the metatarsal with one hand while placing an upward force on the base of the proximal phalanx with the opposite hand (Fig. 1-27). If pain is produced it is positive for intra-articular pathology. If the base of the proximal phalanx also dislocates when this maneuver is attempted, the test is positive for loss of integrity of the collateral and suspensory ligaments and attenuation if not rupture of the flexor plate. With time this insufficiency will result in subluxation or dislocation of the MTPJ with resultant digital deformity.

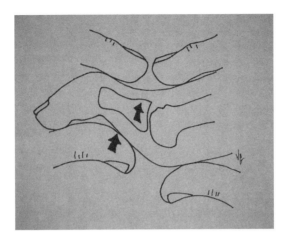

Figure 1-27: Diagram demonstrating the performance of the MTPJ Luxation Test.

Diagnostic Anesthetic Blocks and Arthrogram:

If there is still a doubt about the location or source of pain (intra- versus extra-articular, which or how many interspaces are involved), then diagnostic anesthetic injections can be performed. They can be performed as a diagnostic arthrogram if mixed with a radiopaque dye (Fig. 1-28). The idea is to inject the anesthetic into the area of discomfort while allowing for skin sensation to remain intact. If the pain in the joint is eliminated, and yet normal sensation is felt, and upon radiographic evaluation all the dye remains in the joint; then, it can safely be assumed that the source of pain is from inside the joint.

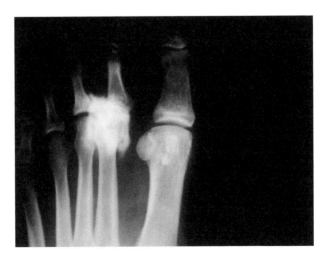

Figure 1-28: AP X-ray view demonstrating a diagnostic arthrogram of the second MTPJ.

Exhibit I: Metatarsalgia Evaluation Form

INVOLVED RAY	1st R	2nd R	3rd R	4th R	5th R	Side	Side	1st L	2nd L	3rd L	4th L	5th L
Non-Weight Bearing:												
Observe for Dactylitis												
Dorsal Edema												
MTPJ MOTION PAIN												
Dorsiflexion / plantarflexion												
Dorsiflexion Only at End ROM												
Plantarflexion at End ROM												
MTPJ Distraction Pain												
Retrograde ROM Pain												
Creptius												
Resisted DF Pain												
Resisted PF pain												
MTPJ LUXATION TEST	pos/neg	pos/neg	pos/neg	pos/neg	pos/neg			pos/neg	pos/neg	pos/neg	pos/neg	pos/neg
MTPJ Dislocatable												
MTPJ Dislocated												
PALPATION PAIN												
Dorsal MTPJ												
Extensor Tendon												
Plantar MTPJ												
Flexor Tendon												
Flexor Sulcus												
IM Space												
Lateral Squeeze Test												
Met. Neck / Shaft						yes/no	yes/no					
Tuning Fork Test						yes/no	yes/no					
SESAMOIDITIS SYMPTOMS:												
Sesamoid Load ROM Pain												
Resisted PF pain												
NEUROMA SYMPTOMS:												
Mulder's Click												
Distal Hypesthesia												
Distal Hyperesthesia												

Digital Evaluation (Exhibit II)

Non – Weight Bearing Portion:

Deformity Classification:

Define the level and extent of pathology by establishing which toes, which joints and which planes are involved. This will allow classification of the digital deformity.

Sagittal plane deformities are classified into three categories based upon which forefoot joints are involved and whether or not the joint is extended or flexed. The claw toe deformity involves all three joints, extended at the MTPJ and flexed at the PIPJ and DIPJ. It can involve all digits but mostly toes 2 to 4. The hammer toe deformity involves two joints, extended at the MTPJ and flexed at the PIPJ. It rarely affects all digits and occurs mostly in toes 2 and 3. The mallet toe deformity involves one joint, the DIPJ, and it is flexed.

- Claw toe: MTPJ, PIPJ, DIPJ; digits 2, 3, 4, 5
- Hammertoe: MTPJ, PIPJ; digits 2, 3, 4
- Mallet Toe: DIPJ; digits 2, 3, 4

Strictly transverse plane digital deviation is classified as either an adductus or abductus and is further described by the level of the deformity which most often is the MTPJ:

- Digital Adductus: MTPJ; PIPJ; DIPJ
- Digital Abductus: MTPJ; PIPJ; DIPJ

Combination transverse plane and frontal plane deformities are classified as clinodactyl or digits which demonstrate an adductovarus deformity. The fifth and fourth digits are most often affected involving the DIPJ and PIPJ as well as the MTPJ in the transverse and frontal plane. This deformity is often found in association with flexor stabilization.

- Clinodactyly, adductovarus: fourth and fifth digits

Lesion/Pain Location:

Describe the location and extent of any discomfort and correlate with areas of any associated mechanically-induced hyperkeratosis and/or nail plate thickening.

- PIPJ: Dorsal (HD/pain); Medial (HM/pain); Lateral (HM/pain)
- DIPJ: Dorsal, Medial, Lateral
- End of toe: DHD; nail plate thickened; painful; onychophosis; onychocrypto sis
- Plantar metatarsal head: tyloma; tyloma with IPK; porokeratosis

Reducibility of Deformity:

Determine the reducibility of the deformity in the sagittal plane by evaluating the involved joints (DIPJ, PIPJ, MTPJ) in order to classify the deformity:

- flexible (totally reducible).

- semi – rigid (partially reducible).

- rigid (non-reducible).

- The Kelikian Push – Up test is performed to determine sagittal plane reducibility of a dorsally contracted MTPJ as follows: If while a dorsally directed pressure is placed against the plantar aspect of the metatarsal head the toe straightens, the test is negative and indicates reducibility of the MTPJ (Fig. 1-29).

If, however, when this manipulation is performed the proximal phalanx remains contracted at the MTPJ, the test is positive indicating a non-reducible deformity. This implies that the proximal phalanx is being prevented from properly realigning with the metatarsal head. It occurs because of structure disorders which can be extrinsic as well as intrinsic to the joint.

Extrinsic disorders may consist of contracture of the dorsal skin, capsule, and extensor tendons mainly the extensor digitorum brevis (EDB).

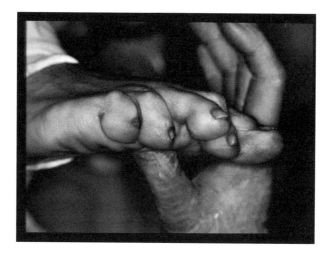

Figure 1-29: Clinical photograph demonstrating the performance of the Kelikian Push Up test. The test is negative as the MTPJ contracture reduces and the toe straightens.

Intrinsic disorders consist of collateral ligament contracture, capsulodesis of the plantar capsule to the plantar aspect of the metatarsal head secondary to chronic anterior displacement of the flexor plate, and finally, a misshapen osteochondral form of the metatarsal head such that no normal articulation of the MTPJ may be obtained.

Tendon and Skin Contracture:

Along with joint reducibility, the dorsal/plantar skin and extensor/flexor tendon to each toe are evaluated for "tightness" or contracture by accessing the tension within the tissue. Usually the more prominent the extensor tendon appears on top of the metatarsals, the greater and more significant the extensor contracture. Dorsal skin contracture becomes a factor when the skin has secondarily adapted to a shortened position. This is found in longstanding presentations such as a second or third dislocated MTPJ or with claw toe deformity of all digits. Plantar digital skin contracture is found in long standing claw toe or mallet toe deformities. In rare cases, a mini-"Z" plasty lengthening of the skin needs to be performed (Chapter 3).

Contracture of all extensor tendons should raise suspicion of an ankle equinus with associated extensor substitution.

Thickness of the skin of the plantar sulcus at the base of the toe can prevent relocation of the digital deformity causing a poor toe purchase. It is sometimes a factor with long standing second or third toe contracture and needs to be excised.

Linear Relationships:

Evaluate the relative digital length pattern to determine if the metatarsal and digit is short, normal, or long. An excessively long metatarsal can be clinically evaluated by performing the Kelikian Push Up test and noting what the toe does in the transverse plane. If while placing a dorsally directed force beneath the metatarsal head in question, the toe adducts or abducts, most likely the metatarsal is long and the MTPJ is unstable. Any clinical impression of length abnormality is confirmed on X-ray.

MTPJ Stability:

Determine the stability (integrity) of the MTPJ by noting toe alignment or separation, subluxation, or dislocation in all planes. If the toe is not dislocated, evaluate sagittal plane instability by determining if subluxation or dislocation has occurred by performing the MTPJ Luxation Test (Modified Lachman) as described above.

Transverse plane MTPJ instability is observed by noting digital splaying, excessive abduction or adduction of the proximal phalanx upon the metatarsal head during rest, weight bearing, or when performing the Kelikian Push Up Test.

Associated Deformities:

Evaluate for associated deformity(ies) which are contributing to the digital deformity.

Observe for a Hallux Abductus Deformity and if found note the hallux-to-second toe relationship. Does the hallux have contact or no contact with the second toe? Does it over ride or under ride the second toe? Evaluate for ROM of the first MTPJ to determine the presence of hallux limitus or rigidus which may be causing transfer metatarsalgia.

Determine the position of the first ray to the second metatarsal by performing a test which evaluates first ray excursion.

Root First Ray Excursion Test: (Fig. 1-30 A, B).

The test determines the first ray position to see if it is normal, structurally elevated, or structurally plantar-flexed when compared to the second metatarsal. The test measures in millimeters the total first metatarsal excursion in the direction of dorsiflexion (A) and the total excursion in the direction of plantarflexion (B). Normal is when the measurement is equal and not excessive. Structural deformity exists if there is more excursion in one direction. If there is excessive motion, evaluation for stability of the first ray is needed.

Determine the stability or instability of the first ray as needed. If, when performing the Root Excursion Test, excessive motion occurs in both directions, the first ray is further accessed to determine if the excessive motion is a normal variant unique to the individual or due to an unstable proximal joint [metatarsal cuneiform (MC); cuneiform navicular (CN) joint] resulting in "hypermobility" of the first ray.

Hicks Dynamic Load Test (Fig. 1-31).

This test evaluates for sagittal plane stability/instability at the MC and CN joints. It is performed by engaging the windlass mechanism by dorsiflexing the hallux and then performing the excursion test. If the excessive motion decreases with this maneuver as compared to when performing the Root Excursion Test, the proximal joints are stable. If, however, the excursion remains excessive especially in dorsiflexion, one or more of the proximal joints are unstable.

Hallux Retrograde Test:

This test evaluates for transverse plane stability/instability at the MC joint. If, while placing a retrograde force of the hallux onto the first metatarsal, the IM angle increases, the MC joint is unstable or hyper-mobile in the transverse plane.

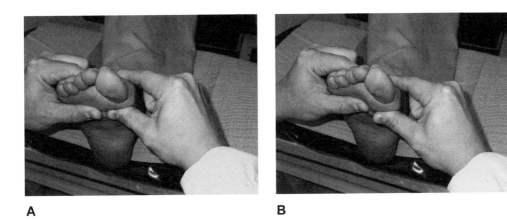

A   B

Figure 1-30: Clinical photograph demonstrating the performance of the Root First Ray Excursion Test. **A:** First ray in maximum dorsiflexed position. **B:** First ray in maximum plantarflexed position.

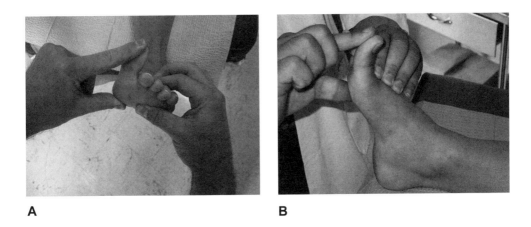

A   B

Figure 1-31: **A:** Clinical photograph demonstrating a frontal plane view of the performance of the Hicks Dynamic Load Test when engaging the windlass mechanism while then performing the first ray excursion. **B:** Clinical photograph demonstrating sagittal plane view of the above.

Tailor's Bunionette Deformity:

Note the presence of a bunionette deformity of the fifth ray and evaluate it as described in Chapter 9.

Ankle ROM:

- Ankle Equinus:

Evaluate for ankle equinus by determining the amount of ankle dorsiflexion with the leg extended. Ankle dorsiflexion at age 10 is measured at 15 degrees and at age 15 at 10 degrees. Any dorsiflexion measurement less than this is classified as an equinus. If an equinus is present, determine if it is a gastrocnemius or combined gastroc soleus equinus by determining the amount of dorsiflexion with the knee flexed. If dorsiflexion is still limited, determine if there is an osseous equinus by taking a stress lateral x-ray. An equinus will create abnormal ground reactive forces upon the forefoot which will result in abnormal pronation and instability and in advance presentations, compounds metatarsalgia.

Weight Bearing Evaluation:

Static Stance:

Observation:

Observe for deformity change from non-weight-bearing appearance to weight-bearing in the relaxed calcaneal stance position (RCSP), to the appearance in neutral calcaneal stance position (NCSP). Note if the deformity remains the same, increases or decreases. Also note the digital purchase or toe-to-ground contact in both RCSP and NCSP and evaluate the relative digital length pattern.

Medial Column Flexibility:

Perform the Hubscher maneuver to see if the medial column is flexible by observing the arch rise as the hallux is dorsiflexed or rigid. If no change in the level of the arch is observed, this indicates a fixed or non reducible deformity (Fig. 1-32).

Dynamic Stance: Gait Evaluation

Evaluate the angle and base of gait for symmetry and note if the feet are abducted, adducted or straight. Observe for biomechanical faults noting tendon contracture and abnormal function such as a premature heel-off or midtarsal break, which is associated with an ankle equinus. Extensor substitution is also observed with equinus; in this case, during swing the extensor tendons contract to dorsiflex the foot at the ankle in order for the forefoot to clear the ground, but in so doing also dorsiflex the toes (Fig. 1-33). The extensor tendons and amount of toe dorsiflexion are more pronounced when there is an ankle equinus. This can also occur with a painful plantar forefoot and cause an antalgic gait as the extensor tendons contract to keep the forefoot from touching the ground. The gait is observed for flexor stabilization which occurs during late stance as the toes are grasping the ground in attempt to gain better stability in a pronated foot (pes planus). An adductovarus rotation of the fourth and fifth toes is noted due to the flexor longus tendon pulling on the toes from a more medial direction as the forefoot abducts as a result of abnormal pronation (Fig. 1-18 A). Flexor substitution also occurs during late stance phase. It results from a weak triceps surae and is due to the long flexor tendons substituting to help plantarflex the foot. The foot supinates as the digits contract in the sagittal plane with a claw toe deformity. There is no adductovarus of toes four and five (Fig. 1-34). It is associated with a pes cavus deformity and an underlying neurological dysfunction should be ruled out. It is the least common presentation.

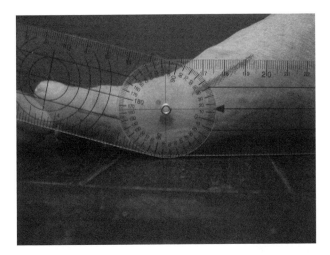

Figure 1-32: Clinical photograph demonstrating the performance of the Hubscher Maneuver in order to evaluate for medial column flexibility. This can be performed while evaluating first MTPJ ROM measurement.

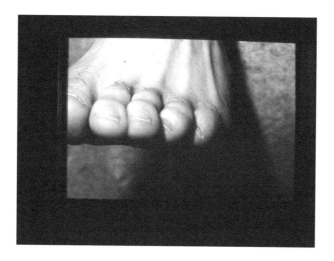

Figure 1-33: Clinical photograph demonstrating extensor substitution by noting prominent extensor tendons and dorsal contracture of MTPJ during swing phase of gait.

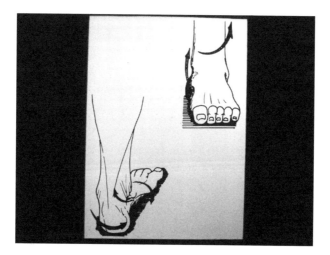

Figure 1-34: Diagram demonstrating flexor substitution for a weak triceps surae. Note the supinated position of the foot and no adductovarus of toes.

Exhibit II: Digital Evaluation Form

NON-WEIGHT BEARING EVALUATION:						RIGHT	LEFT					
INVOLVED RAY	1st R	2nd R	3rd R	4th R	5th R			1st L	2nd L	3rd L	4th L	5th L
DIGITAL EVALUATION:						SIDE	SIDE					
DEFORMITY CLASSIFICATION												
Hammer Toe												
Claw Toe												
Mallet Toe												
Digital Abductus Level:												
MTPJ												
PIPJ												
DIPJ												
Digital Adductus Level:												
MTPJ												
PIPJ												
DIPJ												
Digital Aducto Varus												
LESION / PAIN LOCATION												
PIPJ:												
Dorsal HD/Pain												
Medial HM/Pain												
Lateral HM/Pain												
DIPJ:												
Dorsal HD/Pain												
Medial HM /Pain												
Lateral HM/Pain												
Terminal Phalanx:												
Distal HD / Pain												
Nail Plate Thick												
Onychophosis: Medial Border												
Lateral Border												
Onychocryptosis												
Medial												
Lateral												
Plantar Metatarsal Head:												
Tyloma												

Exhibit II–continued

NON-WEIGHT BEARING EVALUATION:						RIGHT	LEFT					
INVOLVED RAY	1st R	2nd R	3rd R	4th R	5th R			1st L	2nd L	3rd L	4th L	5th L
DIGITAL EVALUATION:						SIDE	SIDE					
Tyloma / IPK												
Porokeratosis												
Verrcuae												
REDUCIBILITY												
PIPJ:												
Flexible												
Semi Rigid												
Rigid												
DIPJ:												
Flexible												
Semi Rigid												
Rigid												
MTPJ Contracture:												
Kelikian Push Up Test:												
Sagittal Plane	pos/neg	pos/neg	pos/neg	pos/neg	pos/neg			pos/neg	pos/neg	pos/neg	pos/neg	pos/neg
Extensor Tendon Tight												
Flexor Tendon Tight												
Dorsal Skin Contracture												
Plantar Skin Contracture												
Plantar Skin Bulk Excessive												
LINEAR RELATIONSHIPS												
Metatarsal Length: Normal												
Short												
Long												
Kelikian Push Up Test:												
Transverse Plane	pos/neg	pos/neg	pos/neg	pos/neg	pos/neg			pos/neg	pos/neg	pos/neg	pos/neg	pos/neg
Digital Length: Normal												
Short												
Long												
Tailor's Bunionette												
Hallux Abductus												
2nd Digit Abutting												

Exhibit II–continued

NON-WEIGHT BEARING EVALUATION:						RIGHT	LEFT					
INVOLVED RAY	1st R	2nd R	3rd R	4th R	5th R			1st L	2nd L	3rd L	4th L	5th L
DIGITAL EVALUATION:						SIDE	SIDE					
ASSOCIATED DEFORMITIES												
2nd Digit Underriding												
2nd Digit Overriding												
Hallux Limitus/ Rigidus												
FIRST RAY:												
Metatarsus Elevatus: Structural												
Root Excursion Test:	Up:___	Down:___		Neutral:___				Up:___	Down:___		Neutral:___	
Met. Elevatus: Hypermobile												
Hicks Dynamic Load Test	pos/neg							pos/neg				
Hallux Retrograde Test	pos/neg							pos/neg				
Ankle Equinus	yes/no							yes/no				
Gastrocnemius												
Soleus												
Osseous												
WEIGHT BEARING EVALUATION:												
STANCE:												
No Toe Purchase:												
RCSP Deformity Increases:												
NCSP Deformity Decreases:												
Hubscher Maneuver:	pos/neg							pos/neg				
GAIT EVALUATION:												
Extensor Substitution	yes/no							yes/no				
Flexor Stabilization	yes/no							yes/no				
Flexor Substitution	yes/no							yes/no				
Early Heel Off	yes/no							yes/no				
Mid Tarsal Break	yes/no							yes/no				

Radiographic Evaluation (Exhibit III)

Plain film X-ray evaluation utilizing lesion markers as needed is essential in evaluating the level and extent of the deformity. Standard AP and lateral views are obtained while the patient is in the angle and base of gait one foot at a time. A medial oblique (MO) view is included if a metatarsal stress fracture is in the differential diagnosis.

AP View:

Evaluate the AP view for transverse plane relationships by noting the following:

- **Digital Deformity Classification**
  Hammertoe
  Claw Toe
  Mallet Toe
  Clinodactyly

- **Lesion Marker Location:**
  Prominent Condyle (medial/lateral)

- **Linear Relationships: Normal, long, short**
  Metatarsals
  Phalanges

- **Positional Relationships (Digit): Abductus/adductus**
  MTPJ level
  PIPJ level
  DIPJ level

- **MTP Joint Condition:**
  Subluxation
  Dislocation
  Erosive Changes

- **Metatarsal head condition**
  Enlarged
  Malformed

- **IM Angles**

- **Metatarsus Primus Adductus**

- **Metatarsus adductus**

- **First Ray Stability (Hypermobility) by noting any subluxation**
  Metatarsal Cuneiform joint
  Cuneiform Navicular joint
  Intercuneiform joint (cuneiform split)

Lateral View:

Evaluate the lateral view for sagittal plane relationships by noting the following:

- **Digital Deformity Classification**
  Hammertoe
  Claw Toe
  Mallet Toe

- **Lesion Marker Location**

- **Linear Relationships**
  Second Metatarsal Length
  First Metatarsal Length

- **Positional Relationships**
  First Metatarsus Elevatus

- **First Ray Stability by noting joint subluxation**
  Metatarsal Cuneiform joint
  Cuneiform Navicular

Plantar Axial View:

Evaluate the plantar axial view for frontal plane relationships by noting the following:

- **Relative Metatarsal Head Position**
  This cannot be used to determine the absolute relationship of the position of the metatarsal head, as the longest toes when dorsiflexed in the positioning device will plantarflex the metatarsal the most.

- **Prominent Condyle (plantarly)**

- **Accessory Bone (plantarly)**

- **Soft Tissue Interface**
  Foreign Body

Exhibit III: Radiographic Evaluation

X-RAY EVALUATION:	1st R	2nd R	3rd R	4th R	5th R		1st L	2nd L	3rd L	4th L	5th L
INVOLVED RAY											
ANTERIOR POSTERIOR VIEW											
LESION MARKER LOCATION											
Proximal Phalanx:											
Head											
Base											
Intermediate Phalanx											
Distal Phalanx											
LINEAR RELATIONSHIPS											
Metatarsal Length: Normal											
Short											
Long											
Proximal Phalanx: Normal											
Short											
Long											
Intermediate Phalanx: Normal											
Short											
Long											
TRANSVERSE PLANE EVAL											
Metatarsus Adductus											
Metatarsus Primus Adductus											
First Metatarsal Cuneiform Joint											
Unstable (cuneiform split)											
Stable											
Digital Deformity											
Hammer Toe											
Claw Toe											
Digital Abductus: MTPJ											
PIPJ											
DIPJ											

Exhibit III–continued

X-RAY EVALUATION:	1st R	2nd R	3rd R	4th R	5th R	1st L	2nd L	3rd L	4th L	5th L
Digital Adductus: MTPJ										
PIPJ										
DIPJ										
Digital Aducto Varus										
Metatarso Phalangeal Joint:										
Subluxed										
Disclocated										
Erosions										
Misshapen										
Sesamoids; Tibial / Fibular										
Arthritic										
Subluxed										
Dislocated										
Fractured										
Bi, Multipartite										
LATERAL VIEW										
SAGITTAL PLANE EVAL										
Metatarsus Elevatus										
First Metatarsal Cuneiform Joint										
Unstable										
Dorsal Spurs										
Arthritic										
Second Metatarsal Length										
Normal:										
Short:										
Long:										
Digital Deformity										
Hammertoe										
Clawtoe										
Mallet Toe										
PLANTAR AXIAL VIEW										
FRONTAL PLANE EVAL										
Relative Met Head Position										
Elevated										
Depressed										

Exhibit III–continued

X-RAY EVALUATION:	1st R	2nd R	3rd R	4th R	5th R		1st L	2nd L	3rd L	4th L	5th L
Prominent Plantar Condyle											
Accessory Bone											
Sesamoids: Tibial / Fibular											
Arthritic											
Subluxed											
Dislocated											
Fractured											
Bi, Multipartite											
Soft Tissue Interface: FB											

Conclusions:

A metatarsalgia differential diagnosis can be established based upon the anatomy of the painful area categorizing the pathology into intra-articular; peri-articular, extra-articular, osseous, and skin disorders (Exhibit IV).

Surgical management of metatarsalgia consists of procedures which address the presenting problem and their sequelae.

Metatarsal structural and functional deformities are addressed with procedures which attempt to neutralize or eliminate an abnormal force or a pressure point either by shortening the central metatarsal, elevating (off - loading) the metatarsal or by performing partial metatarsal head resections with or without joint implantation.

Digital deformities creating retrograde force and prolapse or depression of the central metatarsal heads are surgically addressed at the same time as the metatarsal surgical procedure.

Severe arthrosis of isolated MTPJs is treated with joint destructive procedures such as partial metatarsal head resection with or without an implant; with involvement of multiple MTPJs a pan metatarsal head resection is performed.

Nerve entrapments are treated with neurolysis or neurectomy.

When performing reconstructive surgery on medial column digits one, two, and three, the goal should be to provide stability to the MTPJ and toe in order to obtain a proper digital lever for function of the windlass mechanism. This approach can sometimes be applied to the fourth toe as well, but not the fifth.

When performing surgery on lateral column digits four and five, the goal is to eliminate pressure points by removing bone and creating flexibility. Arthroplastic or total phalangectomy procedures are performed to accomplish this goal.

Significant load transfer to the central metatarsals from a dysfunctional first ray and/or ankle equinus creating transfer metatarsalgia needs to be addressed at the same time as the lesser metatarsal/digital procedures. This often requires custom foot orthotics or procedures to stabilize the first ray as well as to lengthen the Achilles tendon as needed.

The remainder of this text details how to surgically address the various causes of metatarsalgia and digital deformities based upon evaluation as just described.

Exhibit IV: Metatarsalgia Differential Diagnosis

1. **Intra-articular**
    A. Synovitis from a mechanical dysfunction
        1. MTPJ stress syndrome
            a. Pre-dislocation phase
            b. Dislocation phase (early)
    B. Synovitis from a systemic disorder
        1. Sero-positive arthropathy
            a. Rheumatoid arthritis
        2. Sero-negative arthropathy
            a. Crystal induced arthropathy (gout, pseudo-gout)
            b. Reiter's Syndrome
            c. Psoriatic arthropathy
            d. Ankylosing spondylitis
    C. Chondral disorder
        1. Traumatic chondritis from compression trauma
        2. Osteochondritis – sesamoiditis
        3. Osteochondral defect
        4. Arthritis
    D. Neuroarthropathy
    E. Infection: Septic Arthritis
        1. Contiguous
        2. Hematogenous

2. **Periarticular**
    A. Ligament strain
    B. Flexor plate/ligament rupture
        1. MTPJ stress syndrome
            a. Dislocation phase

    C.   Capsulitis/Joint effusion

    D.   Tendinitis/tenosynovitis

        1.   Extrinsic: flexor longus; extensor longus

        2.   Intrinsic: flexor brevis; extensor brevis

3.   **Extra-articular**

    A.   Intermetatarsal space inferior to intermetatarsal ligament (IML)

        1.   Neuritis

        2.   Morton's neuroma

        3.   Neurillemoma (schwannoma)

        4.   Paccinian corpuscle tumor

        5.   Infection

    B.   Intermetatarsal space superior to IML

        1.   Bursitis

        2.   Ganglion

        3.   Lipoma

        4.   Infection

    C.   Submetatarsal space

        1.   Subcutaneous bursitis/fibrosis

        2.   Extra osseous chondroma

        3.   Rheumatoid Nodule

        4.   Infection

4.   **Osseous**

    A.   Stress fracture (distal shaft)

    B.   Tumor

        1.   Enchondroma

        2.   Osteochondroma

        3.   Intraosseous glomus tumor

        4.   Ewing's Sarcoma

        5.   Metastatic

    C.   Avascular necrosis (Freiberg's infraction) (Second metatarsal head)

    D.   Neuroarthropathy

    E.   Infection: Osteomyelitis

5. **Plantar Skin**

    A.   Mechanically induced associated with a prolapsed metatarsal

        1.   Tyloma

        2.   Tyloma with intractable plantar keratoma (IPK)

        3.   Epidermal inclusion cyst

        4.   Ulceration

        5.   Porokeratosis plantaris discretum

    B.   Verrucae plantaris

    C.   Mosaic verrucae

    D.   Pitted keratolysis

    E.   Foreign body

6. **Digital Skin**

    A.   Mechanically induced associated with a digital deformity:

        1.   Heloma dura

        2.   Heloma molle

        3.   Onychophosis (nail groove callus)

        4.   Onychauxis

        5.   Onychocryptosis

        6.   Ulceration

    B.   Verrucae plana (flat wart)

    C.   Synovial (mucinous) cyst

7. **Other**

    A.   Proximal nerve entrapment – referred pain

        1.   Tarsal tunnel syndrome

        2.   Radiculopathy

    B.   Vascular: ischemic pain

    C.   Vascular: phlebitis

References:

Bhatia D, Myerson MS, Curtis MJ, Cunningham BW, Jinnah RH. Anatomical restraints to dislocation of the second metatarsophalangeal joint and assessment of a repair technique. *J Bone Joint Surg* 76:1371-1375, 1994.

Bojsen-Moller F, Flagstad KE. Plantar aponeurosis and internal architecture of the ball of the foot. *J Anat* 121:599-611, 1976.

Bojsen-Moller F. Anatomy of the forefoot, normal and pathologic. *Clin Orthop* 142:10-18, 1979.

Bojsen-Moller F, Lamoreux L. Significance of free dorsiflexion of the toes in walking. *Acta Orthop Scand* 50:471-479, 1979.

Bossley CJ, Cairney PC. The intermetatarsophalangeal bursa: Its significance in Morton's metatarsalgia. *J Bone Joint Surg Br* 62:184-187, 1980.

Carlson RE, Fleming LL, Hutton WC. The biomechanical relationship between the tendoachilles, plantar fascia and metatarsophalangeal joint dorsiflexion angle. *Foot Ankle Int* 21:18-25, 2000.

Davitt JS, Kadel N, Sangeorzan BJ, Hansen ST Jr, Holt SK, Donaldson-Fletcher E. An association between functional second metatarsal length and midfoot arthrosis. *J Bone Joint Surg Am* 87:795-800, 2005.

Deland JT, Lee KT, Sobel M, DiCarlo EF. Anatomy of the plantar plate and its attachments in the lesser metatarsal phalangeal joint. *Foot Ankle* 16:480-486, 1995.

Ford LA, Collins KB, Christensen, JC. Stabilization of the Subluxed Second Metatarsophalangeal joint: Flexor tendon transfer versus primary repair of the plantar plate. *J Foot Surg* 37: 217-222, 1998.

Grebing BR, Coughlin MJ. Evaluation of Morton's theory of second metatarsal hypertrophy. *J Bone Joint Surg Am* 86:1375-1386, 2004.

Grebing BR, Coughlin MJ. The effect of ankle position on the exam for first ray mobility. *Foot Ankle Int* 25:467-475, 2004.

Hicks JH. The mechanics of the foot: II. The plantar aponeurosis and the arch. *J Anat* 88:25 – 30, 1954.

Hughes J, Clark P, Klenerman L. The importance of the toes in walking. *J Bone Joint Surg Br* 72:245-251, 1990.

Jarrett BA, Manzi JA, Green D. Interossei and lumbricales muscles of the foot: An anatomical and functional study. *J Am Podiatry Assoc* 70:1-13, 1980.

Jenkin WM. Central Metatarsophalangeal Joint Arthrosis: Evaluation and Surgical Management. Musculoskeletal Disorders of the Lower Extremities. LM Oloff, Ed., WB Saunders Co., Philadelphia, Pa., 1994.

Mann RA, Mizel MA. Monarticular nontraumatic synovitis of the metatarso-phalangeal joint: A new diagnosis. *Foot Ankle* 6:17 - 21, 1985.

McGlamry ED. Floating toe syndrome. *JAPA* 72:561-568, 1982.

Migues A, Slullitel G, Bilbao F, Carrasco M, Solari G. Floating-toe deformity as a complication of the Weil osteotomy. *Foot Ankle Int* 25:609-613, 2004.

Morris JL. Biomechanical implications of hammertoe deformities. *Clinics in Pod Med & Surg* 3:339-349, 1986.

Morton DJ. The Human Foot: Its Evolution, Physiology and Functional Disorders, pp. 154-211. Columbia University Press, New York, NY, 1935.

Rodgers MM, Cavanagh PR. Pressure distribution in Morton's foot structure. *Med Sci Sports Exerc* 21:23-28, 1989.

Roukis TS, Landsman AS. Hypermobility of the first ray: a critical review of the literature. *Foot Ankle* 42:377-390, 2003.

Sarrafian SK. <u>Anatomy of the Foot and Ankle</u>. JB Lippincott, Philadelphia, Pa., 1993.

Sarrafian SK, Topouzean LK. Anatomy & physiology of the extensor apparatus of the toes. *JBJS* 51A:669-679, 1969.

Taub J, Steinberg M. Porokeratosis plantaris discreta. *Int J Dermatol* 9:1-4, 1970.

Yao L, Cracchiolo A, Farahani, K, Seeger LL. Magnetic resonance imaging of plantar plate rupture. *Foot Ankle* 17:33-36, 1996.

Yao L, Do HM, Cracchiolo A, Farahani K. Plantar plate of the foot: Findings on conventional arthrography and MRI imaging. *AJR* 163:641-644, 1994.

Hallux Hammertoe

2

Albert E. Burns, DPM, FACFAS

Introduction:

Hallux hammertoe or hallux malleus is a structural deformity with flexion contracture at the hallux interphalangeal joint and hyperextension at the first metatarsophalangeal joint. It occurs when there is compromise of the intrinsic muscles resulting in interphalangeal joint and first metatarsophalangeal joint instability. Instability of the first metatarsophalangeal joint occurs whenever there is loss of function of the flexor hallucis brevis, as would occur with the simultaneous excision of the tibial and fibular sesamoids. This loss of stability could be iatrogenic, traumatic or systemic.

Iatrogenic causes include:

1. Hallux varus either congenital or secondary to overcorrection of a hallux abductovalgus deformity where the hallux goes into adductus and dorsiflexion and there is a secondary flexion contracture at the hallux interphalangeal joint in an attempt to achieve hallux purchase.

2. Loss of function of the flexor hallucis brevis secondary to a Keller procedure (arthroplasty of the first metatarsophalangeal joint) or Keller procedure with hemi-implant or total hinge implant where resection of the base of the proximal phalanx was extensive enough to eliminate the insertion of the flexor hallucis brevis. The loss of the antagonist of the extensor hallucis longus at the first metatarsophalangeal joint results in dorsiflexion at that level and a secondary flexion contracture at the hallux interphalangeal in an attempt to achieve hallux purchase.

3. Excessive shortening of the first metatarsal will create "slack in the line" and thus instability at the first metatarsophalangeal joint due to the lack of adequate retrograde pressure and therefore, the development of flexion contracture of the hallux.

Traumatic causes include:

Hallux hammertoe would develop with any direct or indirect severance of the insertion of the flexor hallucis brevis muscle insertion.

Systemic causes would include neuromuscular disorders:

A Hallux hammertoe is usually found with neuromuscular disorders, specifically Charcot Marie Tooth disease. Intrinsic muscle weakness results in instability of the first metatarsophalangeal joint, allowing the extensor hallucis longus and flexor hallucis longus to become deforming forces extending the first metatarsophalangeal joint and flexing the hallux interphalangeal joint. The long-term results of these abnormal forces are the development of callosities plantar to the first metatarsal head, dorsal to the hallux interphalangeal joint and at the tip of the hallux. The foot is gradually changed into a pes cavus foot type that becomes fixed with time and can ultimately result in degenerative changes of the hallux interphalangeal joint, the first metatarsophalangeal joint and the first metatarsal and medial cuneiform articulation.

Paralysis of the anterior tibial muscle has also been implicated in the development of a hallux hammertoe; the paralysis allows the unopposed pull of the peroneus longus, causing aberrant first metatarsal plantarflexion. Due to increased pressure on the plantar surface of the first metatarsal head and dorsal surface of the hallux, this could potentially lead to ulceration in the neuropathic patient. The extensor hallucis longus, which extends the first metatarsophalangeal joint putting retrograde pressure to plantarflex the first metatarsal, will also increase pressure to the plantar surface of the first metatarsal. For these reasons the muscle balance and stability of the entire first ray should be taken into consideration in the management of the clawed hallux.

Conservative Treatment:

Conservative treatment modalities are directed at alleviating the pain associated with this structural deformity from such problems as joint synovitis, tenosynovitis, simple shoe irritation and painful callosities. The palliative care is also preventive, in attempting to obviate the development of ulceration, which could then progress to soft tissue infection and osteomyelitis. This would involve routine palliative care such as debridement of calluses and appropriate padding to protect the areas of irritation. It can also involve shoe modification and even custom molded shoes. For the patient population with an underlying neuromuscular condition, the use of custom molded shoes to both protect the foot and to provide stability to the foot is routine. If ulcerations have already developed, the appropriate wound care and off-weighting of the areas of break down is part of the care.

Surgical Treatment:

Hallux hammertoe is virtually never an isolated condition; when considering surgery, a variety of factors must be considered. The degree of flexibility and rigidity, any dynamic muscle imbalance and the degree of joint degeneration of all the structures and joints of the first ray must be evaluated. The evaluation of any underlying neuromuscular condition and its progression must be completely evaluated in order to prognosticate the long term success of any surgical intervention.

In a hallux varus, whether congenital or iatrogenic, the etiology of the hallux varus must be determined in order to achieve the proper correction. This may involve muscle rebalancing procedures, osteotomies and fusions. Hallux interphalangeal arthrodesis is usually part of the hallux varus repair, since the flexion contracture is fixed and/or there are degenerative changes of the hallux interphalangeal joint. With the hallux hammertoe secondary to a first metatarsophalangeal joint arthroplasty with or without a hemi-implant or total hinge implant, fusion of the hallux interphalangeal joint along with a flexor tendon transfer may be all that is needed in order to straighten the hallux and achieve hallux purchase. The difficulty in this situation comes with the fixation, since an intramedullary screw is not possible and the loss of bone and/or the presence of an implant stem may preclude the use of diagonally placed screws. In this instance the use of crossed K-wires or small staples may be the most appropriate fixation technique. Hallux interphalangeal joint fusion and flexor tendon transfer may again be all that is needed in correcting a hallux hammertoe that is secondary to an excessively shortened first metatarsal. This will transfer the function of the flexor hallucis longus from the hallux interphalangeal joint to the first metatarsophalangeal joint and make it a direct antagonist to the extensor hallucis longus at that level. The fusion will, therefore, simultaneously straighten the hallux and achieve hallux purchase.

For the neuromuscular foot where there is a flexible cavus, the modified Jones procedure has proved to be effective in correction of the clawing and relief of pain with a high degree of patient satisfaction. Jones originally described the transfer of the extensor hallucis longus tendon to the neck of the first metatarsal solely, but the procedure has morphed into also including a hallux interphalangeal fusion to minimize flexion caused by unopposed flexor hallucis longus tendon (Fig. 2-1). Arthrodesis of the hallux interphalangeal joint would obviously be indicated when there is pain due to traumatic arthritis, and the goal of the hallux interphalangeal joint fusion is to relieve pain and provide a stable lever on which the flexors and extensors can function. Both the first metatarsophalangeal joint and the first metatarsal and medial cuneiform articulation also need to be evaluated for the presence and degree of traumatic arthritis for consideration of possible arthrodesis of these joints.

There are several adjunct procedures that have been suggested to supplement the modified Jones. Due to the loss of active dorsiflexion at the first metatarsophalangeal joint, transplanting the extensor digitorum longus slip of the fifth digit to the base of the hallux proximal phalanx has been described. The potential complications associated with this procedure and the lack of any real problem associated with the decreased active dorsiflexion at the first metatarsophalangeal joint except through the action of the extensor hallucis brevis, has led the surgery department faculty at the California School of Podiatric Medicine to discourage this procedure. The unopposed pull of the peroneus longus tendon is not addressed with the modified Jones procedure,

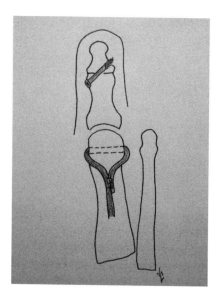

Figure 2-1: Clinical drawing representing the modified Jones procedure. This is the primary procedure used to address hallux hammertoe. The extensor hallucis is transferred to the first metatarsal to elevate it and the hallux interphalangeal joint is fused.

so peroneus longus tendon transfer to the peroneus brevis tendon has been advocated. This transfer, however, has a significant risk factor for elevation of the first metatarsal and the subsequent development of hallux limitus, and it cannot be recommended due to the likelihood of overcorrection. A fixed deformity of plantarflexion of the first ray is not addressed with the modified Jones procedure, so the utilization of a dorsiflexing osteotomy of the first metatarsal, fusion of the first metatarsal and medial cuneiform articulation, or a dorsiflexing osteotomy of the medial cuneiform should be considered to correct this.

An alternative procedure to the modified Jones is the transfer of the flexor hallucis longus tendon to the base of the proximal phalanx (Fig. 2-2). It has been described as the sole procedure with a flexible hallux hammertoe or concomitantly with a hallux interphalangeal joint arthrodesis when there is a fixed deformity at this joint. The procedure has the advantage of not weakening or removing the extensor hallucis longus tendon as a motor unit to the hallux and of not requiring a hallux interphalangeal fusion in a flexible deformity. However, the procedure does not address the plantarflexion of the first ray. The modified Jones procedure remains the procedure of choice and is recommended by the surgery department faculty at the California School of Podiatric Medicine.

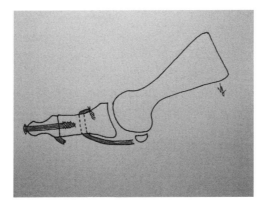

Figure 2-2: Clinical drawing representing the flexor hallucis longus transfer procedure to the base of the proximal phalanx of the hallux. This has been proposed as an alternative to the modified Jones procedure and may be done either with or without an arthrodesis of the hallux interphalangeal joint, depending on whether there is fixed deformity at that level.

Clinical indications for hallux interphalangeal fusion with or without a flexor tendon transfer:

1. Hallux hammertoe that is a fixed deformity.
2. Degenerative joint disease of the hallux interphalangeal joint.
3. Hallux hammertoe associated with hallux varus, assuming concomitant procedures are done to correct the hallux varus.
4. Hallux hammertoe secondary to a first metatarsophalangeal arthroplasty with or without hemi-implant or total hinge implant.
5. Hallux hammertoe secondary to excessive shortening of the first metatarsal, assuming the first metatarsal is evaluated for a concomitant procedure to assure the first ray will maintain its weight bearing capacity.

Clinical indications for the modified Jones procedure:

1. Hallux hammertoe, either flexible or fixed.
2. Hyperextension of the first metatarsophalangeal joint.
3. Plantarflexion of the first metatarsal that is flexible. (In a fixed deformity, an adjunctive dorsiflexing osteotomy of the first metatarsal, a fusion of the first

metatarsal and medial cuneiform articulation or a dorsiflexing osteotomy of the medial cuneiform should be performed.)

4. Degenerative arthritis of the hallux interphalangeal joint.

5. Degenerative arthritis of the first metatarsophalangeal joint would be indication for a first metatarsophalangeal joint fusion in lieu of the extensor hallucis longus transfer.

6. Degenerative arthritis of the first metatarsal and medial cuneiform joint would be indication for fusion of that joint and obviate the need for the extensor hallucis longus tendon transfer.

7. Weakness or paralysis of the anterior tibial muscle.

8. Callosities present plantar to the first metatarsal head, dorsal to the hallux interphalangeal joint and at the tip of the hallux.

Surgical Procedure:

Hallux interphalangeal fusion:

A serpentine incision that starts at the first metatarsophalangeal joint medial to the extensor hallucis longus tendon and extends distally to the hallux interphalangeal joint where it traverses transversally to the lateral side of the hallux, then extends out distally along the distal phalanx. The dissection is carried through the subcutaneous tissue to the level of the extensor hallucis longus tendon. Care should be taken to protect the two dorsal neurovascular bundles. The extensor hallucis longus tendon is incised transversely at the hallux interphalangeal joint and reflected proximally to the midshaft of the proximal phalanx. The capsule and supporting ligaments of the hallux interphalangeal joint are incised, delivering the head of the proximal phalanx into the wound, but making sure to protect the flexor hallucis longus tendon. The bone is cut so that there is no angular deviation in either the transverse or sagittal planes. Whatever angular correction that is desired is usually achieved by the resection of bone off the head of the proximal phalanx.

If a flexor tendon transfer is to be used, it can then be performed at this time. Either the flexor tendon can be split and brought around the proximal phalanx or a Kuwada technique can be performed as described in Chapter 6.

Fixation of the arthrodesis site would include but not be limited to the use of Kirschner wires, stainless steel wire, staples, thermoplastic staples and bone screws. K-wires are a simple and effective way of fixing the fusion site, using 0.062 inch pins. It is accomplished by using two pins in a crossed fashion advancing them from distal to proximal. Each pin should pass through the cortex of the distal phalanx, cross the fusion site and exit at the midpoint of the proximal phalanx (Fig. 2-3). Stainless steel wire may be used, but the wire should pass through both the dorsal and plantar cortices

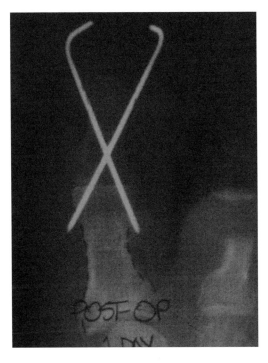

Figure 2-3: Postoperative X-ray illustrating the crossed pin technique for the fixation of the hallux interphalangeal joint fusion.

of the phalanges, not just the dorsal cortex. This should be done with two wires, either parallel to each other or crossing like an "X." K-wires and stainless steel wire could also be used together to create a tension band technique of fixation. Mini staples or small pneumatic-driven staples may also be used to internally fix the fusion site. K-wires, stainless steel wire and standard staples do not, however, provide any compression at the arthrodesis site. Thermoplastic staples like the OSStaple provide the ease of insertion and interfragmentary compression (Fig. 2-4).

The most prevalent method of internally fixing this fusion site, however, is with bone screws. This is most commonly done with either a 4.0 mm cancellous screw or a 3.5 mm fully threaded cancellous screw. When using the 4.0 mm cancellous screw, a drill hole is made through the distal phalanx with a 2.5 mm drill bit from proximal to distal. A small stab incision is made at the tip of the hallux to allow the drill bit to exit. The drill bit is removed, the resected joint surfaces are held flush and the 2.5 mm drill bit is reinserted through the distal phalanx drill hole from distal to proximal, using the drill hole in the distal phalanx as a drill guide to drill a guide hole into the proximal phalanx. The distal end of the distal phalanx should be countersunk to help prevent

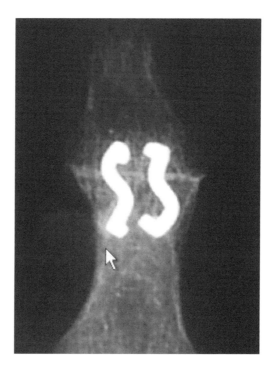

Figure 2-4: Postoperative X-ray illustrating hallux interphalangeal joint fusion with OSStaple™ fixation.

microfracturing and to reduce the protuberance of the head of the screw. A 3.5 mm cancellous tap is used to create a few threads at the distal end of the distal phalanx. The screw is advanced through the distal phalanx until it starts to emerge at the proximal end of that bone. The tip of the screw is then aligned with the guide hole in the proximal phalanx and the screw is advanced until the fusion site is compressed (Fig. 2-5). The length of the screw used depends on whether the surgeon wants to engage the distal or proximal metaphyseal bone of the proximal phalanx with the threads of the screw. A fully threaded 3.5 mm cancellous screw may be used in the exact same technique with the addition of overdrilling the distal phalanx with a 3.5 mm drill bit (Fig. 2-6, 2-7). Another alternative is to use a 4.0 mm cannulated cancellous screw, where a guide pin is driven in first for temporary fixation and the screw is passed right over the pin (Fig. 2-8). With all of these screw techniques, intraoperative radiographs or fluoroscopy should be taken to assure that the screw threads are engaging metaphyseal bone and that they are not violating the first metatarsophalangeal joint. Even with countersinking, however, the head of the screw is protuberant, predictably irritating to the patient and regularly needs to be removed. The advent of the smaller cannulated screws makes it possible to use one or two

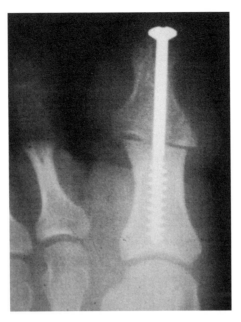

Figure 2-5: Postoperative X-ray illustrating hallux interphalangeal joint fusion with 4-0 cancellous screw fixation.

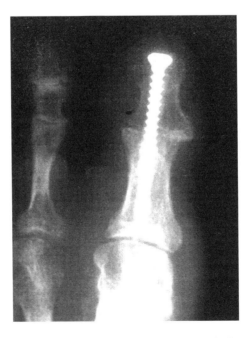

Figure 2-6: Postoperative X-ray illustrating hallux interphalangeal joint fusion with 3.5 cancellous screw fixation with threads engaging the metaphyseal bone of both the head and the base of the proximal phalanx.

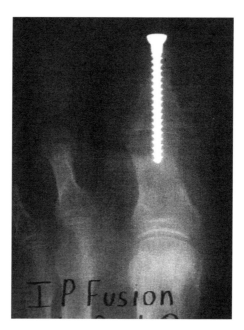

Figure 2-7: Postoperative X-ray illustrating hallux interphalangeal joint fusion with 3.5 cancellous screw fixation with threads engaging only the metaphyseal bone of the head of the proximal phalanx.

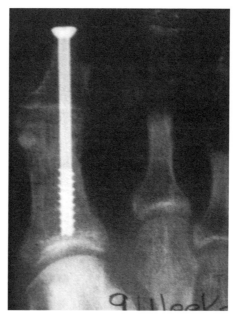

Figure 2-8: Postoperative X-ray illustrating hallux interphalangeal joint fusion with 4.0 cannulated cancellous screw fixation.

screws to cross the hallux interphalangeal joint transversely. This is the method favored by the surgery department faculty of the California School of Podiatric Medicine. Either the 2.4 or the 2.0 mm cannulated OsteoMed screws are used. One screw is passed from distal medial to proximal lateral and the other screw is passed from proximal medial to distal lateral, and they are stacked in the sagittal plane. If just one screw is used, it is passed from proximal medial to distal lateral. This technique has the further advantage of being able to be used if simultaneous fusion of the first metatarsophalangeal joint is required (Fig. 2-9). After adequate lavage, the deep tissues are closed with 3-0 or 4-0 absorbable suture and the skin is closed with 4-0 or 5-0 non-absorbable suture.

Jones procedure: The serpentine incision described for the hallux interphalangeal fusion is extended proximally medial to the extensor hallucis longus tendon to the level of the distal one-third of the first metatarsal (Fig. 2-10). The dissection,

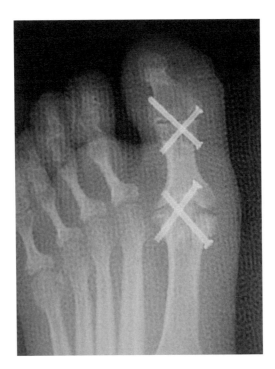

Figure 2-9: Postoperative X-ray of simultaneous hallux interphalangeal joint fusion and first metatarsophalangeal fusion using crossed cannulated 2.4 mm screws at the hallux interphalangeal joint and crossed 3.0 mm screws at the first metatar-sophalangeal.

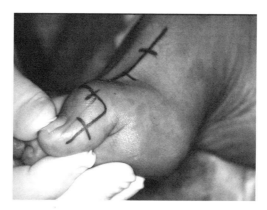

Figure 2-10: The incision for the modified Jones procedure parallels the extensor hallucis longus tendon medial to the tendon and is serpentined across the hallux interphalangeal joint to facilitate the fixation of the hallux interphalangeal joint arthrodesis.

exposure and preparation of the hallux interphalangeal joint are as described previously. Dissection is continued along the medial and lateral aspect of the head and neck of the first metatarsal, creating an artificial plane between the deep fascia and the periosteum. A drill hole is made from medial to lateral through the middle of the neck of the first metatarsal with a 2.0 mm drill bit and progressively enlarged to 3.5 mm (Fig. 2-11). Suture is passed through the end of the extensor hallucis tendon and a Keith needle is used to pull the tendon through the drill hole. With the foot in a neutral position to the leg and the first metatarsal maximally dorsiflexed the tendon of the extensor hallucis longus is put on tension and sutured onto itself with a 3-0 polyester suture (Fig. 2-12). This creates a sling out of the tendon through the neck of the first metatarsal. Attention is redirected back to the hallux interphalangeal joint to complete the fusion in the same fashion as previously described.

Pragmatically, the hallux hammertoe is most often seen with the cavus foot and the plantarflexion of the first ray is most likely to be a fixed deformity. Therefore, the extensor hallucis longus tenosuspension procedure is contraindicated. If the plantarflexion of the first ray is part of a global or total cavus, it will be corrected with the procedure used to correct the cavus deformity. If the plantarflexion is a local problem isolated to the first ray, then it is corrected with a first metatarsal dorsiflexing osteotomy, an arthrodesis of the first metatarsal and medial cuneiform articulation, or a dorsiflexing osteotomy of the medial cuneiform. Unless there is significant degenerative arthritis of the first metatarsal and medial cuneiform articulation, the surgery department of the California School of Podiatric Medicine prefers doing a dorsiflexing osteotomy of the first metatarsal. Exposure is accessed by extending the

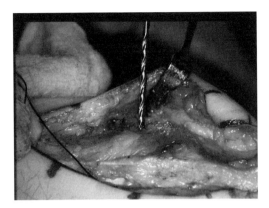

Figure 2-11: A hole to pass the tendon of the extensor hallucis longus is drilled through the neck of the first metatarsal. It is gradually enlarged and does not require opening the first metatarsophalangeal joint unless the joint is opened for another reason.

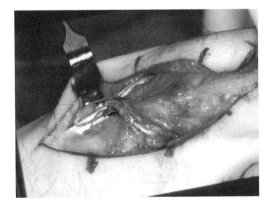

Figure 2-12: The extensor hallucis longus tendon is passed through the first metatarsal neck and sutured back on itself forming a sling to hold the first metatarsal dorsiflexed.

previously described incision proximally along the dorsomedial aspect of the first metatarsal to the level of the medial cuneiform. Dissection is carried down by layers and the base of the first metatarsal is exposed subperiosteally. There are four methods typically used to fashion the osteotomy. The classical method is to do an osteotomy in the transverse plane with the base dorsal and the apex plantar, maintaining a cortical hinge at the plantar cortex (Fig. 2-13). The second is a modification of the first where the osteotomy is oblique running from distal dorsal to proximal plantar again with the base dorsal and the apex plantar, maintaining a plantar cortical hinge (Fig. 2-14). The advantage of this is that is lends itself to fixation with one or two bone screws in a lag technique. The third method is to make an oblique osteotomy from proximal medial to distal lateral that is through and through and gives the advantage of being able to rotate the distal segment to whatever level is determined to be most appropriate intraoperatively (Fig. 2-15). This osteotomy can also be fixed with bone screws, but has the inherent disadvantage of being unstable. It is the method most likely to displace with premature weight bearing. The fourth method is a sagittal "Z" osteotomy that again allows the metatarsal head to be moved in the sagittal plane to the appropriate level. Fixation is achieved with two cortical lag screws passed from medial to lateral (Fig. 2-16). Closure is achieved as previously described (Fig. 2-17).

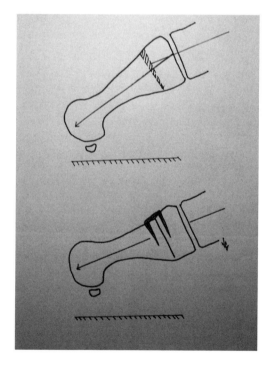

Figure 2-13: A dorsal wedge osteotomy to elevate the first metatarsal may be performed in a traditional fashion at the base of the first metatarsal with the base dorsal and the apex plantar.

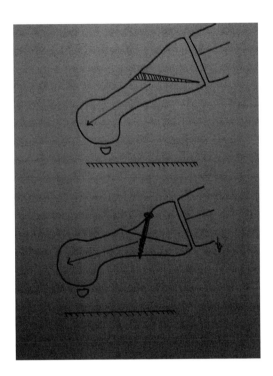

Figure 2-14: The dorsal wedge osteotomy to elevate the first metatarsal may be performed obliquely with the base dorsal distal and the apex plantar proximal in order to accommodate screw fixation.

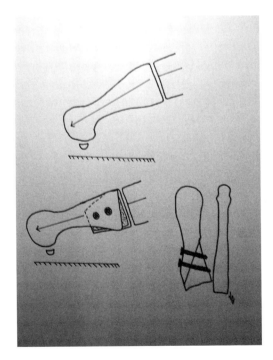

Figure 2-15: A through and through osteotomy of the first metatarsal may be performed from proximal medial to distal lateral to elevate the first metatarsal by rotating the distal segment dorsally and fixing the osteotomy with two lag screws.

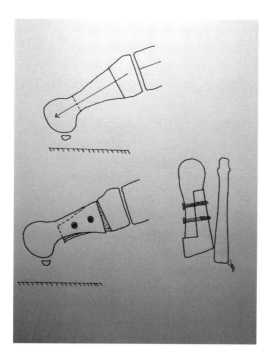

Figure 2-16: A sagittal plane "Z" osteotomy of the first metatarsal may be performed that will allow elevation of the head of the first metatarsal and provide more stability than the straight through and through oblique osteotomy. It is fixed with two lag screws passed from medial to lateral.

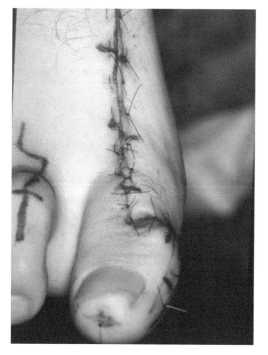

Figure 2-17: An intraoperative photograph illustrating the closure of the modified Jones procedure.

Postoperative Management:

The postoperative management varies depending on the combination of procedures is used. This is specific to the weight bearing and immobilization status of the patient.

1. Arthrodesis of the hallux interphalangeal joint and the first metatarsophalangeal joint do not require non-weight bearing, but three weeks of non-weight bearing with mobilization of the foot is recommended. This would apply whether the two procedures are done separately or together. The ability to mobilize the foot is dependent on whether a fixation technique that creates compression was used or not. After that, protected weight bearing in a postoperative shoe is continued until there is radiographic evidence of union, which is usually at six to eight weeks postoperatively.

2. A dorsal wedge osteotomy of the first metatarsal, fusion of the first metatarsal and medial cuneiform articulation and a dorsiflexion osteotomy of the medial cuneiform all require six to eight weeks of non-weight bearing. The ability to mobilize the extremity is again dependent on whether a fixation technique that creates compression was used or not. In order to build up the bone strength, protected weight bearing in a postoperative shoe for another two to three weeks is used after that whether there appears to be boney union or not.

3. The extensor hallucis longus tendon transfer requires immobilization for four weeks; although non-weight bearing in not required, it is recommended for that period of time. After that, the patient is progressed to partial weight bearing and muscle strengthening exercises for an additional three to four weeks.

4. Immediate postoperative X-rays are taken for all procedures.

5. The patient should return at one week postoperative for a dressing change and evaluation for infection. If there is an infection present the appropriate treatment should be instituted, but the weight bearing and mobilization status would continue to be dictated by the procedures performed.

6. The patient would return at two weeks for suture removal.

7. Serial radiographs are taken approximately every three weeks to evaluate for arthrodesis and osteotomy site healing.

8. If there are external fixation devices, the patient is instructed on how to do pin care with hydrogen peroxide and cotton swabs twice a day, after the sutures have been removed.

9. K-wires are pulled at six weeks unless there is a problem that would require their earlier removal.

Inherent Complications:

1. Catching the great toe when walking barefoot is a common complaint of patients who have had the modified Jones procedure. This is usually described as a minor problem, but should it be significant, it might require a first metatarsophalangeal joint fusion at a later date.

2. Hallux limitus with overcorrection of the elevation of the first ray. This is possible with all of the procedures described, but is primarily associated with the peroneus longus tendon transfer, which is why we do not recommend it. With the other procedures it can often be controlled with a functional orthotic. Failing this, then another procedure to make structural correction or a first metatarsophalangeal fusion of a degenerative joint would be indicated.

3. Metatarsalgia of the lesser metatarsophalangeal joints could also result with overcorrection of the elevation of the first ray. The use of a functional orthotic can usually control this, but additional corrective surgery of the first ray may be required.

4. Stress fractures of the lesser metatarsals. The patient is immobilized in a postoperative shoe for three to four weeks to allow for fracture healing followed by the same treatment describe for metatarsalgia.

5. Transfer lesions to the lesser metatarsal heads can also occur with overcorrection of the first ray. Palliation and orthotics can be used to control the problem, but failure of these can also result in the need for additional surgery of the first ray.

6. Non-union of an arthrodesis site which would require additional non-weight bearing, the use of a bone stimulator, or revision surgery with or without the use of bone graft.

7. Irritation at the tip of the hallux from the head of the bone screw is a common problem and requires the removal of the screw after the hallux interphalangeal fusion is complete.

8. Hallux flexus when the hallux interphalangeal joint is not fused for a flexible hallux hammertoe and the flexor hallucis longus continues to contract over time. For this reason we recommend hallux interphalangeal fusion in either a flexible or fixed deformity of hallux hammertoe.

Clinical Pearls:

1. The extensor hallucis longus tendon transfer should be done extraperiosteally rather than subperiosteally in order to decrease the risk of avascular necrosis.

2. The hole fashioned into the neck of the first metatarsal for the extensor hallucis longus tendon transfer procedure should be progressively enlarged in order to decrease the risk of fracturing the metatarsal.

3. With the elevation of the first metatarsal, no matter which method is selected, it is better to err toward slight under-correction rather than slight overcorrection because of all of the problems associated with an elevated first ray.

4. Regardless of whether the hallux hammertoe deformity is flexible or fixed, we recommend arthrodesis of the hallux interphalangeal joint.

5. For the fixation of the hallux interphalangeal joint arthrodesis, we recommend the use of the small crossing screws or the thermoplastic staples. These give the advantage of interfragmentary compression without the potential irritation problems associated with standard screws.

6. Although controversial in the literature, we recommend a minimum of three weeks of non-weight bearing with any of the procedures described in order to get the highest likelihood of bone healing, except for an isolated hallux IPJ arthrodesis.

References:

Breusch SJ, Wenz W, Doderlein L. Function after correction of a clawed great toe by a modified Robert Jones transfer. *J Bone Joint Surg (Br)* 82-B:250-254, 2000.

Burns AE. Surgical Procedures of the Hallux. McGlamry's Comprehensive Textbook of Foot and Ankle Surgery. Banks A, et al, Ed., Lippincott Williams & Wilkins, Philadelphia, Pa., 2001.

Burns AE. Surgical Procedures of the Hallux. McGlamry's Forefoot Surgery. Banks A, et al, Ed., Lippincott Williams & Wilkins, Philadelphia, Pa., 2004.

DeSteiger RN, Menelaus MB. Hallux Interphalangeal Extensus. *J Pediatric Orthop* 13:797-798, 1993.

Elias FN, Yuen TJ, Olson SL, Sangeorzan BJ, Ledoux WR. Correction of Clawed Hallux Deformity: Comparison of the Jones Procedure and FHL Transfer in a Cadaver Model. *Foot & Ankle International* 28:369-376, 2007.

Forrester-Brown MF. Tendon Transplantation for Clawing of the Great Toe. *J Bone Joint Surg (Am)* 20:57-60, 1938.

Franke JP, Turf R, Tirone M. Arthrodesis of the Hallux Interphalangeal Joint Using a Diagonally planed 2mm Cortical Bone Screw. *J Foot Surg* 28:466-470, 1989.

Gerbert J. Digital Arthrodesis. *Clin in Podiatry* 2:81-94, 1985.

Gerbert J. Chapter 16: Hallux Limitus/Hallux Rigidus. Textbook of Bunion Surgery Gerbert J, Ed., 3rd edition, Saunders, Philadelphia, Pa., 2001.

Jenkin WM. Chapter 17: Hallux Varus. Textbook of Bunion Surgery Gerbert J, Ed., 3rd edition, Saunders, Philadelphia, Pa., 2001.

Kadel NJ, Donaldson-Fletcher EA, Hansen ST, Sangeorzan BJ. Alternative to the modified Jones Procedure: Outcomes of the Flexor Hallucis Longus (FHL) Tendon Transfer Procedure for Correction of Clawed Hallux. *Foot & Ankle International* 26:1021-1026, 2005.

Langford J, Fenton CF. Hallux Interphalangeal Arthrodesis. *J Am Podiatry Assoc* 72:155-157, 1982.

Mills GP. The Etiology and Treatment of Claw Foot. *J Bone Joint Surg (Am)* 6:142-149, 1924.

Olson SL, Ledoux WR, Ching RP, Sangeorzan BJ. Muscular Imbalances Resulting in a Clawed Hallux. *Foot & Ankle International* 24:477-485, 2003.

Shives TC, Johnson KA. Arthrodesis of the Interphalangeal Joint of the Great Toe - An Improved Technique. *Foot & Ankle* 1:26-29, 1980.

Steensma MR, Jabara M, Anderson JG, Bohay DR. Flexor Hallucis Longus Tendon Transfer for Hallux Claw Toe Deformity and Vertical Instability of the Metatarsophalangeal Joint. *Foot & Ankle International* 27:689-692, 2006.

Wagner LC. The Operative Correction of Extreme Flexion Contraction of the Great Toe. *J Bone Joint Surg (Am)* 16:914-918, 1934.

Arthrotomy, Exostectomy, Arthroplasty, Syndactylism and Skin Plasties of Lesser Digits

3

Joel R. Clark, DPM, FACFAS

Introduction:

This chapter will deal with isolated digital procedures other than arthrodesis (Chapter 4) and implants (Chapter 5) for digits two through five. We will cover extensor and flexor tenotomies, arthrotomies of the PIPJ, arthroplasties, intermediate phalangectomy, syndactylism, partial ostectomies, and "V-Y" and "Z" plasties. Our method of clinical evaluation of lesser digits can be found in Chapter 1.

Soft Tissue Releases Digits Two through Four

In this section we will present isolated soft tissue releases for reducible digital deformities of toes two through four. The pathomechanics and evaluation of digital deformities is found in Chapter 1. We will discuss extensor tenotomy, flexor tenotomy and extensor tendon realignment. For flexor tendon transfer and soft tissue management of the dislocated lesser metatarsal-phalangeal joint, the reader is referred to Chapter 6.

Extensor Longus and Brevis Tenotomy:

Indications:

- An elderly patient in whom the PIPJ contracture is chronically irritated by shoe gear and the digit reveals some reducibility.
- Need to perform a minimal procedure for a contracted digit due to a medically compromised patient
- Laterally or dorsally deviated digit secondary to fibrosis from a prior surgery.

Advantages:

- Minimal post-operative recovery allowing immediate propulsive gait.
- Usually can be performed via a minimal incisional approach.

Disadvantages:

- In most cases does not correct the underlying pathology.
- May not achieve sufficient resolution of symptoms.

Inherent Complications:

- Weakness of the involved digit.
- Need for additional surgery.

Procedure:

A stab incision is made at the level of the metatarsal phalangeal joint. The blade is inserted through the incision passing below the extensor longus and brevis. The blade is rotated so the cutting edge is directed dorsally, keeping the handle perpendicular to the original incision. While plantarflexing the toe at the metatarsal phalangeal joint, both tendons are incised. The skin incision is closed with one or two simple interrupted sutures. The procedure may also be performed with a longer 2-3 cm incision centered just proximally to the metatarsal phalangeal joint. The extensor longus tendon is isolated and using a slide technique the longus tendon is lengthened and the brevis tendon transected. The skin is closed and dressed as per the surgeon's preference.

Post-operative Management:

Any shoe large enough to accommodate the bandages may be used. Generally, sutures may be removed in one to two weeks depending on the incision type, with the patient returning to normal activities as tolerated. We will often employ a crest-buttress pad or similar splint for three to four weeks following suture removal to maintain the alignment of the digit.

Flexor Tenotomy:

Indications:

- An elderly patient in whom a contracture at the PIPJ and/or DIPJ is chronically irritated by shoe gear or irritation at the distal tip of the digit with signs of some reducibility.
- Need to perform a minimal procedure for a contracted digit due to a medically compromised patient.
- Laterally or dorsally deviated digit secondary to fibrosis from a prior surgery.

Advantages:

- Minimal post-operative recovery allowing immediate propulsive gait.
- Usually can be performed via a minimal incisional approach.

Disadvantages:

- In most cases does not correct the underlying pathology.
- May not achieve sufficient resolution of symptoms.

Inherent Complications:

- Weakness of the involved digit.
- Painful plantar scar.
- Need for additional surgery.

Procedure:

If a skin contracture is present, then a plantar incision should be made at the level of the involved joint (Fig. 3-1). If no skin contracture exists, then the incision may be made on either the plantar medial or plantar lateral side of the digit. The transverse

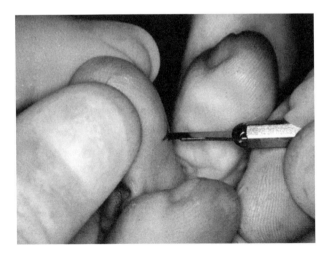

Figure 3-1: Clinical photograph of a plantar stab incision for a flexor tenotomy at the PIPJ.

plantar stab incision is made directly under the involved proximal or distal interphalangeal joint. The blade is advanced and with the toe straightened into a corrected position, the flexor longus and brevis may both be incised if desired at the proximal joint and the flexor longus at the distal joint. If a plantar capsular contracture is present, the blade is advanced and the capsule released. If no plantar skin contracture is present, a longitudinal incision may be made on either side of the toe just below the tendon. The blade is advanced until it is across the tendon(s) and rotated dorsally while the toe is straightened, incising one or both tendons depending on the location and the surgeon's determination of the etiology of the contracture. The blade may then be further directed dorsally to release the plantar capsule. If the flexor brevis was not incised at the proximal joint, then the blade must be reinserted above the brevis to release the plantar capsule. If a plantar skin contracture was present, the plantar incision is not sutured. The skin is closed and dressed as per the surgeon's preference.

Post-operative Management:

Any shoe large enough to accommodate the bandages may be used. Suture may be removed generally in one to two weeks with the patient returning to normal activities as tolerated. We will often employ a crest-buttress pad or similar splint for three to four weeks following suture removal to maintain the alignment of the digit.

Extensor Trifurcation Lock with PIPJ Arthrotomy:

Indications:

- Isolated flexible contracture of the PIPJ unless other procedures are performed to correct additional pathology.
- Absence of pain at the PIPJ with motion.
- Normal to short digit. (An abnormally long digit would be contraindicated.)
- A dorsal heloma dura may be present at the PIPJ.

Advantages:

- No osseous involvement.
- Minimal post-operative recovery.
- Allows for immediate ambulation.

Disadvantages:

- Cannot be performed on a long digit unless an osseous procedure is also performed to create shortening.
- Requires meticulous dissection.
- The procedure does not lengthen a shortened extensor longus tendon.

Inherent Complications:

- Chronic edema (dactylitis) which may require a steroid injection in which the digit is anesthetized and then an acetate steroid is injected into the site of maximum edema.
- Stiff PIPJ.

Procedure:

A longitudinal incision is made centered over the proximal interphalangeal joint. A heloma dura over the PIPJ can be ellipsed if present. The incision is deepened to the level of the extensor tendon. The central slip of the extensor tendon is removed from its attachment to the base of the intermediate phalanx. The medial and lateral slips of the extensor tendon are freed and brought together over the PIPJ, reducing the flexible PIPJ contracture, and sutured together with an absorbable suture (Fig. 2-2 A-C). The skin is closed and dressed as per the surgeon's preference.

Post-operative Management:

The patient is placed in a post-operative shoe. Sutures may generally be removed in two weeks with the patient returning to normal activities as tolerated.

Arthroplasty:

In this section, we will present arthroplasties of the proximal interphalangeal joint of digits 2-5 and the distal interphalangeal joints of digits 2-4. We generally are not performing an arthroplasty of the PIPJ on the second digit as an isolated procedure, but rather in combination with other procedures such as a flexor tendon transfer (see Chapter 6) with K-wire fixation to create more stability than an arthroplasty alone. The third digit PIPJ arthroplasties are more commonly performed but once again, may frequently be combined with techniques to create a more stable post-operative digit as described above. Arthroplasties of the PIPJ of the fourth and fifth and the DIPJ of the second, third and fourth are frequently performed as an isolated procedure.

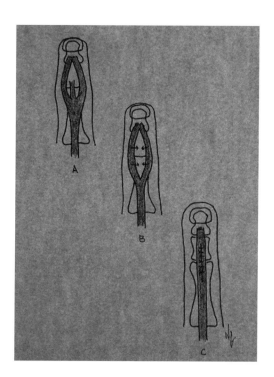

Figure 3-2: A: Diagram of the extensor tendon with its central slip inserting into the base of the intermediate phalanx and the medial and lateral slips passing distally to the base of the distal phalanx. **B:** Diagram showing the central slip removed from the intermediate phalanx. **C:** Diagram showing the medial and lateral slips brought together and sutured with an absorbable suture to reduce the flexible contracture.

PIPJ Arthroplasty:

Indications:

- A semi-reducible or rigid deformity of the PIPJ.
- A varus rotated toe may be present.
- A heloma dura over the PIPJ may be present.
- A heloma molle may be present.
- Pathology may exist at the MTPJ requiring additional procedures.
- An elongated digit may be present.

Advantages:

- Quality of the bone stock is not a factor.
- Allows correction in sagittal, transverse and frontal planes.
- Can be easily stabilized with temporary K-wire fixation.
- Maintains flexibility at the PIPJ.
- Allows shortening of the digit.
- Can be easily combined with other associated procedures in the digit and/or the MTPJ.
- Allows immediate post-operative propulsive ambulation and return to regular foot gear in two to three weeks.

Disadvantages:

- As an isolated procedure does not correct contractures at the MTPJ.
- As an isolated procedure in the second and third digits does not create inherent stability.

Inherent Complications:

- Chronic edema (dactylitis) which may require a steroid injection as described in the Extensor Trifurcation Lock section.
- Weakness of the digit.
- Lack of toe purchase.
- Shortening of the digit.

Procedure:

When a sagittal plane deformity is present, a linear incision is made centered over the PIPJ. If a heloma dura is present, two semielliptical incisions are made (Fig. 3-3) excising as much of the lesion as possible and the skin and deep fascia is removed to the level of the extensor tendon. If varus rotation is present as typically seen in a fifth digit, we use an elliptical incision starting dorsally over the intermediate phalanx and running distal dorsal-medial to proximal plantar-lateral (Fig. 3-4). We make the incision more vertical to the long axis of the toe based on the severity of the varus rotation. In addition, if a heloma dura is present, the incision should be oriented to excise as much of the lesion as possible. The skin is then removed. The extensor long tendon is then transected just proximal to the PIPJ. On the second digit we will sometimes divide the tendon longitudinally, reflecting it to either side of the PIPJ. A dorsal transverse capsulotomy is made and the head of the proximal phalanx is freed of all soft tissue attachments. With the extensor longus tendon dissected proximally or

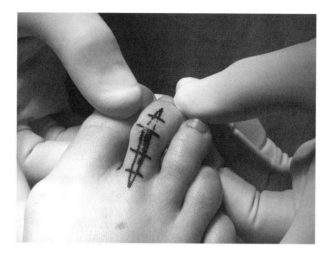

Figure 3-3: Clinical photograph of the two semielliptical incisions we typically use for a PIPJ arthroplasty.

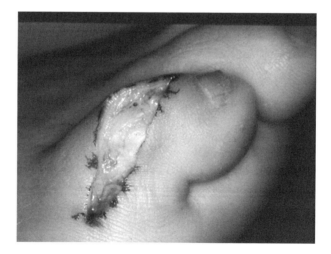

Figure 3-4: Clinical photograph. In a fifth digit, we use an elliptical incision starting dorsally over the intermediate phalanx and running distal dorsal-medial to proximal plantar-lateral. We make the incision more vertical to the long axis of the toe based on the severity of the varus rotation. In addition, if a heloma dura is present, the incision should be oriented to excise as much of the lesion as possible.

reflected to either side of the joint, the head of the proximal phalanx is delivered dorsally and resected perpendicular to the shaft of the phalanx. The toe is manipulated to assure that adequate bone was removed and that the stump of the proximal phalanx is not abutting the base of the intermediate phalanx. The phalanx is inspected for any remaining spicules and the toe is evaluated to assure that all contractures are reduced and the toe is in normal alignment

On the fifth digit we will frequently also perform a hemi-phalangectomy of the intermediate phalanx. A blade is inserted plantarly under the intermediate phalanx and then rotated around the lateral side to the dorsal surface. The dorsal lateral surface of the intermediate phalanx is then resected. This reduces the frequency of a reoccurrence of the dorsal lateral heloma dura as the toe drops back following the head resection on the proximal phalanx.

The wound is flushed. If the extensor tendon has been transected or divided longitudinally, it is reapproximated with an absorbable suture. The skin is closed and dressed as per the surgeon's preference.

Post-operative Management:

The patient is placed in a post-operative shoe. X-rays are taken at one week to access the arthroplasty site. Sutures may generally be removed in two weeks with the patient returning to normal activities as tolerated. The toe may continue to be splinted with a Darco Digital Splint™ or similar device for an additional two to four weeks when necessary.

DIPJ Arthroplasty:

Indications:

- Semi-reducible or rigid deformity of the DIPJ.
- An excessively long intermediate phalanx may be present.
- A heloma dura may be present over the DIPJ or at the distal end of the toe.
- A mucin cyst may be present.

Advantages:

- Quality of the bone stock is not a factor.
- Allows correction in sagittal, transverse and frontal planes.
- Can be easily stabilized with temporary K-wire fixation.
- Maintains flexibility at the DIPJ.
- Allows shortening of the digit.
- Can be easily combined with other associated procedures in the digit and/or the MTPJ.

- Allows immediate post-operative propulsive ambulation and return to regular foot gear in two to three weeks.

Disadvantages:

- Does not allow for stability at this level of the digit.
- Usually requires a special transverse incisional approach.

Inherent Complications:

- Chronic edema (dactylitis) which may require a steroid injection as described in the Extensor Trifurcation Lock section.
- Weakness of the digit.
- Lack of toe purchase.

Procedure:

A "U" shaped or smile incision is made centered over the DIPJ (Fig. 3-5). The width dorsally is proportional to the amount of bone to be removed. The arms of the U extend from dorsal aspect to plantar proximal along both sides of the digit. The dorsal portion of the incision is incised deep to bone while the incisions along the sides of the toe are only through the skin. For ease of removal, we make a longitudinal incision centrally on the toe and dissect the tissue to either side. All tissue is removed dorsally down to bone and as the dorsal-medial and dorsal-lateral borders are reached, the dissection removes only the skin to preserve the neurovascular structures on the medial and lateral sides of the toe. The head of the intermediate phalanx is freed of all soft tissue attachments and the extensor longus tendon is reflected proximally off the shaft of the intermediate phalanx. Sufficient bone is removed from the head of the intermediate phalanx. The toe is manipulated to assure that adequate bone was removed and that the stump of the intermediate phalanx is not abutting the base of the distal phalanx. The phalanx is inspected for any remaining spicules and the toe is evaluated to assure that all contractures are reduced and the toe is in normal alignment. The wound is flushed. We prefer to close the incision using one non-absorbable vertical mattress suture dorsally, with the deep arms of the mattress stitch approximating the extensor tendon and skin. The remainder of the incision is closed with simple interrupted sutures.

Post-operative Management:

The patient is placed in a post-operative shoe. X-rays are taken at one week to access the arthroplasty site. Sutures may generally be removed in two weeks with the patient returning to normal activities as tolerated.

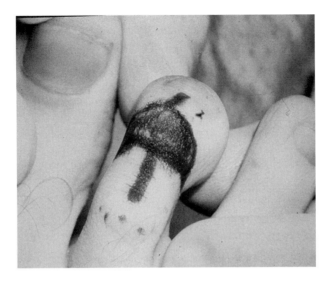

Figure 3-5: Clinical photograph of a "U" shaped or smile incisioncentered over the DIPJ. The width dorsally is proportional to the amount of bone to be removed. The arms of the U extend from dorsal aspect to plantar proximal along both sides of the digit.

Combined PIPJ and DIPJ Arthroplasty:

Indications:

- Excessively long intermediate phalanx.
- A semi-reducible or rigid deformity at the DIPJ and PIPJ.
- A heloma dura may be present over the PIPJ, DIPJ or at the distal end of the toe.
- Pathology may exist at the MTPJ requiring additional procedures.

Advantages:

- Quality of the bone stock is not a factor.
- Allows correction in sagittal, transverse and frontal planes.
- Can be easily stabilized with temporary K-wire fixation.
- Maintains flexibility at the PIPJ and DIPJ.
- Allows shortening of the digit.

- Can be easily combined with other associated procedures in the digit and/or the MTPJ.

- Allows immediate post-operative propulsive ambulation and return to regular foot gear in two to three weeks.

Disadvantages:

- As an isolated procedure does not correct contractures at the MTPJ.

- As an isolated procedure in the second and third digits does not create inherent stability.

Inherent Complications:

- Chronic edema (dactylitis) which may require a steroid injection as described in the Extensor Trifurcation Lock section.

- Weakness of the digit.

- Lack of toe purchase.

- Shortening of the digit.

Procedure:

A linear incision is made from just proximal to the nail matrix over the DIPJ and PIPJ to the base of the proximal phalanx. If a heloma dura(s) is/are present, two semielliptical incisions are made excising as much of the lesion(s) as possible and removing the skin and deep fascia to the level of the extensor tendon. The extensor longus tendon is then transected just proximal to the DIPJ and reflected proximally across the PIPJ to midshaft on the proximal phalanx. The heads of the proximal and intermediate phalanxes are freed of soft tissue attachments and transected perpendicular to the phalanx. The toe is manipulated to assure that adequate bone was removed and that the stump of the proximal is not abutting the base of the intermediate phalanx and the stump of the intermediate phalanx is not abutting the base of the distal phalanx. The phalanxes are inspected for any remaining spicules and the toe is evaluated to assure that all contractures are reduced and the toe is in normal alignment. The wound is flushed. The extensor tendon is reapproximated with an absorbable suture. The skin is closed and dressed as per the surgeon's preference.

Post-operative Management:

The patient is placed in a post-operative shoe. X-rays are taken at one week to access the arthroplasty sites. Sutures may generally be removed in two weeks with the patient returning to normal activities as tolerated. The toe may continue to be splinted with a Darco Digital Splint™ or similar device for an additional two to four weeks when necessary.

Intermediate Phalangectomy:

In selected cases we may elect to perform an intermediate phalangectomy of the digit rather than a head resection at the PIPJ and/or DIPJ. The procedure is most commonly considered when evaluating a fourth or fifth digit where the intermediate phalanx is small. If a heloma dura or heloma molle is present, lesion markers should be used when taking X-rays to asses the osseous pathology underlying the lesion. It may be necessary when performing an intermediate phalangectomy to perform a partial ostectomy on the head of the proximal phalanx to adequately eliminate osseous prominences underlying the lesion. The decision to perform an intermediate phalangectomy verses a resection of the head of the proximal or intermediate phalanx is often based on the surgeons' personal preference and experience with the procedure.

Indications:

- A small intermediate phalanx in which there is contracture at the DIPJ and/or PIPJ.
- Varus rotated fourth or fifth toes.
- Heloma dura may be present.
- Elongated digit may be present.

Advantages:

- Shorten digit.
- Eliminates pathology at the DIPJ and PIPJ.
- Will allow de-rotation of a varus fourth or fifth toes.
- Does not involve cutting bone.

Disadvantages:

- Can only be performed in the presence of a small intermediate phalanx.
- Limited patient population.

Inherent Complications:

- Chronic edema (dactylitis) which may require a steroid injection as described in the Extensor Trifurcation Lock section.
- Excessively shortened toe.
- Significant weakness of the toe.

Procedure:

The appropriate skin incision is used as previously described for an arthroplasty of the digit of digits 2-4 or the fifth digit, although it may be extended slightly more distal to gain access to the DIPJ. The extensor tendon is incised just proximal to the DIPJ and reflected proximally past the PIPJ. A transverse capsulotomy is then made at the DIPJ and the PIPJ. The intermediate phalanx is then freed of its soft tissue attachments and dissected from the wound. If a partial ostectomy is needed on the head of the proximal phalanx, it is now performed. The wound is flushed. The extensor tendon is reapproximated with an absorbable suture. The skin is closed and dressed as per the surgeon's preference.

Post-operative Management:

The patient is placed in a post-operative shoe. Sutures may generally be removed in two weeks with the patient returning to normal activities as tolerated. The toe may continue to be splinted with a Darco Digital Splint™ or similar device for an additional two to four weeks when necessary.

Syndactylism of the Fourth and Fifth Digits:

A syndactylism, or web space advancement, of the fourth and fifth digits is a procedure we use both as a primary procedure when confronted with a painful fibrotic heloma molle of the fourth interspace, or as a salvage procedure for a failed fifth digit. When a longstanding and fibrotic heloma molle is found, our experience is that it will often not resolve with a typical arthroplasty procedure and the patient will continue to develop symptoms in the area. The syndactylism allows the ability to perform the necessary associated osseous procedures while removing the fibrotic heloma molle. The procedure is also used following a failed procedure on the fifth digit in which a flail fifth toe exists and/or a painful heloma molle remains.

Indications:

- A painful, fibrotic heloma molle may be present in the web of the fourth interspace.
- A heloma dura may be present on the dorsal lateral aspect of the fifth digit or on the dorsal aspect of the fourth.
- A contracture at the PIPJ of the fourth toe as well as contracture and/or varus rotation of the fifth toe.
- A semi-reducible or rigid deformity of the PIPJ may be present.
- A flail fifth toe secondary to a prior fifth toe surgery.

Advantages:

- Quality of the bone stock is not a factor.
- Will eliminate a fibrotic heloma molle of the fourth web space.
- Allows for correction of a contacted PIPJ of the fourth toe as well as a contracted and/or varus rotated fifth digit.
- Provides stability to flail fifth digit.

Disadvantages:

- Requires patient acceptance and good patient compliance.
- Potential for dehiscence of the wound.
- Requires meticulous dissection and wound closure.

Inherent Complications:

- Hematoma formation creating wound dehiscence.
- Chronic edema.

Procedure (Fig. 3-6 A-D):

Using an indelible skin scribe, the incision is outlined from the center of the web space along the dorsal medial and plantar medial aspect of the fifth toe coming together just distal to the PIPJ. With the fifth toe held in a corrected alignment, the medial side of the fifth toe is held firmly against the lateral side of the fourth toe. The image on the fifth is transferred as a mirror image to the lateral side of the fourth toe. Once the entire planned skin incision has been remarked and modified at the apexes of the sulcus if necessary, the encompassed skin and all fibrotic tissue is carefully excised from the underlying subcutaneous tissue. If any osseous procedures will be necessary, they are now addressed. To approach the PIPJ of the fourth or fifth toe, a longitudinal incision is made along the midline of the digit to avoid the dorsal and plantar neurovascular structures. Hemostasis must be carefully maintained throughout the procedure avoid a post-operative hematoma. The subcutaneous tissue is retracted and a vertical capsulotomy is made at the level of the PIPJ. The head of the proximal phalanx is freed from its attachments and the distal portion of the toe is distracted in the transverse plane bringing the head of the proximal phalanx into view. The head is resected and the phalanx inspected for any spicules. The wound is flushed. We prefer to close the wound with simple interrupted sutures by placing all sutures before any are tied. We begin on the plantar surface of the wound at the sulcus and place a 5-0 non-absorbable suture and clamp the suture with a hemostat. We continue to lay in our sutures, clamping each with a hemostat and laying the thumb hole of each hemostat in order over another hemostat. When we reach the distal aspect of the wound, we then

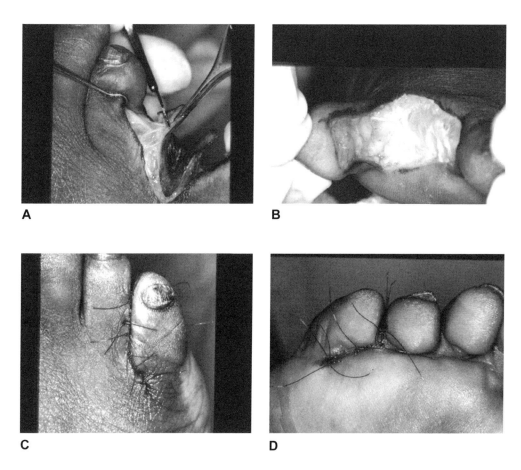

A   B

C   D

Figure 3-6: Clinical photographs: **A:** When performing a syndactylism the entire planned skin incision has been remarked and modified at the apexes of the sulcus. The encompassed skin and all fibrotic tissue are now carefully excised from the underlying subcutaneous tissue. **B:** Careful excision of the encompassed skin and fibrotic tissue. **C:** Closure of the syndactylism site from a dorsal view. **D:** Closure of the syndactylism site from a plantar view.

start on the dorsal proximal aspect placing and clamping each suture as before until are sutures are in place. The clamp holding the hemostats with the plantar sutures is now inverted and we tie each suture in order leaving a relatively long tag to facilitate removal. The same procedure is used on the dorsal hemostat until all sutures are tied. The wound is dressed.

Post-operative Management:

The patient is placed in a post-operative shoe. The patient must be very compliant post-operatively to keep the extremity elevated and limit time walking/standing for the first several days following surgery to minimize the risk of a hematoma. If performed, X-rays are taken at one week to access the arthroplasty site. Sutures may generally be removed in two to three weeks with the patient returning to normal activities as tolerated.

Partial Ostectomies:

We use partial ostectomies as an isolated procedure primarily to treat a heloma molle in a digit where there is no other structural deformity. However, the procedure can be combined with other procedures on the digit as well as the MTPJ when indicated. We prefer to use a small incisional approach to perform a partial ostectomy and have found that it affords better protection to the surrounding soft tissue in the area. We recommend placing a lesion marker on the skin prior to taking the X-rays to more clearly identify the area of osseous pathology. A minimal incision technique using a rotary burr to remove the osseous enlargement is acceptable.

Indications:

- A painful heloma molle at the level of the PIPJ or DIPJ.
- No abnormal structural alignment of the toe is seen unless it will be addressed by other procedures or the patient is aware that the other pathologies will not be corrected.
- A prominent condyle(s) should be seen on X-ray in the area of the lesion marker.

Advantages:

- No shortening of the toe.
- No loss of digital stability.
- Quality of bone stock is not a factor.
- Minimal post-operative management.

Disadvantages:

- Does not correct any abnormal alignment of the toe unless combined with other procedures.
- Are limited to discreet lesions typically a heloma molle on the medial or lateral sides of the PIPJ and/or DIPJ.

Inherent Complications:

- Chronic edema.
- Chronic DIPJ and/or PIPJ capsulitis.
- DJD of the involved DIPJ or PIPJ which may require a future arthroplasty or other digital procedure.

Procedure:

We make a small incision, generally less than 10 mm on the dorsal lateral or dorsal medial side of the toe above the heloma molle. Dissection is carried down along the side of the bone and all soft tissue is freed and retracted exposing the underlying bone. Using a hand rasp, bone forceps, small burr or sagittal saw, the boney prominence is removed. The area is examined to assure that sufficient bone has been removed. The wound is flushed. The skin is closed and dressed as per the surgeon's preference.

Post-operative Management:

The patient is placed in a wide shoe, sandal or post-operative shoe. X-rays are taken at one week to access the ostectomy site. Bandages and sutures are removed in 10 days to two weeks and the patient returns to regular shoes and activities as tolerated.

"V-Y" and "Z" Plasties

These two techniques can be used when a severe skin contracture exists, producing a dorsal dislocation of the digit. They require careful dissection of the skin and subcutaneous tissue as a full thickness flap with careful manipulation and closure to avoid necrosis.

Indications:

- A skin contracture at the MTPJ.
- A contracted scar over the MTPJ may be present.

Advantages:

- Allows for lengthening of skin contractures.
- Can be combined with other procedures at the MTPJ or digit.

Disadvantages:

- Requires patient acceptance and good patient compliance.
- Potential for dehiscence of the wound.
- Requires meticulous dissection and wound closure.

Inherent Complications:

- Hematoma formation creating wound dehiscence.
- Chronic edema.

Procedure:

"V-Y" Plasty: (Fig. 3-7 A-E)

For mild contractures, we have used a "V-Y" incision to gain length. The "V" is placed over the site and in the line of the contracture, with the base of the "V" proximal and the apex distal. The skin is freed along with the underlying subcutaneous tissue and the toe is straightened converting the "V" incision to a "Y." Careful, meticulous dissection must be observed to prevent damage to the apex of the "V." The wound is flushed. We generally use simple interrupted sutures to close the "Y" with an apical stitch at the apex of the "V." The wound is dressed as per the surgeon's preference.

Rotational "Z" Plasty: (Fig. 3-8 A-E)

For more severe contractures, we use a "Z" lengthening technique. The central line of the "Z" flap is oriented along the line of the contracture. The central and side arms of the "Z" must be of equal length and the angle between the arms is typically 60 degrees. This will generally allow approximately a 75 percent increase in length along the line of contracture. The skin flaps are dissected along with the underlying subcutaneous tissue and transposed to accomplish the skin lengthening. Careful, meticulous dissection must be observed to prevent damage to the flaps. Skin hooks should be used to retract and reposition the flaps to avoid damage. The wound is flushed. We generally we use simple interrupted sutures to close the "Z" with an apical stitch at the apex of each flap. The wound is dressed as per the surgeon's preference.

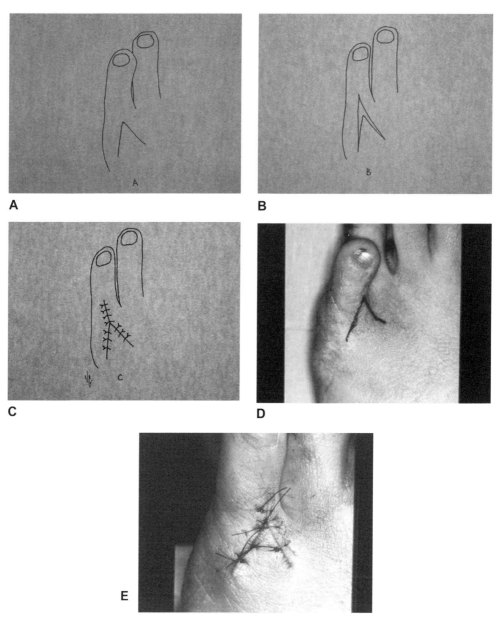

Figure 3-7: A: Diagram showing the "V" placed over the site and in the line of the contracture with the base of the "V" proximal and the apex distal. **B:** Diagram showing the skin being freed along with the underlying subcutaneous tissue and the toe straightened converting the "V" incision to a "Y." **C:** Diagram showing the use of simple interrupted sutures to close the "Y" with an apical stitch at the apex of the "V." **D:** Clinical photograph showing the "V" placed over the site and in the line of the contracture with the base of the "V" proximal and the apex distal. **E:** Clinical photograph showing the use of simple interrupted sutures to close the "Y" with an apical stitch at the apex of the "V."

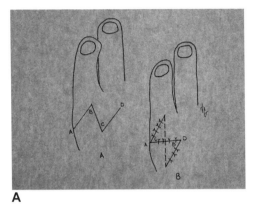

A

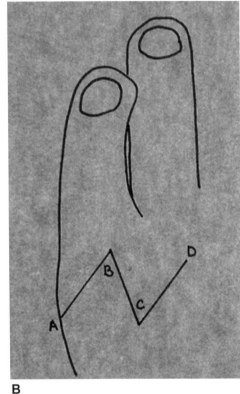

B

Figure 3-8: **A:** Diagram showing the central line, B-C of the "Z" flap is oriented along the line of the contracture. The central arm B-C and side arms A-B and C-D of the "Z" must be of equal length and the angle between the arms is typically 60 degrees. **B:** Diagram showing the skin flaps have been transposed to accomplish the skin lengthening. Apex B is now at D and apex C is now at A. This will generally allow approximately a 75 percent increase in length along the line of contracture shown by the dotted line.

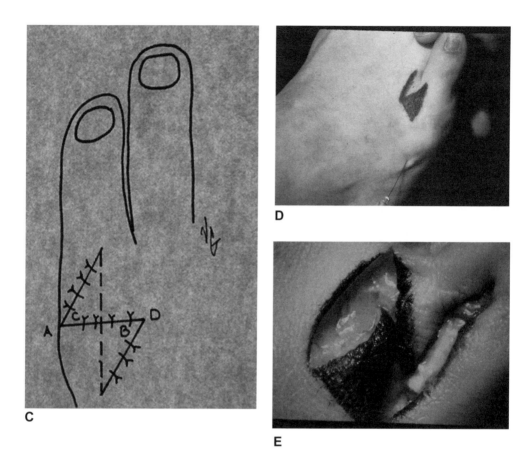

C

D

E

Figure 3-8: C: Clinical photograph showing the planned "Z" lengthening with one portion of the flap highlighted with a skin scribe to better visualize the eventual rotation of the flaps. **D:** Clinical photograph showing the skin flaps dissected along with the underlying subcutaneous tissue. **E:** Clinical photograph showing the skin flaps transposed to accomplish the skin lengthening.

Post-operative Management:

The patient is placed in a post-operative shoe. The patient must be very compliant post-operatively to keep the extremity elevated and limit time walking/standing for the first several days following surgery to minimize the risk of a hematoma. If any osseous procedures were performed, X-rays are taken at one week to access the procedure. Sutures may generally be removed in two to three weeks with the patient returning to normal activities as tolerated.

Clinical Pearls:

The following are tips we believe can be helpful in assisting the surgeon to achieve a more favorable outcome and preventing post-operative complications.

- Do not rely on soft tissue procedures to correct underlying pathology.
- Place lesion markers on the specific lesion prior to taking X-rays to better identify underlying osseous pathology.
- Always verify that sufficient bone has been removed by manipulation of the digit. Following an arthroplasty, manipulate the digit to make certain raw bone does not grind against the base of the adjacent phalanx.
- Generally an arthroplasty on the second and third digits need to be combined with other procedures to create more stability.
- An intermediate phalangectomy should only be performed in the presence of a small intermediate phalanx.
- When a longstanding and fibrotic heloma molle is present in the fourth interspace, consider a syndactylism.
- Limit the use of partial ostectomies to discreet lesions in digits without abnormal alignment.
- Perform a "V-Y" or "Z" plasty when skin contractures are present.
- In the case of unilateral digital pathology it is often helpful to take bilateral X-rays in order to compare osseous structures in the symptomatic and asymptomatic foot (wide head of the proximal phalanx, lateral condyle enlargement, osseous spur, etc.)

References:

Buggiani FP, Biggs E. Mallet toe. *J Am Podiatry Assoc* 66(5):321-326, 1976.

Coughlin MJ. Mallet toes, hammer toes, claw toes and corns: Causes and treatment of lesser-toe deformities. *Postgrad Med* 75(5): 191-198, 1984.

Coughlin, MJ. Operative repair of the mallet toe deformity. *Foot Ankle Int* 16(3): 109-116, 1995.

Coughlin MJ, Doriris J, Polk E. Operative repair of the fixed hammertoe toe deformity. *Foot Ankle Int* 21(2):94-104, 2000.

Coughlin MJ, Kennedy MP. Operative repair of the fourth and fifth toe corns. *Foot Ankle Int* 24(2): 147-157, 2003.

Creer WS. Treatment of hammer toe. *BMJ* 1:527-528, 1935.

Kelikian H, Clayton L, Loseff H. Surgical syndactylia of the toes. *Clin Orthop* 19:207-229, 1961.

Leonard MH, Rising EE. Syndactylization to maintain correction of overlapping fifth toe. *Clin Orthop* 43:241-243, 1965.

Marek L, Giacopelli, Granoff D. Syndactylization for the treatment of fifth toe deformities. *J Am Podiatr Med Assoc* 81(5) 241-252, 1991.

McGlamry ED. Floating toe syndrome. *J Am Podiatry Assoc* 72(11): 561-568, 1982.

Myerson MS, Fortin P, Girard P. Use of skin Z-plasty for management of extension contracture in recurrent claw and hammer toe deformity. *Foot Ankle Int* 15(4):209-212, 1994.

Ross ER, Menelaus MB. Open flexor tenotomy for hammer toes and curly toes in childhood. *J Bone Joint Surg Br* 66(5): 770-771, 1984.

Sarrafian SK. Correction of fixed hammer toe deformity with resection of the head of the proximal phalanx and extensor tendon tenodesis. *Foot Ankle Int* 16(7):449-451, 1995.

Thordarson DB. Congenital crossover fifth toe correction with soft tissue release and Cutaneous Z-plasty. *Foot Ankle Int* 22(6):511-512, 2001.

Fusion of Central Digits

4

William M. Jenkin, DPM, FACFAS

Introduction:

This chapter will present the techniques we utilize for fusion of the proximal interphalangeal joint (PIPJ) and / or the distal interphalangeal joint (DIPJ) of the central toes 2, 3, and 4 as needed in order to correct a digital deformity. We do not recommend fusion of the fifth PIPJ due to the resultant rigidity of the toe causing pressure reactions along the lateral aspect of the fifth digit while wearing shoes. The goal of the digital fusion is to provide a rigid, straight, stable toe, well aligned in all planes, free of pressure points and their resultant mechanically-induced hyperkeratosis (corns, calluses). Biomechanically, a digital fusion will prevent "buckling" of the PIPJ and eliminate the retrograde plantarflexory force of the proximal phalanx on the metatarsal head (Fig. 4-1 A, B). It also helps to stabilize the MTPJ in the sagittal plane by allowing the flexor digitorum longus (extrinsic flexor tendon) to transfer its plantarflexory forces to the proximal phalanx, thereby plantarflexing the entire digit at the MTPJ. This action augments the intrinsic muscles' "pressor" effect of the proximal phalanx onto the walking surface. It helps to neutralize the digital effects of extensor substitution associated with an ankle equinus, flexor stabilization associated with abnormal pronation and flexor substitution associated with gastroc soleus weakness (Fig. 4-2). The reader is referred to Chapter 1 for a complete discussion of the biomechanics of digital deformity.

Indications:

Arthrodesis of the PIPJ and/or DIPJ of the central digits is indicated for the following digital deformities which may be associated with mechanically induced hyperkeratosis or instability of the MTPJ resulting in central metatarsalgia:

- Semi-rigid or rigid hammertoe (PIPJ)
- Semi-rigid or rigid claw toe (PIPJ, DIPJ)
- Semi-rigid or rigid mallet toe (DIPJ)
- Interphalangeal joint arthralgia/arthritis
- Excessively long digit (PIPJ)

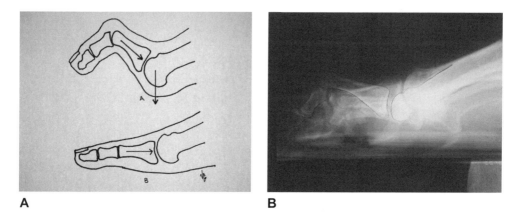

A   **B**

Figure 4-1: A (top): Diagram demonstrating retrograde buckling of the toe upon the metatarsal head with MTPJ and PIPJ contracture. **(bottom):** Diagram demonstrating no retrograde buckling as a result of straight toe from a MTPJ release and fusion of the PIPJ. **B:** Lateral X-ray projection demonstrating hammertoe formation with retrograde buckling of second digit.

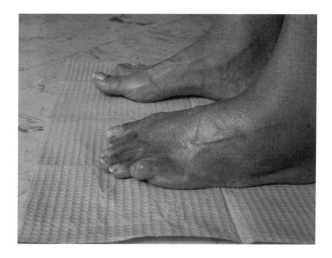

Figure 4-2: Clinical photograph demonstrating digital deformities from the effects of extensor substitution and flexor stabilization on the right foot and the effects of successful PIPJ arthrodesis of toes 2, 3, and 4 on the left foot.

- Hammertoe or claw toe associated with a MTPJ Stress Syndrome
- Hammertoe or claw toe secondary to a neurological etiology
- Iatrogenic or posttraumatic digital malalignment or flail toe

Central digital arthrodesis can be utilized as a substitute for or in conjunction with a flexor tendon transfer as an augmentation procedure when performing a metatarsal shortening osteotomy to prevent MTPJ instability and subsequent floating toe.

Central digital arthrodesis is always indicated when dealing with a digital deformity associated with an underlying neurological dysfunction.

Clinical and Radiographic Evaluation:

The clinical evaluation of the involved digit or digits is described in Chapters 1 and 3. The digit should be evaluated while the patient is both non-weight bearing and weight bearing. In the weight bearing examination the digital pathology should be observed both in a resting calcaneal stance position (RCSP) and a neutral calcaneal stance position (NCSP). If the deformity significantly reduces in the NCSP a functional foot orthotic device may be of assistance.

Conservative Therapies:

Conservative therapy consists mostly of palliative measures which do not solve the problem and are repeated as needed consisting of the following:

- Lesion reduction
- Pressure off pads
- Footgear modification
- Injection therapy with a steroid for acute sub-lesion bursitis

For chronic presentations where the patient is not a surgical candidate, footgear modifications such as stock extra depth shoes or custom shoes which have a deeper toe box to prevent irritation to the digital deformity may be employed.

Surgical Procedures:

Digital arthrodesis procedures are performed using an anesthetic deemed appropriate by the surgeon with or without the assistance of an ankle tourniquet for hemostasis. As previously stated, the procedure is most often performed upon the second and third digits and occasionally the fourth.

Arthrodesis PIPJ

The techniques to be discussed vary by the design of the PIPJ fusion and are as follows: flat end-to-end, peg-in-hole, and a chevron type fusion. Each technique may be augmented by a flexor tendon transfer (see Chapter 6) to assist in maintaining digital purchase. This is especially beneficial when the linear shortening of the toe as a result of bone removal creates laxity of the FDL and FDB tendons. The planar (flat) end-to-end technique provides the surgeon with the greatest flexibility in deciding how much to shorten the digit and allows for transverse plane correction at the level of the PIPJ if needed.

Arthrodesis PIPJ: Planar (flat) End-to-End Technique with K-wire fixation

A linear skin incision is made centered over the PIPJ of the digit unless the MTPJ is to be addressed, in which case the incision is extended proximally over the MTPJ in a serpentine fashion (Fig. 4-3). If multiple digits are involved, multiple incisions are made at the same time (Fig. 4-4). If there is a dorsal corn over the PIPJ, it is incorporated in the incision and ellipsed, taking care to leave enough tissue for closure (Fig. 4-5). The incision is deepened to the level of the extensor expansion over the proximal phalanx. At this level, dissection continuous peripherally and the EDL tendon and PIPJ are identified. A transverse tenotomy is performed in the EDL tendon 0.5 cm proximal to the PIPJ to insure a good tendon tag for EDL re-approximation. The tendon tag is dissected distally to the PIPJ where a transverse capsulotomy is performed exposing the head of the proximal phalanx (Fig. 4-6). The dorsal capsule is further dissected free of its insertion onto the dorsal surface of the intermediate phalanx in order to expose the cartilage on its base, taking care not to disrupt the central slip attachment of the EDL. Once the PIPJ is entered, it is disarticulated by releasing the collateral and suspensory ligament attachments onto the epicondyles on either side of the phalangeal head. The plantar distal part of the capsule insertion into the intermediate phalanx base is freed to further expose the articular cartilage. If the toe is dorsally contracted at the MTPJ, then an extensor recession and a release of the MTPJ are performed as needed (refer to Chapter 6 for a detailed discussion). The head of the proximal phalanx is then stabilized and, using power instrumentation, the predetermined amount of bone is then resected off the head of the proximal phalanx perpendicular to the long axis of the phalanx in all planes, based upon the amount of linear shortening needed (Fig. 4-7). The articular cartilage on the base of the intermediate phalanx is then resected with power instrumentation in the fashion just described exposing subchondral bone (Fig. 4-8). The two resected surfaces are then placed end to end to evaluate for congruity and alignment (Fig. 4-9 A, B). Fine tuning of the joint resection is performed by running the saw blade several times from dorsal to plantar at the fusion site as an assistant lightly compresses the intermediate phalanx onto the proximal phalanx (reciprocal planing). Once satisfactory alignment is

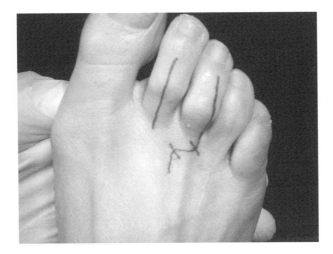

Figure 4-3: Clinical photograph demonstrating linear skin incision centered over PIPJ on second and third toe with proximal extension over third MTPJ with a serpentine design to minimize scar contracture while allowing access to MTPJ.

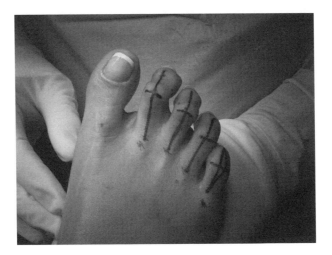

Figure 4-4: Clinical photograph demonstrating multiple skin incisions.

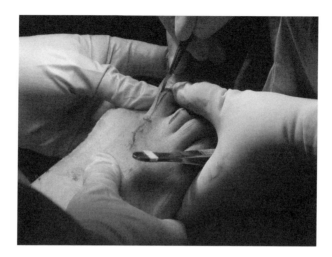

Figure 4-5: Clinical photograph demonstrating controlled depth elliptical skin incision.

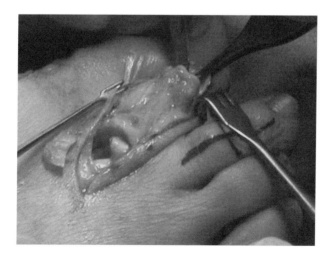

Figure 4-6: Clinical photograph demonstrating performance of dorsal capsulotomy of PIPJ after performing an EDL transverse tenotomy and extensor recession.

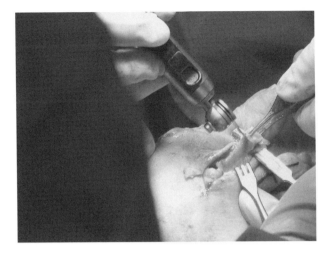

Figure 4-7: Clinical photograph of resection of head of the proximal phalanx while stabilized by forceps.

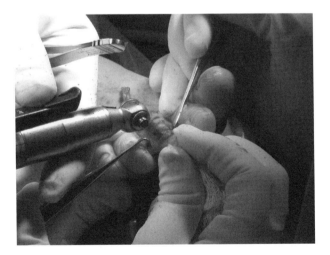

Figure 4-8: Clinical photograph of resection of the base of the intermediate phalanx.

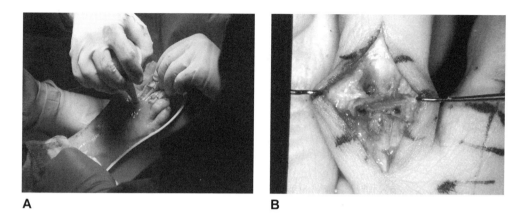

A   **B**

Figure 4-9: A: Photograph of retrograde force being placed on digit to evaluate alignment and congruity of joint resection while being flushed. **B:** Photograph of congruous PIPJ resection.

obtained, a copious lavage is performed. If a flexor tendon transfer is to be performed, the flexor tendon must be harvested at this time (refer to Chapter 6 for details). Fixation is obtained utilizing a .045 or .062 inch, smooth, double-trochar, K-wire. The wire is driven antegrade from proximal to distal through the intermediate phalanx, DIPJ and distal phalanx, exiting out the center portion on the end of the toe, taking care to avoid traumatizing the nail bed (Fig. 4-10). After sufficient pin has been driven out the end of the toe, the K-wire driver is re-attached to the exiting wire and the wire is further drawn out the toe so that only a small portion remains sticking beyond the base of the intermediate phalanx (Fig. 4-11). The digit is aligned and the K-wire is then retrograded into the proximal phalanx at least to its subchondral base (Fig. 4-12 A, B). If the MTPJ had to be released the K-wire can be further advanced across the MTPJ into the corresponding metatarsal at least two to four centimeters (Fig. 4-13). Once placement of the K-wire has been accomplished, it is bent 90 degrees as it exits the end of the toe. The length is trimmed and the end is capped for protection (Fig. 4-14 A, B, C). If a flexor tendon transfer is to be performed, it is completed at this time. The extensor tendon is then sutured end to end without tension at the resected joint level with a 4-0 absorbable suture (Fig. 4-15). If there is tension in the EDL tendon, then a "Z" tendon lengthening should be performed at the MTPJ level (Fig. 4-16). The skin margins are approximated according to the surgeon's preference. We often utilize several buried absorbable sutures and then re-approximate the skin using a combination of simple interrupted sutures with several either vertical mattress or horizontal mattress sutures to insure skin margin eversion.

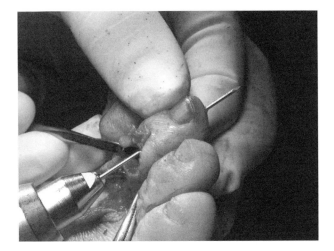

Figure 4-10: Clinical photograph of K-wire being antegraded out the end of the toe.

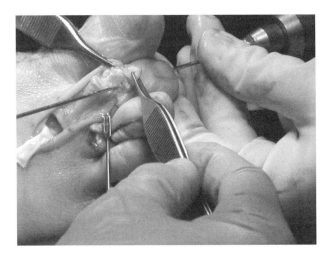

Figure 4-11: Clinical photograph of K-wire being further withdrawn distally.

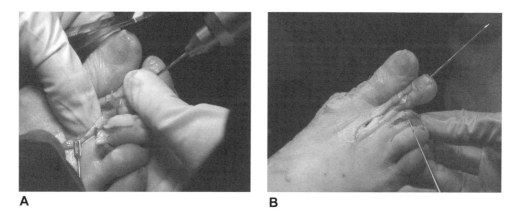

A   **B**

Figure 4-12: A: Clinical photograph of K-wire being retrograded back into the toe.
B: Clinical photograph of K-wire in place across PIPJ fusion site and MTPJ.

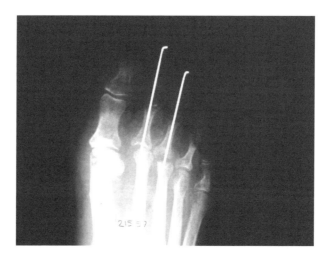

Figure 4-13: AP X-ray view demonstrating K-wires in place across MTPJ.

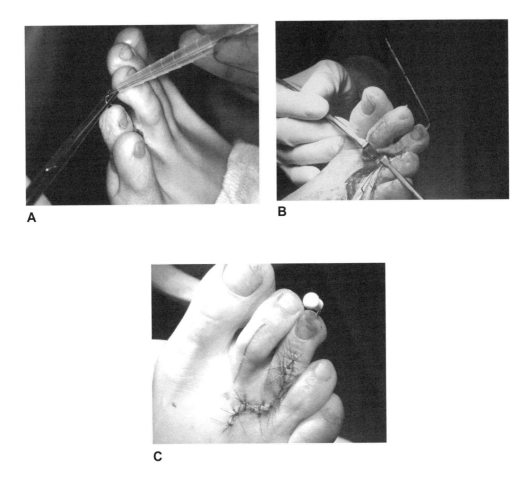

Figure 4-14: A: Photograph of external K-wire being bent with suction tip while stabilized with a forcep as it exits the end of the toe. **B:** Photograph of external K-wire bent at 90 degrees as it exits the end of the toe. **C:** Photograph of external K-wire cut shorter with protective cap in place.

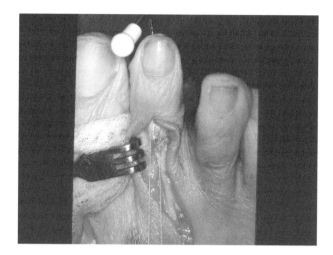

Figure 4-15: Clinical photographgraph of end to end approximation of EDL tendon in toe.

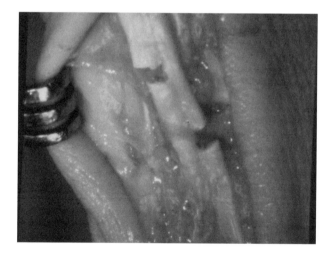

Figure 4-16: Clinical photographgraph of "Z" plasty EDL tendon "slide" lengthening.

Arthrodesis PIPJ: TAPAS ™ (Peg-in-Hole) Technique with K-wire fixation

This is a technique which facilitates cartilage removal from both sides of the PIPJ. The peg-in-hole configuration is created by special instrumentation (TAPAS™) which creates a perfectly congruous stable fit and increases the surface area of cancellous bone to bone contact of resected joint surfaces (Fig. 4-17 A, B, C). This is not to be confused with the peg-n-hole technique popularized by McGlamry where a peg is fashioned out of the distal portion of the proximal phalanx and a hole is fashioned in the intermediate phalanx at which time the peg is impaled into the hole (Fig. 4-18 A, B, C). We have abandoned this technique as it creates excessive digital shortening and a toe which does not purchase the weight bearing surface.

The TAPAS modification is as follows: the PIPJ is exposed and disarticulated as described above. The appropriately sized peg creator is selected and the articular cartilage on the head of the proximal phalanx is removed as the head is fashioned into a peg. Utilizing the hole creator from the TAPAS instrumentation, the cartilage on the base of the intermediate phalanx is now removed as a hole is fashioned to the exact size of the peg (Fig. 4-19 A, B). Once the peg-n-hole has been created, the digit is stabilized by placing a 0.045 K-wire as described above which will cross the PIPJ and the DIPJ as it exits the end of the toe (Fig. 4-20). Closure is once again performed based upon the surgeon's preference.

Arthrodesis PIPJ: Chevron technique with K-wire fixation

This modification of the planar cut creates a chevron or "V" design which provides a greater bone to bone contact surface area between the proximal and intermediate phalanx than an end to end technique. More importantly, by design it will limit any frontal plane rotation of the intermediate phalanx upon the proximal phalanx while allowing sagittal plane plantarflexion of the intermediate phalanx upon the proximal phalanx. (Fig. 4-21 A, B, C, D).

The Chevron modification is as follows: The PIPJ is exposed and disarticulated as described above except that the central slip of the EDL and dorsal tissue on the base of the intermediate phalanx is dissected free. The head of the proximal phalanx is fashioned into the shape of a "V" with the apex distally by removing the medial and lateral condyles. A corresponding V-shaped wedge of bone is then removed from the base of the intermediate phalanx incorporating the articular cartilage on the base. The opposing ends of the V design are approximated and evaluated for congruity. They are modified as needed and fixated with a 0.045 inch K-wire placed as described above across the PIPJ and DIPJ. At this time the intermediate phalanx can be plantarflexed upon the proximal phalanx by slightly bending the K-wire at the level of the PIPJ fusion site to improve digital purchase. As described below in the section for alternative fixation, an absorbable rod is ideal for this method as it is easy to bend. Tendon repair and skin closure are completed as described.

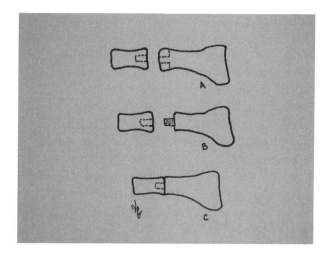

Figure 4-17: A: Sagittal view diagram of the TAPAS™ peg-in-hole PIPJ fusion design. **B:** Sagittal view diagram demonstrating a cancellous bone peg being fashioned out of the head of the proximal phalanx while a hole is created in the base of the intermediate phalanx. **C:** Sagittal view diagram demonstrating completed peg-in-hole PIPJ fusion.

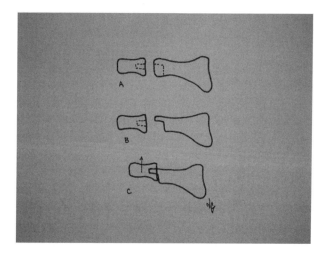

Figure 4-18: A: Diagram of a traditional peg-in-hole arthrodesis. **B:** Diagram of a peg being created out of the distal portion of the proximal phalanx including its dorsal cortex. **C:** Diagram of peg inserted in hole and elevated distal aspect of toe.

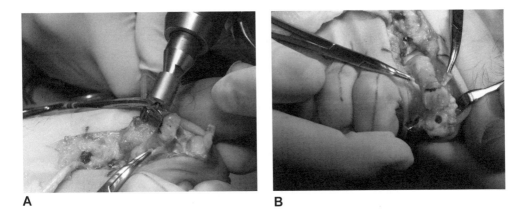

Figure 4-19: A: Clinical photograph of TAPAS instrumentation to remove the cartilage and create a cancellous bone peg out of the head of the proximal phalanx. **B:** Clinical photograph demonstrating a cancellous bone peg protruding out of what remains of the head of the proximal phalanx and a hole in the base of the intermediate phalanx. Mosquito forceps are visible which are attached to the medial and lateral slips of the FDB tendon awaiting the completion of an adjunctive FDB transfer. Additionally, a Weil shortening osteotomy was performed and the head of a screw fixation is visible dorsally on the distal metatarsal head.

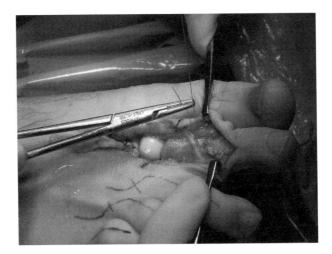

Figure 4-20: Clinical photograph of completed peg-in-hole arthrodesis with adjunctive FDB transfer and external 0.045 inch K-wire in place exiting end of the toe.

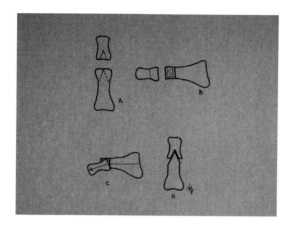

Figure 4-21: Diagram of Chevron PIPJ Arthrodesis **A:** This is a dorsal view showing the planned bone resection from the head of the proximal phalanx and the "V" section of bone to be removed from the base of the intermediate phalanx. **B:** Sagittal plane view showing the apex of the "V" on the proximal phalanx and the bone cut made into the intermediate phalanx. **C:** Sagittal view showing the proximal phalanx inserted into the intermediate phalanx. Note how one can plantarflex the intermediate phalanx to create better toe purchase. **D:** Dorsal view showing the proximal phalanx inserted into the intermediate. Note that this procedure will create shortening.

The Chevron-designed arthrodesis is technically difficult and introduces the complication of one of the wings of the "V" fracturing. The method described can only be performed where the intermediate phalanx is of such size that it can accommodate a wedge of bone being removed from its base. If the intermediate phalanx is a short bone, then it can be fashioned into a wedge with the apex proximal and a corresponding wedge of bone can be fashioned and removed from the head of the proximal phalanx (Fig. 4-22 A, B).

Arthrodesis of the DIPJ: Planar end to end technique with K-wire fixation

Arthrodesis of the DIPJ as an isolated procedure is performed as treatment for a mallet toe deformity involving toes 2, 3 or 4.

A linear skin incision is placed over the DIPJ taking care to avoid the nail matrix beneath the proximal nail fold. An alternate approach is a transverse semi-elliptical incision which removes any redundant dorsal skin resulting from fusing the toe in the corrected position. The incision is deepened down to the level of the DIPJ. A

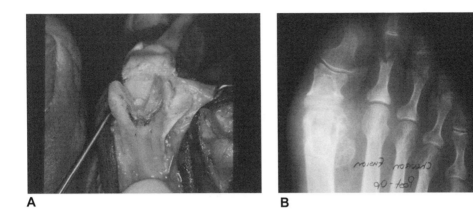

A   **B**

Figure 4-22: A: Clinical photograph of chevron wedge being removed from head of proximal phalanx. **B:** AP X-ray view of "reverse" Chevron arthrodesis.

transverse EDL tenotomy and capsulotomy is performed. The DIPJ is disarticulated by releasing the collateral ligaments (Fig. 4-23). Based upon the amount of shortening desired, a predetermined amount of bone is resected off the head of the intermediate phalanx. The base of the terminal phalanx is exposed and is resected with a rongeur or surgical burr. The DIPJ is aligned in the corrected position. If the distal phalanx is still contracted, the plantar DIPJ capsule is incised exposing the FDL. A transverse tenotomy of the FDL tendon is performed to allow the distal phalanx to straighten. A 0.045 inch K-wire is then placed across the DIPJ as described above for PIPJ fusion. The EDL tendon is evaluated for excessive length and modified as necessary. The end of the tendon is approximated with a 4-0 absorbable suture (Fig. 4-24). The skin is approximated and closed based upon the surgeon's preference.

Arthrodesis of the DIPJ and PIPJ

A combined PIPJ and DIPJ fusion is performed at times in a claw toe deformity. The DIPJ fusion is a planar end to end design and the PIPJ can be of the planar, peg-in-hole, or Chevron design. If the claw toe is associated with a neurological dysfunction, it is advised to fixate the fusion sites with a 0.062 inch external K-wire.

Postoperative Management:

Guarded weight bearing eliminating propulsion is employed for six weeks, either in a prefabricated walker with rocker sole or a postoperative rigid soled shoe. In either case K-wires crossing the MTPJ must be accommodated for by placing quarter inch

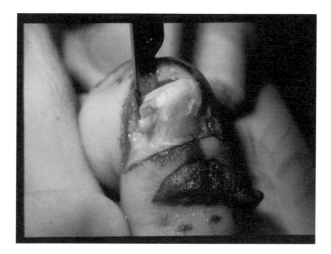

Figure 4-23: Clinical photograph of transverse elliptical incision and DIPJ capsulotomy and disarticulation.

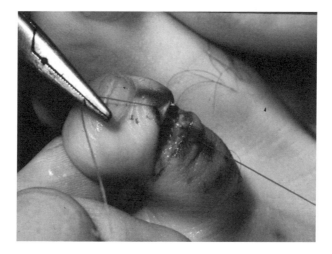

Figure 4-24: Clinical photograph of EDL being approximated at DIPJ level.

adhesive felt in the sole of the device to lessen the bending force at the MTPJ. After six weeks of immobilization, transition to regular footgear as tolerated is instituted.

Bathing restrictions will depend upon the fixation utilized. With an external K-wire, the restriction is enforced until the wire is removed at four to six weeks. With internal fixation bathing is restricted only until the sutures are removed at 14 days.

Postoperative AP and lateral radiographs are obtained the day of surgery or on the first post op visit at seven to 10 days. Repeat X-rays are obtained at three weeks and six weeks to evaluate healing and alignment.

Alternative Fixation Methods:

There are multiple fixation methods to fuse digits and the choice of fixation of the fusion site is a surgeon's preference. There are, however, pros and cons to each. The devices we presently employ are a smooth double trochar .045 or .065 inch external K-wire which exits the end of the toe, or an internal, intramedullary absorbable 2.0 mm PLLA rod (Trim-It Drill Pin™), (Trim-It Spin Pin™).

Technique for utilization of the absorbable pin:

The 2.0 bio-absorbable rod is placed in the digit utilizing the same method as used with a K-wire crossing the PIPJ and DIPJ exiting the end of the toe (Fig. 4-25). It is then retrograded back into the digit until it reaches the level of the subchondral bone at the base of the proximal phalanx. The rod is withdrawn distally by about 5 mm at which time it is trimmed even with distal phalanx. The entire pin is then retrograded back into the distal phalanx using the tamp provided in the set. It is important to place a slight bend in the rod at the DIPJ level to help prevent distal rod migration and to allow for a better toe purchase (Fig. 4-26).

The rod can be modified to just cross the PIPJ (Trim-It Spin Pin™). This method allows the surgeon to place an intramedullary rod the exact length as the combined lengths of the proximal and intermediate phalanx and fuse the PIPJ without crossing the DIPJ. After an arthrectomy of the PIPJ has been performed, the 2.0 bio-absorbable rod which comes attached to a 25 mm metal pin marked with circumferential laser lines spaced 5 mm apart, is placed within the medullary canal of the proximal phalanx. It is retrograded to the subchondral bone at the level of the base of the proximal phalanx. Measurement of this depth is taken (Fig. 4-27). The pin is removed and is then inserted into the medullary canal of the distal phalanx and advanced to the level of the subchondral bone in the head of the intermediate phalanx. Measurement of this depth of insertion is noted (Fig. 4-28). The rod is then further advanced distally out the end of the toe until the metal pin is completely visible. The depth of the proximal and intermediate phalanx is combined to determine the exact length of the rod that will be needed for fixation. A circumferential notch on the portion of the rod closest to the metal pin is located. This notch will ultimately correspond to the level of the head of the intermediate phalanx just proximal to the DIPJ. From this point toward the end opposite the metal pin, the length of rod to be placed across the fusion site is determined.

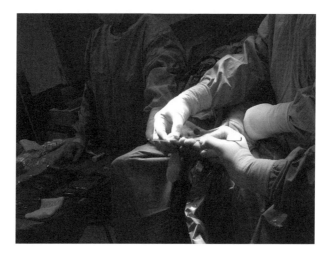

Figure 4-25: Clinical photograph demonstrating Trim-It Drill Pin™ exiting end of toe.

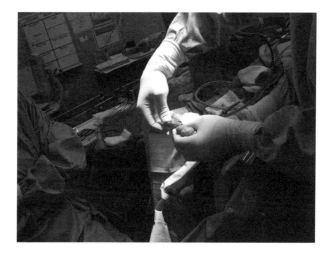

Figure 4-26: Demonstration of bending the rod at the DIPJ level by plantarflexing the distal phalanx on the intermediate phalanx to avoid distal migration of the rod.

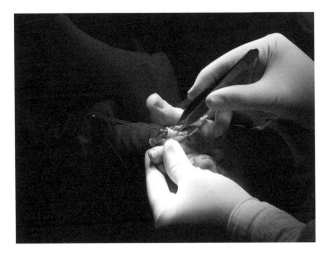

Figure 4-27: Clinical photograph demonstrating proximal phalanx being pre drilled and measured using the Trim-It Spin Pin™.

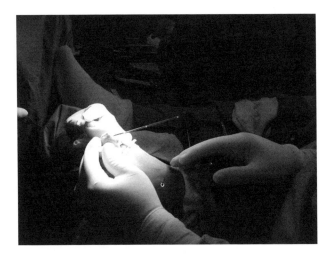

Figure 4-28: Clinical photograph demonstrating intermediate phalanx being pre drilled and measured using the Trim-It Spin Pin™.

The rod is cut on an angle leaving a tapered end (Fig. 4-29 A, B). The metal pin portion of the rod exiting the end of the digit is placed in the K-wire driver. The rod is then retrograded into the proximal phalanx (Fig. 4-30). The rod is firmly grasped with mosquito forceps within the PIPJ. At the same time the K-wire driver is engaged, causing the rod to break at the structural notch which is located just proximal to the DIPJ (Fig. 4-31). The rod is then slightly bent at the level of the PIPJ. The repair is then completed as discussed above.

The advantages of the K-wire are as follows:

1. It is a temporary fixation device which will be removed at some time post operatively.
2. It is easily removed in the office.
3. In addition to crossing the DIPJ and PIPJ it can cross the MTPJ to help maintain the relocated position of a dislocated MTPJ.

The disadvantages of the external K-wire are as follows:

1. External exit of pin serves as a portal for potential pin tract infection.
2. Bathing restriction until pin removed.
3. Poor patient acceptance: inconvenient, unsightly.
4. Pin "fracture"/ retention.
5. Pin failure causing early removal.
6. The so-called "pin ferry" syndrome: pin is prematurely extracted by bed clothing during sleep.

The advantages of the internal PLLA (polylactide) rod:

1. Internal placement makes the fixation non-visible.
2. No external portal on the end of the toe decreasing infection potential.
3. No bathing restriction beyond suture removal because there are no portals.
4. High patient acceptance.
5. The rod can be bent in the sagittal plane allowing for a flexed toe fusion as needed.
6. The rod can be used to cross both PIPJ and DIPJ (Trim-It Drill Pin™).
7. This fixation method allows the surgeon to fuse the PIPJ and also cross the intact DIPJ which "stiffens" the joint and can help to minimize a mallet toe formation.
8. Allows for fusion of both joints if so desired.

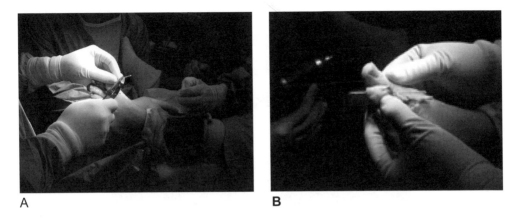

A   B

Figure 4-29: A: Photograph of pin being trimmed at an angle. **B:** Photograph of "trimmed" pin exiting end of toe.

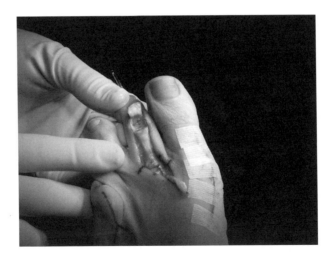

Figure 4-30: Photograph of pin exiting from base of intermediate phalanx as it is being inserted into the proximal phalanx.

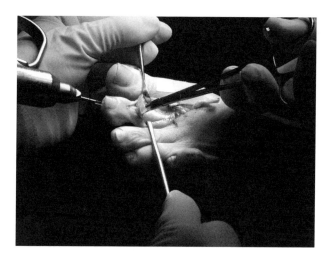

Figure 4-31: Photograph of pin being stabilized at the level of the PIPJ while the pin exiting the end of the toe is spun with the K-wire driver fracturing the pin at the notch located proximal to the DIPJ.

The disadvantages of the internal PLLA (polylactide) rod:

1. Does not allow for stabilization across MTPJ if needed.
2. May create excessive bone destruction and a post surgical dactylitis as material undergoes degradation (Fig. 4-32 A, B).
3. Pin may migrate distally out the end of the toe. This can be minimized by bending the rod at the DIPJ level by slightly plantarflexing the distal phalanx upon the intermediate phalanx. The use of the Trim-it Spin Pin™ which only crosses the PIPJ will negate this potential problem.

Inherent Complications and Management:

*   Digital Malalignment
    -   Malalignment post-arthrodesis of the PIPJ can occur at several levels. If the digit deviates in either the transverse or sagittal plane at the PIPJ and the fusion is complete, a revisional arthrodesis must be performed to better align the toe. If the mal-alignment at the PIPJ is reducible, it is secondary to a non-union and either a revisional arthrodesis or digital implant arthroplasty (refer to Chapter 5) must be performed to

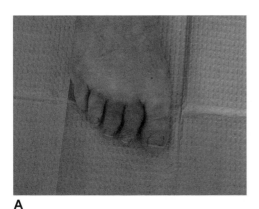 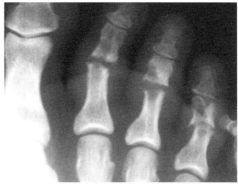

A   B

Figure 4-32: A: Post surgical dactylitis involving second and third toes. **B:** AP X-ray view demonstrating failed fusions and excessive bone destruction and loss as a result of the degradation process of a resorbable rod of PLA placed internally to fixate the PIPJ of the second, third, and fourth toes.

provide stability. If the digit deviates in the transverse plane at the level of the MTPJ and this deviation increases with the Kelikian Push-Up Test, a shortening metatarsal osteotomy is indicated.

- A mallet toe can develop after a successful PIPJ fusion due to FDL contracture. This can be prevented by performing a FDL transfer at the time of PIPJ fusion (Fig. 4-33). The mallet toe deformity can be treated with a FDL transfer if this was not performed at the time of the original surgery. In selected cases involving a geriatric, sedentary patient, a FDL tenotomy and plantar capsulotomy at the level of the DIPJ can be performed.

- Poor toe purchase
    - If the end of the toe does not purchase the ground and there is a dorsal contracture of the extensor tendon, an EDL tendon lengthening just proximal to the extensor expansion along with a tenectomy of the EDB tendon and a MTPJ dorsal capsulotomy is indicated (Fig. 4-34).

- Excessive digital shortening
    - If the digit is excessively short, a digital lengthening can be performed by inserting a bone graft along with performing a revisional arthrodesis at the PIPJ (Fig. 4-35 A, B).

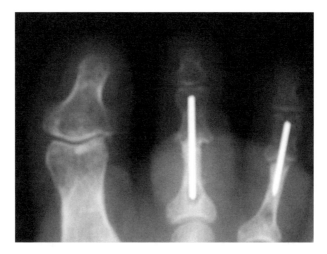

Figure 4-33: AP X-ray view demonstrating PIPJ fusion with an internal 0.062 inch threaded K-wire fixation with a FDL transfer to base of proximal phalanx through a drill hole in order to treat a claw toe deformity without fusing the DIPJ.

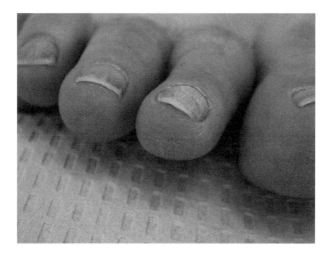

Figure 4-34: Clinical photograph demonstrating poor toe purchase following arthrodesis of the PIPJ on toes 2 and 3.

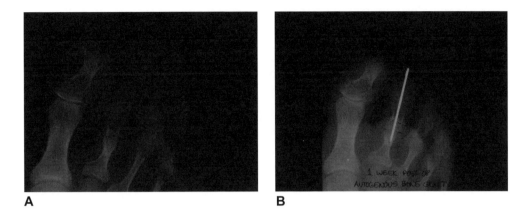

A   **B**

Figure 4-35: A: AP X-ray demonstrating the result of excessive bone removal during a previous PIPJ arthrodesis causing a short second toe. **B:** AP X-ray demonstrating restoration of digital length by performing a digital lengthening with autogenous bone graft.

- Retained K-wire
    - If a portion of the K-wire remains within the metatarsal due to pin fracture, most of the time no attempt is made to retrieve it unless it migrates and becomes symptomatic. If this occurs it is removed.
- Dactylitis
    - If a post surgical dactylitis occurs and remains eight weeks post operatively, injection therapy with an acetated steroid is performed at the base of the digit after the digit has been anesthetized. A compressive dressing is applied daily for several weeks. This injection may be repeated once or twice but multiple injections may result in digital tissue atrophy.

Clinical Pearls:

- Arthrodesis is best utilized in medial column toes 2 and 3 to create stability and enhance the ability of the windlass mechanism to create re-supination of the foot.
- Arthrodesis is sometimes utilized in the fourth toe especially with claw toe deformity.

- Arthrodesis should always be utilized in a patient with an underlying neurological dysfunction.

- Arthrodesis of both PIPJ and DIPJ should be considered in a claw toe deformity if a FDL transfer is not going to be performed.

- Arthrodesis should not be utilized in the fifth toe.

- When inserting an absorbable rod, the metal portion of the rod should be seated in the K-wire driver to avoid shearing or twisting of the rod itself.

- When inserting an absorbable rod, pre-drilling with a 0.045 inch K-wire will lessen the chance of damaging the rod especially in the patient with "hard" bone.

- Internal K-wires placed in the digits tend to migrate necessitating another surgery for their removal and therefore are not recommended (Fig. 4-36 A, B, C).

- A transverse plane digital deformity at the MTPJ level of the second and third toes which increases with performance of the Kelikian Push-Up test suggests consideration for the need for a metatarsal shortening or medial displacement osteotomy as an adjunctive procedure to the digital arthrodesis.

- Protect the K-wire if it crosses the MTPJ by modifying the postoperative shoe to prevent bending of the wire.

- Caution should be used with mechanical fixation devices which provide an instantaneous fusion as they may also instantly fail and can be extremely difficult to remove (Fig. 4-37 A, B, C).

References:

Coughlin MJ, Polk E. Operative repair of the fixed hammertoe deformity. *Foot Ankle Int* 21:94-103; 2000.

Gerbert J. Digital arthrodesis. *Clin Podiatric Med Surg* 3:77-93; 1986.

Goforth WP, et al. Lesser – metatarsal medial displacement osteotomy for the treatment of digital transverse plane deformities. *J Am Podiatr Med Assoc* 95(6): 550-555; 2005.

Konkel KF, et al. Hammer Toe Correction using an absorbable intramedullary pin. *Foot Ankle Int* 28:916-920, 2007.

Mahan KT, Downey MS, Weinfeld GD. Autogenous bone graft interpositional arthrodesis for the correction of flail toe: a retrospective analysis of 22 procedures. *J Am Podiatr Med Assoc* 93(3): 167 – 173; 2003.

McGlamry ED. Floating toe syndrome. *JAPA* 72(11): 561-568; 1982.

Pietrazak WS, Lessek TP, Perms SV. A bioabsorbable fixation implant for use in proximal interphalangeal joint (hammer toe) arthrodesis: biomechanical testing in a synthetic bone substrate. *The Journal of Foot & Ankle Surgery* 45(5):288-294; 2006.

Schilefman BS, Fenton CF, McGlamry ED. Peg in hole arthrodesis. *JAPA* 73(4): 187 195; 1983.

Soomekh DJ. Correction of deformities of the lesser digits. *Foot & Ankle Specialist* 1(1):81-83; 2008.

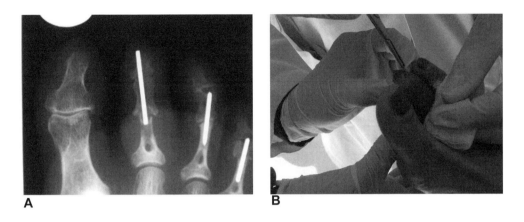

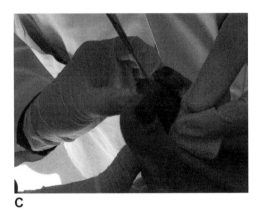

Figure 4-36: A: AP X-ray view showing distal migration of an internally place 0.062 inch threaded K-wire out the end of the toe. Note the holes at the base of proximal phalanges on toes 2, 3 and 4 where the FDL was transferred. **B:** Clinical photograph showing a Kelly hemostat being placed on the protruding internally placed K-wire which has migrated. **C:** Clinical photograph of removal of the protruding K-wire which had migrated out the end of the toe.

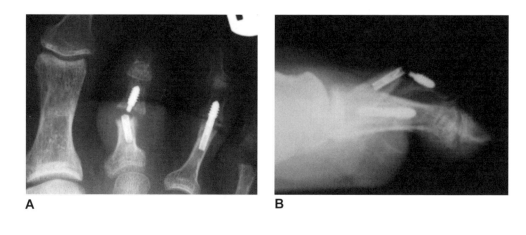

A   B

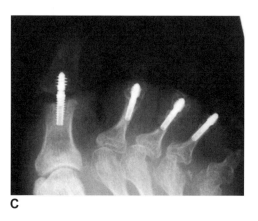

C

Figure 4-37: A: AP X-ray view demonstrating failure of Stay Fuse™ fixation to lock within second toe PIPJ. **B:** Lateral X-ray view demonstrating failure of Stay Fuse™ fixation to lock within second toe PIPJ. **C:** AP X-ray demonstrating successful placement of Stay Fuse™ fixation in PIPJ of toes 2, 3, and 4 and failure to engage bone in head of proximal phalanx of Hallux.

Digital and Lesser MTPJ Implants

5

Joel R. Clark, DPM, FACFAS

Digital Implants

Introduction:

Digital implants have been available for more than 25 years. They have been used in place of digital arthroplasties or arthrodesis procedures of the proximal interphalangeal joint primarily in the second digit, but on occasion in digits three and four. We have also used an implant in the fifth digit for stability in lieu of a syndactylism or for a "floppy digit." This chapter will discuss the following digital implants being used by the surgery department faculty: the Weil Digital Implant™ by Wright, the Sgarlato Ship Implant™, the Futura Flexible Digital Implant™ and the InterPhlex Implant Spacer™ by OsteoMed.

The decision to use a digital implant rather than perform a traditional arthroplasty or arthrodesis is often the surgeon's preference in the treatment of a semi rigid or rigid digital deformity. All of the above implants, with the exception of the Futura Flexible Digital Implant™, are solid spacers with no hinge component. Motion occurs between the implant body and flexible stems within the modularly canal of the phalanx. We have observed that all provide equal stability in the transverse plane but that the hinged system by Futura does provide slightly more sagittal plane flexibility at the PIPJ.

Advantages over PIPJ arthroplasty are:

1. More intrinsic stability.

2. Maintains the length of the digit.

3. Better toe purchase.

Advantages over PIPJ arthrodesis are:

1. Immediate postoperative propulsive ambulation and return to regular foot gear in two to three weeks.

2. No need for internal or external fixation devices.

3. Maintain proximal interphalangeal joint motion.

4. Maintains the length of the digit.

Disadvantages:

1. Possible reaction to the implant material.
2. Need adequate bone stock to receive the implant stem.
3. Reoccurrence of deformity.
4. Chronic digital edema.

Clinical Evaluation:

The same general criteria is used for selection of a digital implant as for a digital arthroplasty as discussed in Chapter 3 and an arthrodesis as discussed in Chapter 4.

Procedure:

A dorsal linear incision is made centered over the proximal interphangeal joint of the digit. If a dorsal hyperkeratotic lesion is present it can be excised by two semielliptical incisions (Fig. 5-1). Dissection is carried down to the level of the extensor tendon which is incised transversely just proximal to the joint, or divided longitudinally and retracted to either side of the joint. Using power equipment to avoid possible microfractures to the phalangeal shaft, the head of the proximal is then resected. We typically do not resect any bone from the base of the intermediate phalanx to serve as a better buttress against the implant (Fig. 5-2). Therefore, whatever shortening is required should be taken from the proximal phalanx. The digit should now be evaluated to assure that no remaining contractures exist at the metatarsal phalangeal joint and if present refer to Chapter 6 for correction of the deformity. Holes are fashioned into the medullary canal of the proximal phalanx and through the articular cartilage into the base of the intermediate phalanx. The drills and broaches specific to the implant brand selected can be used to create the holes (Fig. 5-3 A-C). Care must be taken to avoid fracture or braking through the cortex of either bone. Once the holes are created a trial sizer is used to select the appropriate implant size (Fig. 5-4 A, B). The implant should rest just beyond the cortical margins of both phalanxes if possible and with the foot loaded, maintain the toe in proper alignment in all three planes. Any additional procedures, such as flexor tendon transfers, should be performed prior to inserting the actual implant and the toe reevaluated with the sizer to assure proper digital alignment and reduction of all deformities. Once satisfactory correction is achieved, the wound is flushed copiously and the actual implant is inserted. It should be transferred from the package into a saline or lactated ringer's solution to reduce static charges on the implant material and inserted in the digit using atraumatic forceps. The extensor tendon is repaired and the skin approximated. The surgical site is dressed in the same manner as one would do for an arthroplasty.

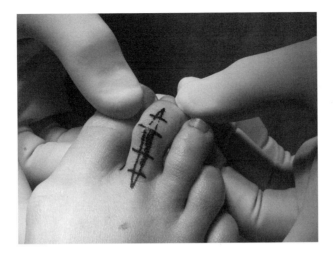

Figure 5-1: Clinical photograph of two semielliptical incisions centered over the PIPJ.

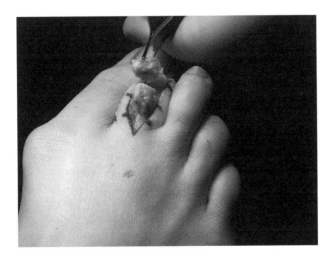

Figure 5-2: Clinical photograph of resection of the head of the proximal phalanx. Typically, no bone is removed from the base of the intermediate phalanx.

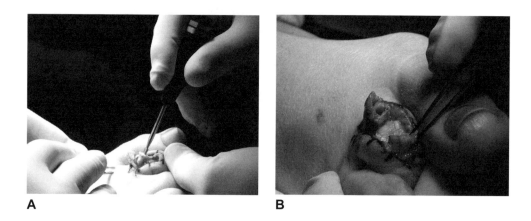

A   B

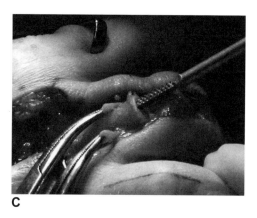

C

Figure 5-3: Clinical photographs: **A:** A rectangular broach used with the Sgarlato Ship Implant™ inserted into the proximal phalanx. **B:** Note the rectangular opening created in the shaft of the proximal phalanx and the articular cartilage preserved on the base of the intermediate phalanx. **C:** The round broach used with the Futura Flexible Digital Implant™. Mosquitoes are clamped onto the flexor brevis tendon in preparation for a transfer following insertion of the digital implant.

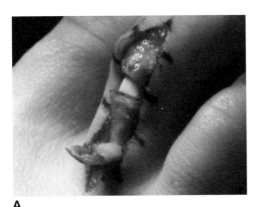 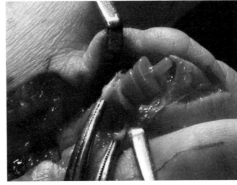

A   B

Figure 5-4: A: Clinical photograph of the trial sizer for the Sgarlato Ship Implant™ inserted in the PIPJ. **B:** Clinical photograph of the trial sizer for the Futura Flexible Digital Implant™ inserted into the PIPJ.

Post Operative Management:

The patient is placed in a post operative shoe and allowed to ambulate. Bandages are changed at weekly intervals and sutures are removed at 14 days. X-rays are taken within the first postoperative week to access the implant position (Fig. 5-5 A-E). The patient is allowed to return to regular shoe gear and activities as soon as possible following suture removal.

Inherent Complications:

1. Dactylitis of the involved digit which will usually respond to a compressive dressing and/or physical therapy. If the condition persists, it may require an acetate steroid injection after anesthetizing the digit.

2. Excessive fibrosis (encapsulization) at the joint. This generally will reduce with time but may require removal of the implant and leaving the toe with an arthroplasty.

3. Implant failure has not been a complication we have seen with digital implants. However, failure of the phalanx to support the implant stem has occurred when the cortex of the proximal phalanx has been damaged while reaming the canal for the implant stem. This may require removal of the implant and leaving the toe with an arthroplasty or performing an arthrodesis.

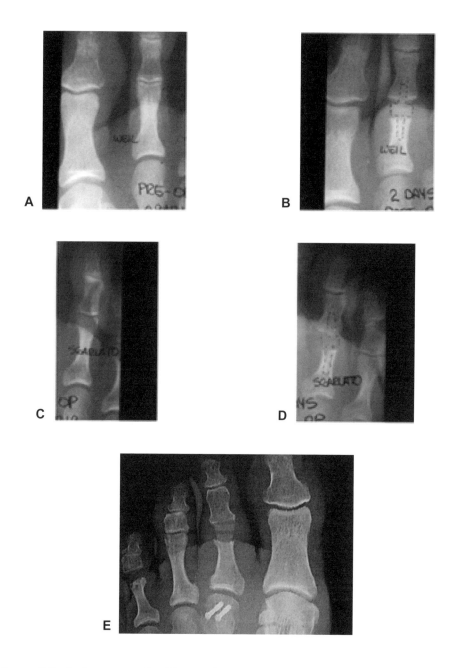

Figure 5-5: A: A preoperative X-ray prior to insertion of the Weil Digital Implant™. **B:** A postoperative X-ray with the Weil Digital Implant™ in the PIPJ. **C:** A preoperative X-ray prior to insertion of the Sgarlato Ship Implant™. **D:** A postoperative X-ray with the Sgarlato Ship Implant™ in the PIPJ. **E:** A postoperative X-ray with the Futura Flexible Digital Implant™ inserted into the PIPJ.

4. Reoccurrence of the deformity. This generally is a failure to properly reduce all associated deformities at the time of the original procedure. Once those deformities have been identified, they should be corrected and the implant should not typically need to be removed.

5. Bone resorption at the implant/bone interface which is usually the result of insufficient bone removed prior to implant insertion. If symptomatic, the implant can be removed, more bone resected and the implant reinserted or left as an arthroplasty.

Clinical Pearls:

1. Make sure that all associated deformities of the metatarsal phalangeal joint and associated tendon contractures have been properly identified and corrected.

2. Select an implant size that is appropriate to that specific toe. Too large an implant will increase the bulk around the site of insertion.

3. Have adequate bone stock present of the involved digit.

4. Allow a few millimeters of pistoning of the implant to occur after insertion.

5. Use a compressive taping of the digit following suture removal for one to two weeks to reduce postoperative edema.

6. Be sure the patient understands that an artificial joint spacer will be used and that it may require removal in the future.

Lesser MTPJ Implants

Introduction:

Lesser metatarsal phalangeal joint (MTPJ) implants are available as double stemmed units such the LMP™ hinged implant by Futura and the InterPhlex™ implant spacer by OsteoMed, or as a hemi implant such as the Cobalt Chrome Toe MP™ joint by BioPro or Cannulated Hemi Implant System™ by Vilex. (The latter is used for either the metatarsal head or the base of the proximal phalanx -- not both.) (Fig. 5-6 A-D). These implants are indicated in lieu of a partial ostectomy of the metatarsal head or metatarsal head resection. Most commonly, we have used these implants in the second or third MTPJ and rarely the fourth. We have not used MTPJ implants in the fifth. The decision to consider the use of a MTPJ implant is the surgeons' preference as well as the choice of the design.

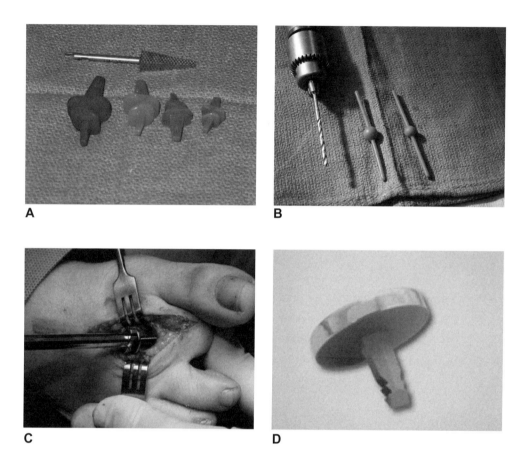

Figure 5-6: Clinical photographs: **A:** The LMP™ implant sizers and broach by Futura. **B:** The sizers and drill for the InterPhlex™ implant spacer by OsteoMed. **C:** The Canulated Hemi Implant System™ by Vilex. **D:** The Cobalt Chrome Toe MP™ joint by BioPro.

Advantages over partial or complete head resection procedures:

1. More intrinsic stability with some implant designs (Total Hinged/Spacer).
2. Better toe purchase with some implant designs (Total Hinged/Spacer).
3. Maintains the length of the digit.
4. Can preserve intrinsic attachments to the base of the proximal phalanx.
5. Can preserve the collateral suspensory ligaments to the plantar plate thus providing more stability to the metatarsal head with some implant designs (Hemi).

6. Maintains the plantar condyles under the metatarsal head with some implant designs (Hemi).

7. No need for internal or K-wire fixation. However, the cannulated hemi implant by Vilex would allow the insertion of a K-wire through the implant if desired.

Disadvantages:

1. Possible reaction to the implant material.

2. Requires adequate bone stock to receive the implant stem(s).

3. Possible reoccurrence of deformity.

Clinical Evaluation:

• The patient should have pain with range of motion of the MTPJ.

• A previous Freiberg's infraction or DJD of the MTPJ will be present.

• A complete dislocation of the MTPJ or an unstable MTPJ may be present from previous surgery or trauma.

• AP X-rays are taken to confirm the DID of the MTPJ and to evaluate the bone stock.

Procedure:

A dorsal serpentine incision is made over the involved MTPJ extending as far distally and proximally as necessary (Fig. 5-7 A). After the initial incision, blunt and sharp dissection is performed to the level of the joint capsule (Fig. 5-7 B). Depending on any associated deformities the extensor digitorum longus and the extensor digitorum brevis may be retracted, tenotomized or lengthened as necessary. We typically make a longitudinal incision through the capsule to expose the base of the proximal phalanx and the metatarsal head. All soft tissue contractures must be released if present.

The Double Stemmed Implants:

If the LMP™ hinged implant by Futura will be used, we prefer to preserve the base of the proximal phalanx and remove bone from the head of the metatarsal (Fig. 5-8 A-D). If the InterPhlex™ implant spacer by OsteoMed is used, we will often remove the base of the proximal phalanx as well as a portion of bone from the metatarsal head. Using the appropriate instrumentation, a hole made in the medullary canal of the metatarsal and through the cartilage on the base of the proximal phalanx (Fig. 5-9 A, B). A trial sizer is inserted into the void and checked for proper fit (Fig. 5-10 A-D). The MTPJ should be loaded to assure that all associated deformities have been corrected and that no jamming occurs with range of motion. Once satisfied, the wound is copiously flushed and the appropriate size implant is inserted. The joint capsule is closed making sure that the implant is completely incased. Subcutaneous tissue and skin are closed and the wound bandaged

The Hemi Implant:

The hemi implant can be used to resurface the metatarsal head or to resurface the base of the proximal phalanx. The Cobalt Chrome Toe MP™ joint by BioPro replaces the base of the proximal phalanx; the Cannulated Hemi Implant System™ by Vilex can be used on either the metatarsal head or the base of the phalanx, but not both. When the hemi system is used to resurface the metatarsal head, minimal bone is removed preserving the plantar condyles and the suspensory ligaments to the plantar plate. The BioPro implant utilizes a drill and broach to create an opening into the medullary canal of the proximal phalanx and a trial sizer is inserted into the void and checked for proper fit. The MTPJ should be loaded to assure that all associated deformities have been corrected and that no jamming occurs with range of motion. Once satisfied, the wound is copiously flushed and the appropriate size implant is inserted. With the Vilex implant for the metatarsal head, once appropriate bone has been removed, a sizer is used to determine the appropriate implant based on the diameter of the metatarsal head remaining. The implant should be just slightly larger in diameter than remaining head. Once the correct size implant has been chosen, a K-wire is inserted into the center of the remaining metatarsal head and down the shaft.

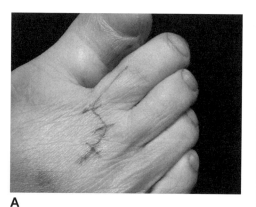 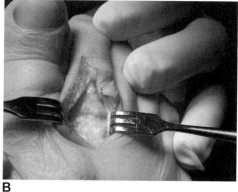

A   B

Figure 5-7: Clinical photographs: **A:** A typical dorsal serpentine incision centered over the MTPJ. **B:** Dissection is carried down to the joint capsule where a longitudinal incision is made exposing the base of the proximal phalanx and the metatarsal head.

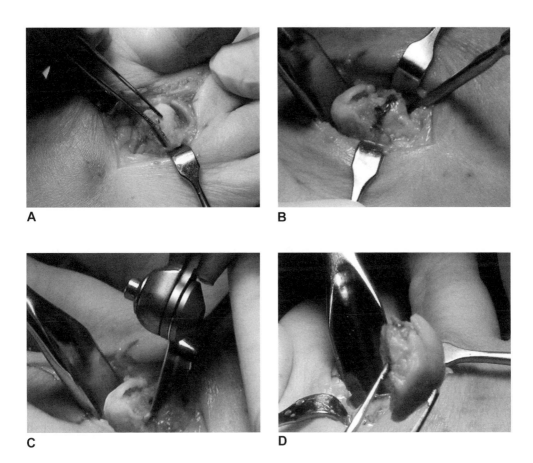

Figure 5-8: Clinical photographs: **A:** Depending on the pathology and laxity desired while preserving the base of the proximal phalanx a relatively small amount of the metatarsal head can be resected. **B:** The metatarsal head in this case had extensive degeneration. The amount of bone to be resected is marked on the metatarsal head. **C:** A sagittal saw is used to remove the metatarsal head. **D:** The resected portion of the metatarsal head showing the extensive articular damage.

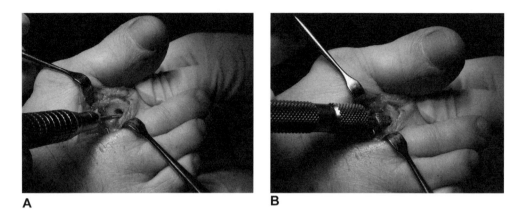

A   **B**

Figure 5-9: Clinical photographs: **A:** A side cutting burr is used to begin the hole in the base of the proximal phalanx. **B:** The appropriate broach for the implant selected is then used to create the hole in the phalanx.

The wound is copiously flushed and the appropriate size cannulated implant is placed over the K-wire. Using an instrument designed to fit over the implant and secure it, the implant is screwed into the metatarsal head and shaft. The K-wire is removed and the MTPJ is loaded to assure that all associated deformities have been corrected and that no jamming occurs with range of motion.

When the Vilex hemi implant is used to resurface the base of the proximal phalanx, the articular cartilage is resected preserving as much of the base as possible. A sizer is used to determine the appropriate implant based on the diameter of the phalangeal base remaining. The implant should be just slightly larger in diameter than remaining base. A K-wire is inserted centrally through the remaining base of the proximal phalanx and advanced distally into the medullary canal of the proximal phalanx. The wound is copiously flushed and the appropriate size cannulated implant is placed over the K-wire and using an instrument designed to fit over the implant and secure it, the implant is screwed into the proximal phalanx. The K-wire is removed and the MTPJ is loaded to assure that all associated deformities have been corrected and that no jamming occurs with range of motion. If K-wire fixation of the digit or the MTPJ is desired the K-wire can inserted through either of the Vilex implants. The joint capsule is closed making sure that the implant is completely incased. Subcutaneous tissue and skin are closed and the wound bandaged.

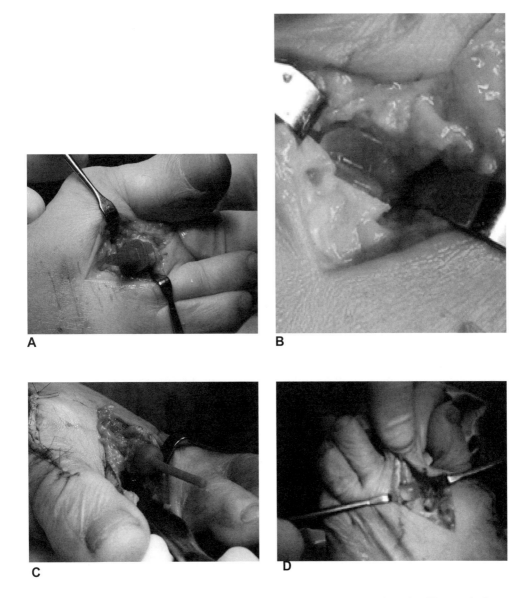

Figure 5-10: Clinical photographs: **A:** The LMP™ implant sizer by Futura being inserted in the MTPJ to check for proper fit. **B:** The LMP™ implant by Futura inserted in the MTPJ. **C:** The sizer for the InterPhlex™ implant spacer by OsteoMed inserted in the MTPJ to check for proper fit. **D:** The InterPhlex™ implant by OsteoMed inserted in the MTPJ.

Post Operative Management

The patient is encouraged to maintain a propulsive gait and can be allowed to ambulate in just bandages or a postoperative shoe when needed for protection. Bandages are changed at weekly intervals and sutures are removed at 14 days. X-rays are taken within the first postoperative week to access implant position (Fig. 5-11 A-E). The patient is allowed to return to regular shoe gear as soon as possible following suture removal. Active range of motion is encouraged and referral to physical therapy is made when necessary.

Inherent Complications:

1. Chronic edema which will usually respond to compressive dressings and physical therapy.

2. Excessive fibrosis (encapsulization) may develop at the MTPJ. This will generally resolve with time but may require removing the implant and leaving the MTPJ with a partial ostectomy and/or base resection.

3. Implant failure or bone resorption at the implant stem(s) may occur. Generally this will indicate that insufficient bone was removed and will require removal of the implant, additional bone resection and reinsertion of the implant.

4. Reoccurrence of the deformity. This generally is a failure to properly reduce all associated deformities at the time of the original procedure. Once those deformities have been identified, they should be corrected and the implant retained.

Clinical Pearls:

Make sure that all associated deformities have been identified and corrected.

1. Utilize a serpentine incision across the MTPJ.

2. Allow a few millimeters of pistoning of the implant to occur after insertion of the total joint implants.

3. Load the foot with the sizer to determine that all contractures have been released and put the joint through a range of motion to assure that no impingement occurs prior to inserting the actual implant.

4. Have adequate bone stock to accept the stem of the implant.

5. Be sure the patient understands that an artificial joint or spacer will be used and that it may require removal in the future.

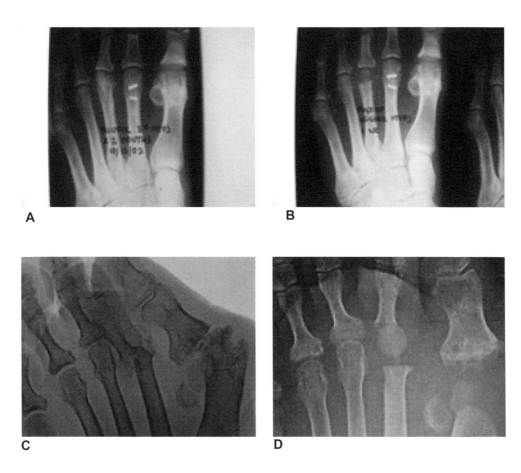

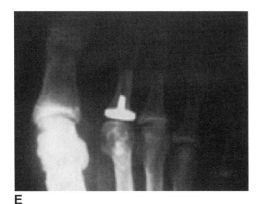

Figure 5-11: A: Preoperative X-ray prior to the insertion of the LMP™ implant by Futura. **B:** Postoperative X-ray with the LMP™ implant by Futura inserted in the MTPJ. **C:** Preoperative X-ray prior to the insertion of the InterPhlex™ implant by OsteoMed. **D:** Postoperative X-ray with the InterPhlex™ implant by OsteoMed inserted in the MTPJ. **E:** Postoperative X-ray with the Cobalt Chrome Toe MP™ joint by BioPro inserted in the base of the proximal phalanx.

References:

Biologically Oriented Prostheses. BioPro, 17 Seventeenth Street, Port Huron, Mich., 48060.

Cracchiolo A, Kitaoka HB, Leventen EO. Silicone implant arthroplasty for the second metatarsophalangeal joint disorders with and without hallux valgus deformitities. *Foot Ankle* 9(1):10-18; 1988.

Fox IM, Pro AL. Lesser metatarsophalangeal joint implants. *J Foot Surg* 26(2):159-163; 1987.

Gerbert J. Digital Implantation. *Clin Podiatric Med Surg* Jan:3(1):95-102; 1986.

Gerbert J, Benedetti L. Swanson design finger joint implant utilized in the proximal interphalangeal joints of the foot: A preliminary study. *J Foot Surg* 22(1):60-65; 1983.

Mednick DI, et al. Comparison of total hinged and total non-hinged implants for the lesser digits. *J Foot Surg* 24(3):215-218; 1985.

Nexa Orthopedics Inc., Futura, 11035 Roselle Street, San Diego, Calif. 92121.

OsteoMed Corporation, 3885 Arapaho Road, Addison, Texas 75001.

Silberman J, Kanat IO. Total joint replacement in digits of the foot. *J Foot Surg* May-Jun:23(3):207-12; 1984.

Sgarlato Labs, 2315 S. Bascom Avenue Suite 200, Campbell, Calif. 95008.

Sgarlato TE. Implants for lesser toes. *J Foot Surg* 22(3):247-250; 1983.

Sgarlato TE. A new implant for the metatarsophalangeal joint. *Clin Podiatry* Apr:1(1):69-77; 1984.

Sgarlato TE. Sutter double-stem silicone implant arthroplasty of the lesser metatarsophalangeal joints. *J Foot Surg* 28(5):410-413; 1989.

Sgarlato TE, Tafuri SA. Digital implant arthroplasty. *Clin Podiatric Med Surg* Apr:13(2):255-62; 1996.

Shaw AH, Alvarez G. The use of digital implants for the correction of hammer toe deformity and their potential complications and management. *J Foot Surg* 31(1):63-74; 1992.

Silberman J, Kanat IO. Total joint replacement in digits of the foot. *J Foot Surg* 23(3):207-212; 1984.

Sollitto RJ, Werner MS. A preliminary report on the status of implants for the lesser toes. *J Foot Surg* Nov-Dec:24(6):453-5; 1985.

Vilex Incorporated, 345 Old Curry Hollow Road, Pittsburgh, Pa. 15236.

Wright Medical Technologies, 5677 Airline Road, Arlington, Texas 38002.

Soft Tissue Management of the Dislocated Lesser Metatarsal-Phalangeal Joint

6

Joshua Gerbert, DPM, FACFAS

Introduction:

A dorsal contracture or dislocation of lesser MTPJ is a very common pathological finding and is dynamic. Once the dislocation begins it will progress over time, advancing from a flexible manually reducible deformity to a rigid non-reducible deformity. In many of these cases, the dislocation is not just in a pure dorsal plane but often it is dislocated on the transverse plane as well. In order to effectively treat this condition, one must determine the etiology(ies). In most instances there is one primary etiology along with one or more secondary factors. Our method for the clinical evaluation of the lesser MTPJ can be found in Chapter 1.

The following is a list of primary etiologies for a lesser MTPJ dislocation:

1. Long standing hallux abductus with bunion deformity producing second MTPJ dislocation (Fig. 6-1).

2. Hypermobile first ray producing chronic second MTPJ stress syndrome with eventual second MTPJ dislocation (Fig. 6-2).

3. Abnormally long lesser metatarsal producing chronic MTPJ stress syndrome with eventual MTPJ dislocation. (Transverse plane dislocation along with dorsal subluxation is very common with a long metatarsal.) (Fig. 6-3).

4. Abnormally long lesser digit resulting in hammertoe formation and abnormal retrograde forces resulting in an MTPJ dislocation (Fig. 6-4).

5. Trauma to the glenoid plate/rupture of the plantar MTPJ capsule.

6. Chronic inflammation (metabolic or mechanical) of the involved MTPJ creating disruption of the collateral ligaments with subsequent MTPJ dislocation.

The following is a list of secondary factors for a lesser MTPJ dislocation:

1. Contracted extensor digitorum longus and/or brevis tendon.

2. Prior dorsal linear incision over the MTPJ.

3. Abnormal foot mechanics during gait (see Chapter 1).

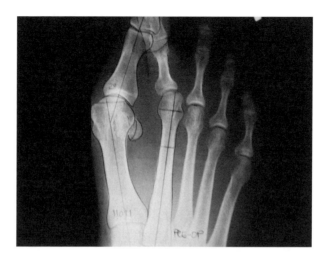

Figure 6-1: AP X-ray view showing a long standing hallux abductus with bunion deformity with a secondary medial/dorsal dislocation of the second digit.

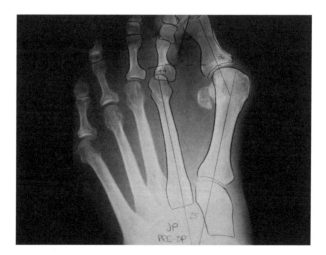

Figure 6-2: AP X-ray view showing a patient's foot with a hypermobile first ray with a bunion deformity and a secondary dorsal/medial dislocation of the second digit and mild dislocation of the third digit.

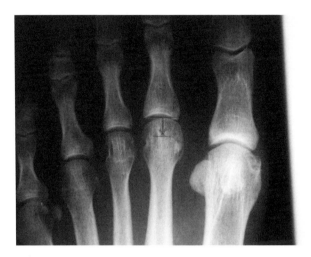

Figure 6-3: AP X-ray view showing an abnormally long second metatarsal relative to the length of the first metatarsal.

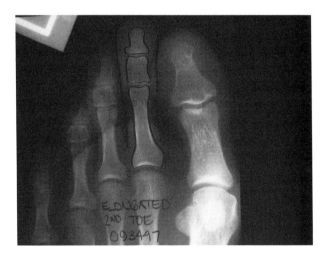

Figure 6-4: AP X-ray view showing an abnormally long proximal phalanx of a second digit.

Clinical Evaluation:

In the early stages of a painful lesser MTPJ stress syndrome without obvious signs of a MTPJ dislocation or hammertoe, which in the vast majority of cases will eventually progress to a dislocated joint, one can easily mistake the pain to be the result of an inter-metatarsal nerve entrapment or a neuroma. All too often a patient has undergone a surgery to release the transverse metatarsal ligament or remove the inter-metatarsal nerve only to have the original symptoms continue. The following are the steps we utilize to evaluate a patient who presents with pain in the lesser MTPJ area with or without obvious signs of an MTPJ dislocation or hammertoe formation.

- Direct dorsal/plantar palpation of the involved MTPJ in an attempt to elicit well localized pain in the involved MTPJ.

- Manual subluxation of the MTPJ in a sagittal plane direction (modified Lachman's test). If pain is produced then the test is considered positive.

- Retrograde force of the involved digit onto the metatarsal head which will produce symptoms if the synovial tissue is inflamed and/or there is degenerative disease of the MTPJ.

- Manual loading of the plantar aspect of the involved MTPJ to determine whether the involved digit deviates on the transverse plane and to determine the flexibility of the joint (Kelikian Push-Up Test).

- Evaluation of any contracture of the involved digit (flexibility versus rigidity) which could be producing retrograde forces on the MTPJ.

- Detailed first ray evaluation if symptoms are located in second MTPJ.

- In some cases, intra-articular injection of the involved MTPJ with local anesthetic with or without dye to determine if symptoms are related to the joint pathology versus an adjacent inter-metatarsal nerve entrapment or neuroma. In acute cases with a history of injury, the addition of the dye may allow one to determine whether the plantar capsule/plate has been ruptured (Fig. 6-5); however, due to the rapid healing of synovial tissue, the tear into the capsule may not allow any dye to escape after five or six days following the injury (see Chapter 1).

- Gait analysis to determine the weight bearing position of the involved digit (Fig. 6-6).

- Weight bearing radiographic evaluation (AP, lateral and plantar axial) to determine condition of MTPJ, length of involved metatarsal, length and position of involved digit and structural alignment of adjacent metatarsals.

- MRI or ultrasound to evaluate the plantar capsule/plate for possible disruption which may or may not prove more beneficial than the other clinical exams (Fig. 6-7 A-C).

- Obtain a detailed history of any previous trauma to the involved MTPJ and/ or prior forefoot surgery.

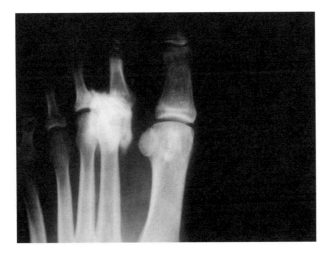

Figure 6-5: AP X-ray view showing contrast media injected into the second MTPJ to evaluate the integrity of the plantar capsule and plate.

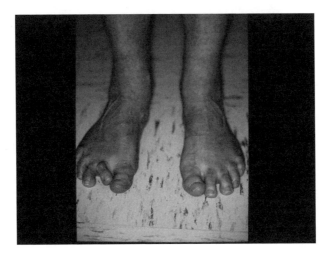

Figure 6-6: Clinical photograph showing weight bearing view of patient showing dorsal/medial dislocation of the second digit of the right foot.

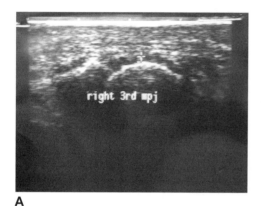

A

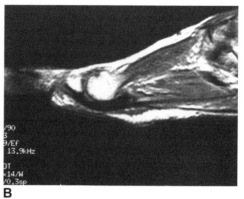

B

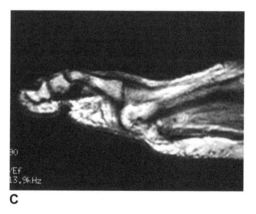

C

Figure 6-7: A: This is a lateral ultrasound view of the plantar aspect of a third metatarsal head and the proximal phalanx of a patient with clinical signs of a plantar plate rupture. The plantar aspect of the metatarsal head is located at the top portion of the photo. Fluid can be noted along the plantar aspect of the metatarsal head. **B:** This is a sagittal MRI view of a fourth MTPJ showing an intact plantar plate and capsule. **C:** This is a sagittal MRI view of a third MTPJ of the same patient showing a complete disruption of the plantar plate and capsule with dorsal dislocation of the proximal phalanx.

This chapter will focus on the soft tissue procedures that can be utilized when treating a lesser MTPJ dislocation. The reader is referred to those chapters (3, 4, 5 and 7) dealing with hammertoe correction, lesser metatarsal osteotomies and lesser MTPJ joint prostheses for information regarding procedures to correct structural deformities. There are very few conservative options for a patient with a painful lesser MTPJ dislocation; however, if the patient cannot undergo a surgical procedure the following can be utilized to reduce symptoms.

Conservative Therapies:

- Removable Budin splint (Fig. 6-8 A-F).
- Removable Darco™ digital splint at night (Fig. 6-9 A, B).
- Intra-articular injection with local anesthetic and a phosphate steroid. (If the MTPJ is not clinically dislocated, then I recommend no more than several injections. The involved digit should be splinted for several weeks following the injection with one of the above devices and the patient's physical activities should be limited to prevent inadvertent rupture of the MTPJ ligaments.)
- Physical therapy to reduce the inflammation.
- Non-steroidal anti-inflammatory medication.
- Utilization of an extra-depth shoe with a rocker-sole or one of the newer specialty shoes with a rocker bottom sole.

Surgical Procedures:

In the Department of Podiatric Surgery at the California School of Podiatric Medicine at Samuel Merritt College, we employ the following soft tissue procedures in trying to correct a lesser MTPJ dislocation in conjunction with any structural procedure that may be necessary. Many of us prefer performing these procedures without the use of an ankle tourniquet in order to better appreciate how the soft tissue contractures respond when severed. It also allows us to appreciate any potential vascular compromise of the involved digit as it is straightened. However, this is a surgeon's preference.

The following are the surgical procedures to be discussed in this chapter:

- Sequential MTPJ release.
- Tightening of the lateral or medial MTPJ capsule depending upon the dislocation occurring on the transverse plane.
- Flexor tendon transfer on the involved digit.
- Removal of plantar ellipse of skin from the sulcus of the involved digit.
- Flexor plate/capsule repair.

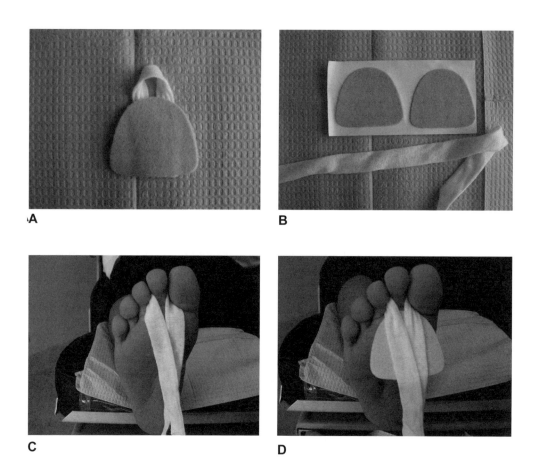

Figure 6-8: These photographs demonstrate the fabrication of a Budin removable splint: **A:** A completed Budin splint used to assist in maintaining a plantargrade position of the involved digit during ambulation. **B:** Materials used are two pieces of moleskin and 5/8 inch Surgitube® gauze. **C:** This photo shows the tube gauze being placed around the involved digit. **D:** This photo shows one piece of mole skin being placed with the adhesive side away from the foot and the tube gauze laid over it.

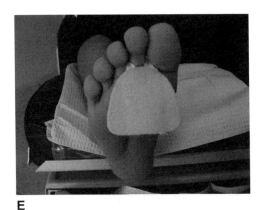

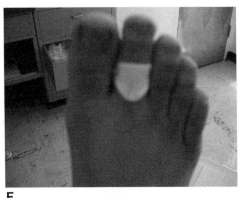

E

F

Figure 6-8: E: This photo shows the second piece of mole skin applied to the first thereby encompassing the tube gauze. **F:** Dorsal view showing the tube gauze around the involved digit following the fabrication of the splint. As the patient ambulates the mole skin pad will slip toward the heel thereby plantarflexing the digit.

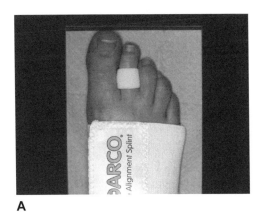

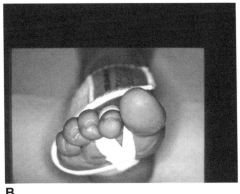

A

B

Figure 6-9: Clinical photographs of Darco™ digital splint: **A:** Dorsal view of a Darco™ digital splint applied to the second digit. **B:** This is a distal view of the foot showing the splint in place and with the second digit being held in a plantarflexed position.

Sequential MTPJ Release:

A dorsal serpentine incision is made over the involved MTPJ extending as far distally and proximally as necessary in order to gain the exposure necessary to perform whatever procedures are needed to correct the deformity(ies) (Fig. 6-10). This type of incision will help prevent any dorsal contracture of the MTPJ as it heals and contracts.

In many cases we prefer to perform this procedure without the use of a pneumatic ankle cuff in order to better judge which soft tissue structures are tight and to what extent the dislocation is being resolved as the soft tissues are released.

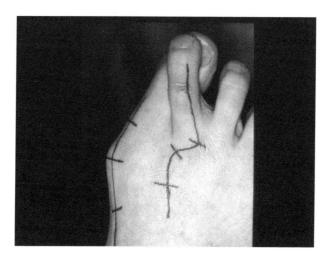

Figure 6-10: Clinical photograph of a dorsal view showing the long serpentine incision having been marked over the second digit and second metatarsal of the right foot.

After the initial incision, one can use sharp and blunt dissection to expose the dorsal aspect of the extensor expansion and the extensor tendons at the level of the MTPJ. The first step is to release the medial and lateral wings of the extensor expansion as far distally and proximally as deemed necessary (Fig. 6-11 A, B). The second step is to evaluate the extensor brevis tendon; if it is tight with the forefoot loaded, then it is tenotomized. The long extensor tendon is then retracted laterally or medially exposing the dorsal aspect of the MTPJ capsule (Fig. 6-12). By distracting the involved digit, one can easily determine the exact location of the MTPJ by the dimpling seen at the joint (Fig. 6-13). A transverse incision is made across the joint (Fig. 6-14). Any pannus formation noted within the joint is removed. The forefoot is then loaded to determine the degree of reduction of the dislocation achieved (Fig. 6-15 A). If further correction is necessary, then the MTPJ collateral ligaments are released (Fig. 6-15 B). It should be noted that both medial and lateral collateral ligaments should be released, even though the transverse plane MTPJ dislocation is medial or lateral. All too often, surgeons will only release the collateral ligaments on the side of the joint that is abnormally tight or dislocated. For example, if the involved digit is dislocated dorsally and medially at the MTPJ, many surgeons will release only the medial collateral ligament. The problem with this is that unless one tightens or at least creates scarring on the opposite site of the joint which has been abnormally stretched, one cannot hope to achieve soft tissue re-alignment of the joint. Once again the forefoot is loaded and the correction of the dislocation is evaluated. In cases with

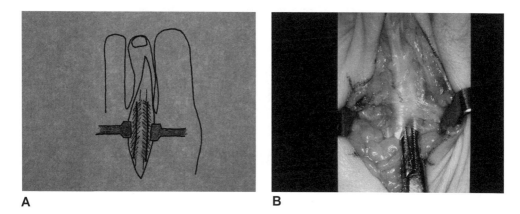

A **B**

Figure 6-11: A: This drawing depicts the extensor tendon and extensor expansion that needs to be severed both medially and laterally. **B:** Clinical photograph of a dorsal intraoperative view showing blunt dissection exposing the lateral portion of the extensor expansion.

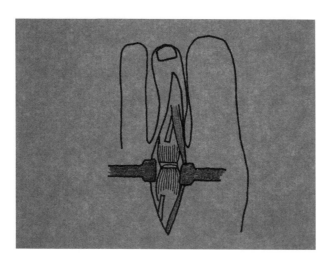

Figure 6-12: This drawing depicts the extensor tendon being retracted medially exposing the second MTPJ. The extensor brevis tendon has been tenotomized.

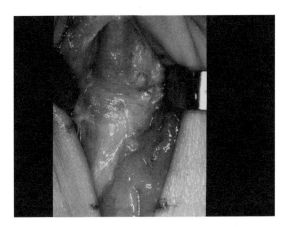

Figure 6-13: Clinical photograph of a dorsal intraoperative view showing the dimpling of the second MTPJ as the digit is distracted.

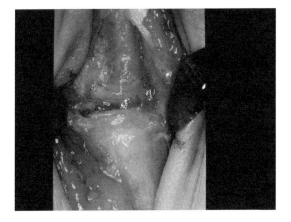

Figure 6-14: Clinical photograph of a dorsal intraoperative view following a transverse MTPJ capsulotomy.

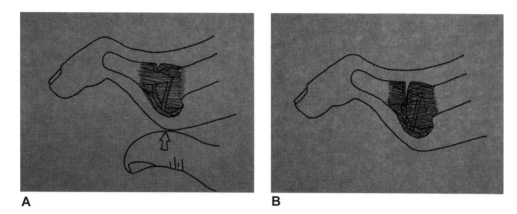

A   **B**

Figure 6-15: A: This drawing depicts a sagittal view of the involved MTPJ following a transverse capsulotomy followed by a Kelikian Push-Up test. **B:** This drawing depicts the collateral ligament having been severed.

significant medial dislocation, the lumbricale tendon may need to be tenotomized. If needed, the next step is to use a McGlamry® metatarsal elevator and release the glenoid plate/capsule that may have become adhesed distally at the joint level with a long standing dorsally dislocated MTPJ (Fig. 6-16 A, B). The last step is to load the

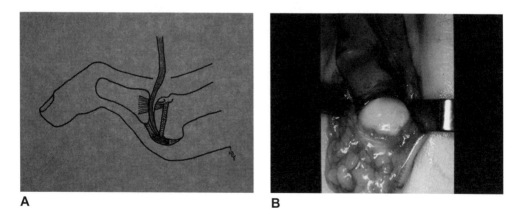

A   **B**

Figure 6-16: A: This drawing depicts the use of a McGlamry® elevator into the MTPJ to free any plantar adhesions. **B:** This is a dorsal intraoperative view showing the McGlamry® elevator being used.

foot and determine whether the extensor digitorum longus tendon is abnormally tight and requires lengthening. However, if one utilized an ankle cuff for hemostasis, the cuff needs to be released prior to determining whether the EDL tendon is abnormally tight (Fig. 6-17 A - C).

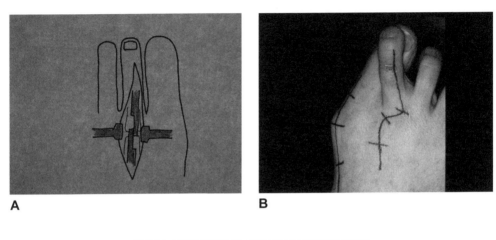

A   B

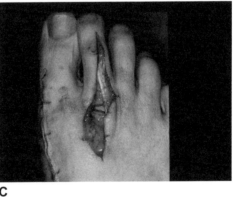

C

Figure 6-17: A: This drawing depicts the lengthening of the extensor digitorum longus tendon as the last step in performing an MTPJ soft tissue release. **B:** Clinical photograph of a preoperative view of a patient with a medial/dorsal dislocation of the second MTPJ. **C:** Clinical photograph of an intraoperative view of this patient with the second digit in a much improved position following a sequential soft tissue release with the forefoot loaded.

Balancing of the MTPJ Capsule:

In cases where there is transverse plane dislocation, once any structural pathology has been corrected such as shortening the involved metatarsal, then the medial and lateral capsular structures along with the collateral ligaments are severed. This is usually already performed when a sequential MTPJ release has been performed for the dorsal dislocation pathology. If the digit is dislocated medially, a section of the lateral capsule and collateral ligament is removed and then sutured to achieve lateral transverse plane correction. If the digit had a lateral dislocation, the section of capsule and collateral ligament would be removed medially and sutured. Just releasing the side of the MTPJ that is contracted will not allow for scarring to occur on the opposite side of the joint in which the capsule and collateral ligament have been abnormally stretched. To determine the amount of capsular tissue to remove from the stretched out side, one should make the vertical capsular cut, have the digit held in the proper transverse plane position and determine how much tissue overlaps and then remove that section. After placing the initial suture across this vertical capsulotomy, the surgeon can cross the stitch and with the foot loaded, observe how much correction is achieved prior to actually tying the stitch. If needed, more tissue can be removed in order to better hold the digit in its proper position. If the capsular tissue is too friable to obtain a good bite with the stitch, a small soft tissue anchor can be inserted into the base of the proximal phalanx and then sutured into the capsular tissue proximally on the metatarsal head (Fig. 6-18). In some instances in long standing transverse plane dislocations, the articular cartilage of the involved metatarsal head may be functionally adapted; therefore, it may be necessary to perform an osteotomy to realign the articular cartilage so that it is in the proper position. This is something that can easily be accomplished when the metatarsal requires shortening (Fig. 6-19 A, B).

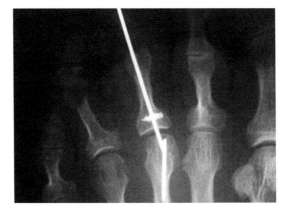

Figure 6-18: This is an AP X-ray view of a patient who had a previous attempt to correct a laterally dislocated third MTPJ with K-wire stabilization. The K-wire broke during the healing process. A second surgery was performed in which a soft tissue anchor was used inserted into the medial aspect of the base of the proximal phalanx to re-enforce the medial capsule.

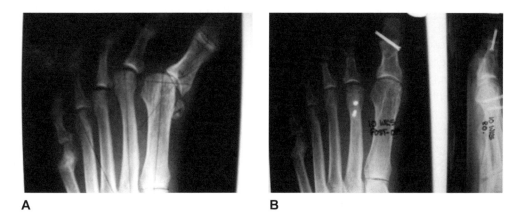

A   **B**

Figure 6-19: A: This is an AP X-ray view showing a severe hallux varus with medial dislocations of the second and third MTPJs. **B:** This is a postoperative X-ray showing the correction of the deformity in which the second MTPJ dislocation was treated via a Weil osteotomy that shortened the metatarsal and the osteotomy was rotated on the transverse plane to allow for better cartilage alignment. A flexor tendon transfer was also utilized.

Flexor Tendon Transfer:

In most cases of lesser MTPJ dislocation, a flexor tendon transfer will be needed to assist in maintaining ground purchase of the involved digit. In cases of acute plantar capsule/plate rupture where an open repair of these structures is performed, a tendon transfer is not needed; however, it has been our clinical experience that a flexor tendon transfer appears to be as effective with less surgical trauma as compared to the open plantar plate repair. When a flexor tendon transfer is performed along with an MTPJ release, we utilize a dorsal serpentine incision extending from the intermediate phalanx proximally, curving over the MTPJ and then extending proximally over the involved metatarsal head to a level that allows adequate exposure for the procedures being performed without causing undo tension on the skin. There is considerable debate over whether one should utilize the flexor digitorum longus (FDL), the flexor digitorum brevis (FDB) or both for the flexor tendon transfer. In our 30 year experience, we have found that for the second digit, using the FDB is sufficient in the majority of cases, provided that it is large enough. For the third digit, it depends upon the size of the FDB encountered; for the fourth digit, we will always use the FDL. Recently, with the advent of small soft tissue anchors, in some cases we have been maintaining the insertion of both FDL and FDB and attaching them to the plantar aspect of the proximal phalanx. This has proven to be very effective in those cases in which only an open arthrotomy of the PIPJ is to be performed. Over the years, the following tendon transfer techniques have been advocated and utilized:

- Girdlestone (1947) transferred the FDL and FDB without performing a PIPJ procedure (Fig. 6-20).

- Sgarlato (1970) transferred the FDL, tenotomized the FDB and performed a PIPJ arthroplasty (Fig. 6-21).

- Kuwada and Dockery (1980) transferred the FDL through a drill hole in the proximal phalanx, kept the FDB intact and did not perform a PIPJ procedure (Fig. 6-22).

- Surgery Department at CSPM (1986) transferred the FDB keeping the FDL intact, and performed a PIPJ arthrotomy, arthroplasty or arthrodesis using a K-wire in most cases through the digit for stabilization during the healing period (Fig. 6-23).

- Surgery Department at CSPM (1991) kept the insertions of the FDL and FDB intact and sutured both tendons to the plantar surface of the head of the proximal and performed either an open arthrotomy, an arthroplasty or an arthrodesis of the PIPJ along with a K-wire in most cases through the digit during the healing period (Fig. 6-24).

- Surgery Department at CSPM (2006) performed the same type of transfer as described above except that a soft tissue anchor was inserted into the plantar aspect of the proximal phalanx which allowed both tendons to be secured to the bone (Fig. 6-25).

Over the years our clinical experience has demonstrated that all of the flexor tendon transfers will be effective provided any underlying structural pathology has been corrected and that adequate soft tissue release is performed at the involved MTPJ.

PIPJ Open Arthrotomy with Flexor Tendon Transfer:

In those cases where the PIPJ of the involved digit is still flexible and the digit is not abnormally long, then an open arthrotomy of the PIPJ is performed to locate the flexor tendons. On the second and sometimes the third digit, the FDB is usually large enough to effectively function as the transfer. If it is not, then the FDL is utilized. On the fourth digit, the FDL is always utilized. Once the PIPJ is opened, the head of the proximal phalanx is retracted dorsally (Fig. 6-26) to expose the plantar capsule which is then removed exposing the FDB. At this level the FDB tendon is split in a linear direction and is attached to the base of the intermediate phalanx. The FDL lies just beneath the FDB and can easily be identified by slipping a curved mosquito hemostat under the FDB and pulling it dorsally to be able to visualize the FDL. At this time the

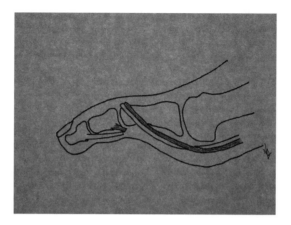

Figure 6-20: This drawing demonstrates a transfer of the FDL and FDB to the head of the proximal phalanx following an open arthrotomy of the PIPJ. The tendons are split and brought around the proximal phalanx and sutured to each other under tension. The FDB is shown shaded.

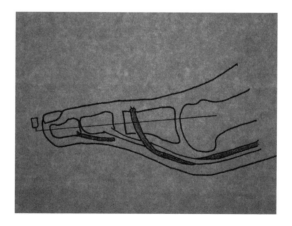

Figure 6-21: This drawing demonstrates a transfer of the FDL, which is shown shaded, to the dorsal aspect of the proximal phalanx following an arthroplasty of the PIPJ. The tendon is split and brought around the proximal phalanx and sutured to each other under tension. The FDB is shown tenotomized.

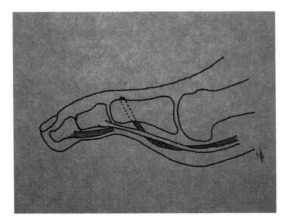

Figure 6-22: This drawing demonstrates a transfer of the FDL, which is shown shaded, to the dorsal aspect of the proximal phalanx following an open arthrotomy of the PIPJ. The tendon is kept whole and brought through a drill hole in the proximal phalanx and sutured to the dorsal surface under tension. The insertion of the FDB is maintained.

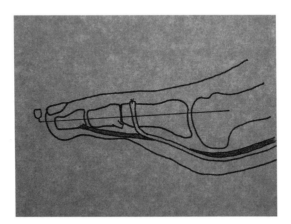

Figure 6-23: This drawing demonstrates a transfer of the FDB to the dorsal aspect of the proximal phalanx following an arthrodesis of the PIPJ. The tendon is split and brought around the proximal phalanx and sutured to each other under tension. The FDL is shown shaded and its insertion is maintained. A K-wire is shown through the digit and across the MTPJ for stabilization during the healing period.

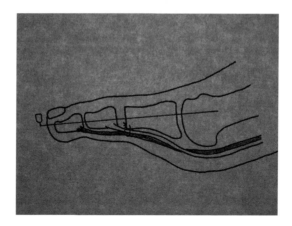

Figure 6-24: This drawing demonstrates a transfer of the FDB and FDL (shaded) in which their insertions are kept intact and both tendons are sutured to the plantar aspect of the proximal phalanx though a drill holes made in the phalanx. In this drawing an arthroplasty had been performed of the PIPJ and a K-wire is shown through the digit and across the MTPJ for stabilization during the healing period.

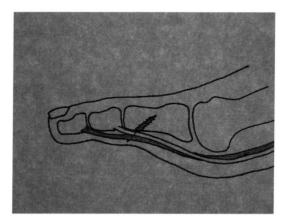

Figure 6-25: This drawing demonstrates a transfer of the FDB and FDL (shaded) in which their insertions are kept intact and both tendons are sutured to the plantar aspect of the proximal phalanx via a soft tissue anchor which has been inserted into the plantar aspect of the phalanx. In this drawing an open arthrotomy had been performed at the PIPJ.

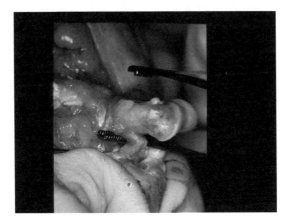

Figure 6-26: Clinical photograph of an intraoperative lateral view showing the freeing of the head of the proximal phalanx.

surgeon must decide whether the transfer will be as shown in Figure 6-25, in which both tendons are secured to the plantar aspect of the head of the proximal phalanx via a soft tissue anchor, or whether a single tendon will be split and brought dorsally over the head of the proximal phalanx. We would rather maintain the insertion of the FDL tendon if at all possible, especially in the second digit, and only use the FDB tendon if we are going to transfer a single tendon. This will prevent the clinical extensus of the distal phalanx that usually occurs approximately six months following the severance of the FDL tendon for a single transfer. If we elect to perform a single tendon transfer using the FDB, the tendon is severed from its insertion on the plantar aspect of the base of the intermediate phalanx by careful dissection. It is already split, but further longitudinal splitting of the tendon will be necessary. Once the tendon is split, a mosquito clamp is attached to each distal end and with the digit held in a corrective position, the tendon is crisscrossed over the head/neck area of the proximal phalanx (Fig. 6-27 A, B) and sutured under physiological tension. We normally utilize several 4.0 absorbable sutures. Care should be taken to make certain that there is no soft tissue between the tendon and the proximal phalanx in order to achieve maximum force on the digit following the transfer. The extensor tendon that has been tenotomized at the PIPJ level is reattached. The foot is then loaded and if the digit now assumes a normal position, the subcutaneous tissue and skin are closed (Fig. 6-28 A, B) and bandages applied maintaining the digit in good position (Fig. 6-29). If the digit still remained elevated, one may need to utilize a K-wire through the digit and across the MTPJ for several weeks until fibrosis occurs to help maintain digital correction and/or a plantar skin plasty which is described later in this chapter.

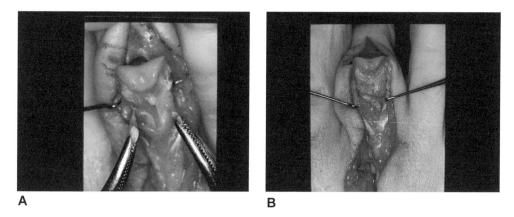

A   B

Figure 6-27: Clinical photographs: **A:** Dorsal intraoperative view showing clamps holding the two cut ends of the split flexor digitorum brevis tendon on either side of the neck area of proximal phalanx. **B:** Dorsal view following the suturing of the extensor digitorum brevis tendon over the neck of the proximal phalanx under physiological tension.

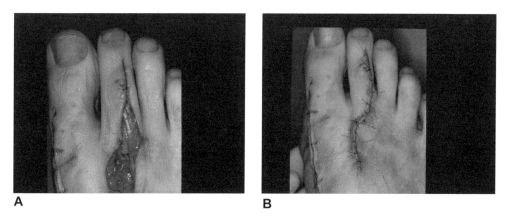

A   B

Figure 6-28: Clinical photographs: **A:** Dorsal intraoperative view following the sequential soft tissue MTPJ release and flexor digitorum brevis transfer and re-attachment of the extensor digitorum longus tendon with the foot loaded prior to skin closure. **B:** The same patient following skin closure and the forefoot loaded in which the second digit now is in a good corrected position. A bunionectomy had also been performed to prevent further pressure to the second digit.

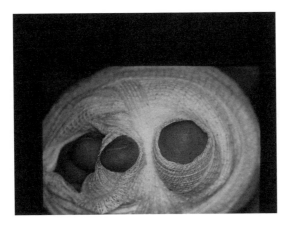

Figure 6-29: Clinical photograph of an intraoperative view showing the postoperative bandaging in which the second digit is maintained in a corrected position in which no K-wire was utilized.

In those cases in which a soft tissue anchor is to be used (Fig. 6-30 A-E) to suture both tendons to the plantar aspect of the proximal phalanx just proximal to the head, the suture is passed through both the FDB and FDL and tied. This then creates an attachment of both tendons to the plantar aspect of the proximal phalanx. A plantar incision on the digit can be used which will allow for good exposure for insertion of the anchor without having to open the PIPJ. A separate dorsal incision can be made over the involved MTPJ in order to perform a soft tissue release of that joint. A K-wire can still be used but due to the anchor it cannot be inserted through the digit as described above. It can be inserted from distal dorsal going through the base of the proximal phalanx into the metatarsal head with the digit being held in the corrective position on the transverse and sagittal planes.

The use of a postoperative shoe or a removable walking boot is needed to eliminate the propulsive phase of gait until one believes that the tendon transfer has healed with sufficient strength. This is usually three to four weeks. A Darco™ digital splint is utilized by the patient at night to maintain the involved digit in the proper sagittal plane alignment once all bandaging has been removed for approximately four to six weeks. X-rays are taken within the first week following surgery and then as needed (Fig. 6-31 A, B).

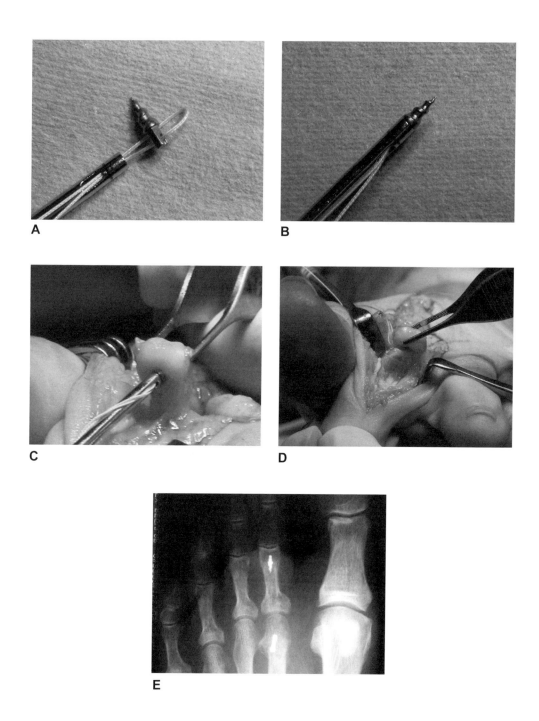

Figure 6-30: A: Clinical photograph of an Arthrex small bone FASTak™ suture anchor with FiberWire. **B:** Clinical photograph of the anchor attached to its inserter. **C:** Intraoperative clinical photograph showing the insertion of the anchor into the plantar aspect of the proximal phalanx. **D:** Intraoperative clinical photograph following insertion of the anchor prior to passing the FiberWire through both the FDL and FDB tendons. **E:** AP X-ray following a PIPJ arthrotomy and a flexor tendon transfer to the plantar aspect of the proximal phalanx using the FASTak™ anchor.

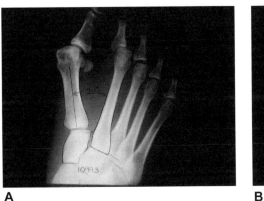
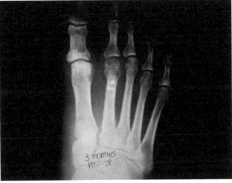

A   B

Figure 6-31: A: Preoperative AP X-ray showing a bunion with a hypermobile first ray, an elongated second metatarsal and a medially/dorsally dislocated second MTPJ. **B:** Three months postoperative X-ray of McBride bunionectomy with first MCJ fusion, Weil osteotomy second metatarsal and PIPJ arthrotomy second digit with flexor digitorum brevis transfer to dorsal aspect of proximal phalanx.

PIPJ Arthroplasty with or without a Digital Implant or PIPJ Arthrodesis with Flexor Tendon Transfer:

In those situations where the involved digital contracture is semi-rigid or rigid or the digit is abnormally long, then one can either utilize a PIPJ arthroplasty with or without digital implant (Fig. 6-32) or a PIPJ arthrodesis along with a flexor tendon transfer (Fig. 6-33 A, B; Fig. 6-34 A, B). The surgical technique for the transfer would be as described above except that for an arthroplasty or arthrodesis, a K-wire is normally used through the digit and across the involved MTPJ. The flexor tendon is not sutured across the phalanx dorsally until the K-wire has been inserted and the surgeon determines that the digit is in a good transverse and sagittal plane position.

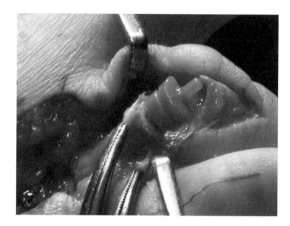

Figure 6-32: Intraoperative clinical photograph in which a digital implant is going to be used in the PIPJ. The clamps are holding the split portions of the FDB tendon that will be used for the transfer.

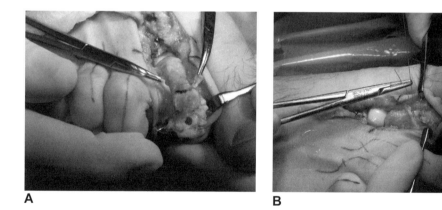

A   B

Figure 6-33: Clinical photographs: **A:** Distal view of a second digit in which a peg-n-hole arthrodesis will be done along with a FDB transfer. The clamps are holding the split ends of the FDB tendon on either side of the proximal phalanx. **B:** Intraoperative view showing the suturing of the FBD tendon slips over the dorsal aspect of the proximal phalanx following the completion of the PIPJ arthrodesis in which a K-wire was used through the digit.

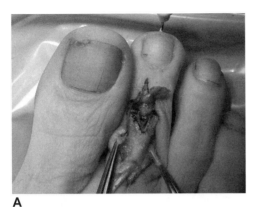
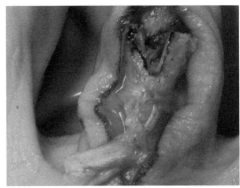

A **B**

Figure 6-34: Clinical photographs: **A:** Dorsal view of a second digit in which a "V" wedge arthrodesis of the PIPJ is to be performed along with a FDB tendon transfer. **B:** Dorsal view following the suturing of the FDB tendon over the dorsal aspect of the proximal phalanx. Note that the FDL tendon has not been re-attached at this time.

The tendon is then sutured under physiological tension using several 4.0 absorbable sutures. For the surgical techniques and postoperative management for an arthroplasty, the reader is referred to Chapter 3; for digital implant procedures Chapter 5; for a PIPJ arthrodesis, Chapter 4; and for a hallux IPJ arthrodesis, Chapter 2.

In many instances, it is necessary to correct a deformity of the first ray in order to more effectively correct the second MTPJ dislocation (Fig. 6-35 A-G; Fig. 6-36 A-F).

If a K-wire was utilized through the digit, then the shoe or walking boot needs to be accommodated with a half inch felt pad extending from the heel to the sulcus of the digits. This raises the entire foot, allowing the digit with wire not to be in contact with the shoe as shown in Chapter 3. This will help to prevent bending of the wire during ambulation. The K-wire is usually removed at the third to fourth week. Radiographs are normally taken within the week following surgery to make certain that the digit is in proper alignment (Fig. 6-37). Further radiographs may be necessary depending upon other adjunctive procedures performed.

Again, a Darco™ digital splint is utilized by the patient at night to maintain the involved digit in the proper sagittal plane alignment once all bandaging has been removed for approximately four to six weeks.

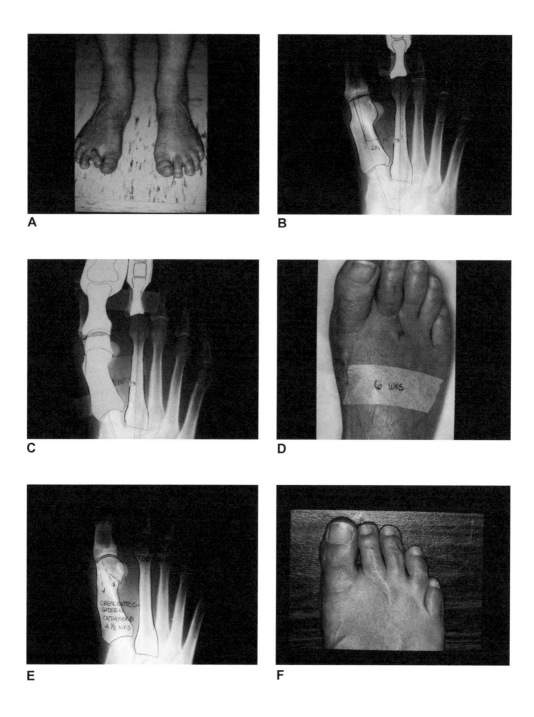

A

B

C

D

E

F

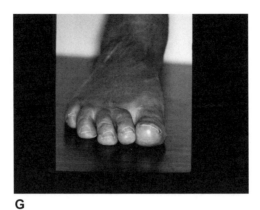

G

Figure 6-35: A: Preoperative clinical photograph of patient with medial/dorsal dislocation of the second digit right foot which developed one year following a first metatarsal head osteotomy procedure to correct a bunion deformity. **B:** AP X-ray showing paper template of second digit placed in its proper position. This maneuver allowed the surgeon to appreciate the over correction of the bunion site and the resulting hallux adductus which in turn created the second MTPJ instability. **C:** AP X-ray showing template for a crescentic osteotomy to re-align the hallux. **D:** Clinical photograph showing dorsal view of the foot at six weeks following the osteotomy of the first metatarsal, a sequential release of the second MTPJ, a PIPJ arthroplasty with a FDB transfer. **E:** AP X-ray view four and a half weeks following the surgery showing the hallux and second digit in good alignment. **F:** Clinical photograph showing dorsal view five years post-op of the same patient showing some medial driftof the second digit but no further dorsal dislocation. **G:** Clinical photograph showing distal view of the same patient showing the alignment of the digits at five years following surgery.

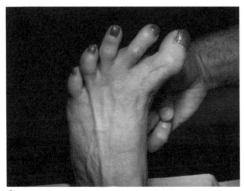

A

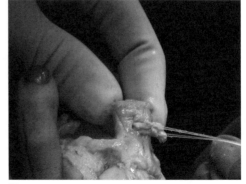

B

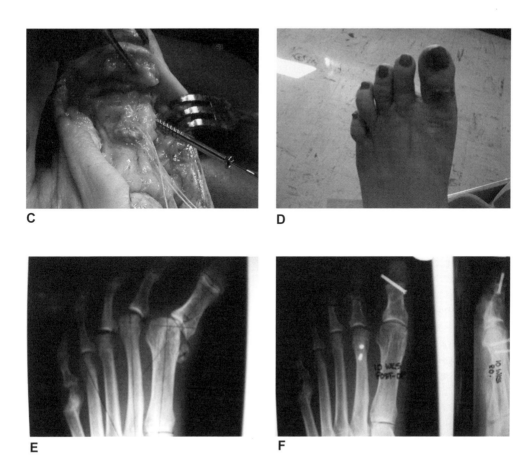

C   D

E   F

Figure 6-36: Clinical photographs: **A:** Preoperative view of a foot with significant hallux varus and medial dislocations of second and third digits. **B:** Intraoperative view showing flexor hallucis longus tendon being pulled through a drill hole made in the proximal phalanx (Kuwada technique). **C:** Intraoperative view showing 2.0 cannulated screw being utilized to fixate the hallux IPJ fusion and the flexor tendon having been sutured to the dorsal tissues under physiological tension. **D:** Postoperative view of the foot at 10 weeks with the digits in significantly better alignment. **E:** Preoperative X-ray showing the severe dislocations occurring at the first, second and third MTPJs. **F:** Postoperative X-ray at 10 weeks showing a hallux IPJ fusion with screw fixation, dorsal hole in the proximal phalanx where FHL tendon was transferred, osteotomy of the second metatarsal in which the bone was shortened and cartilage realigned, and arthroplasties with flexor tendon transfers of the second and third digits.

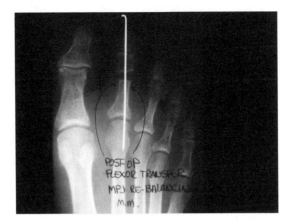

Figure 6-37: Postoperative AP X-ray showing K-wire through digit following a PIPJ arthroplasty with FDB tendon transfer.

Contraindications to Performing a Flexor Tendon Transfer:

In our opinion there are a few instances where performing a flexor tendon transfer would be contraindicated and they are as follows:

- Isolated tendon transfer in a non flexible digit
- Isolated tendon transfer in an abnormally long digit
- FDB tendon transfer with a mallet toe deformity

Plantar Sulcus Ellipse:

For a number of patients with a dorsal dislocation at the MPTJ, once the digit has been relocated to its proper position there is often redundancy of the plantar skin at the sulcus of the digit (Fig. 6-38). Failure to evaluate for this condition may lead to excessive plantar skin which will serve as a buttress to hold the digit off the ground postoperatively. Following relocation of the involved digit, we will load the forefoot and inspect the sulcus for this redundancy. If found, we will ellipse the redundant plantar skin in a semi-elliptical fashion. This maneuver will also aid in holding the involved digit in a good sagittal plane position (Fig. 6-39 A-C). The postoperative management is based upon the other procedures being performed for the dislocation. The sutures from this plantar ellipse are normally removed at the third week.

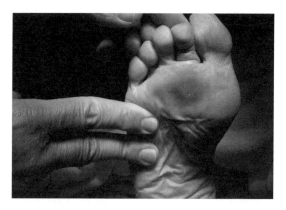

Figure 6-38: Clinical photograph of plantar view of foot with the second digit being held in its anticipated corrected position which creates significant redundant tissue at the plantar sulcus of the toe.

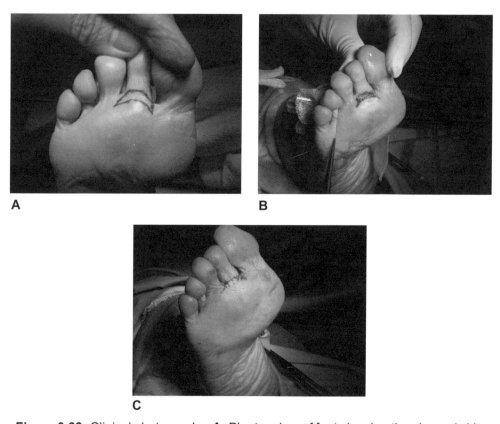

A

B

C

Figure 6-39: Clinical photographs: **A:** Plantar view of foot showing the planned skin ellipse from the sulcus to eliminate the redundant tissue which will occur once the toe is put into it corrected position. **B:** This view shows the skin ellipse removed. **C:** This view shows the plantar ellipse closed using 5-0 non-absorbable sutures.

Plantar Plate Repair:

It has been our philosophy that there are limited indications for performing an isolated plantar plate repair for a dislocated lesser MTPJ. In our clinical experience and after a review of the literature, we do not believe that plantar plate repair is any more effective than a flexor tendon transfer with appropriate digital or metatarsal procedures. The utilization of lesser MTPJ arthrography has been advocated to demonstrate a tear in the plantar plate and that leakage into the flexor tendon sheath is pathognomonic for a plantar plate tear. However, one should appreciate several potential problems with arthrography. First of all, the synovial tissue heals very rapidly, so unless one injects the joint within the first week following the injury there is a good chance that no dye will be seen to leak from the joint even with a plantar plate tear. Secondly, if one penetrates the joint capsule by inserting the needle too far plantar, medial or lateral, dye will be seen to appear to leak outside the joint. Thirdly, there is not sufficient information regarding the normal anatomy of the flexor tendon sheath, its relationship with the plantar plate and capsule structure and whether there is a normal anastomosis that can occur between these two structures. The utilization of an MRI to determine the integrity of the plantar plate is once again open to interpretation and the quality of the imaging study.

Therefore, if we were to decide upon a primary repair of the plantar plate, it would need to be performed on a patient with no digital deformity, no underlying structural pathology of the involved metatarsal, a totally reducible MTPJ as determined by the Kelikian push-up test and a very recent traumatic event.

The actual surgical technique involves a plantar longitudinal incision between the involved metatarsals. As the incision approaches the involved MTPJ, it can be curved over the area and then extended distally onto the base of the involved digit (Fig. 6-40). (Refer to Chapter 1 for pictures of the pertinent anatomical details of this area.) By sharp dissection, the subcutaneous and fat tissue is incised to the level of the flexor tendon sheath. The sheath is incised and the flexor tendons retracted laterally or medially thereby exposing the plantar plate. An obvious tear will be seen and can be sutured using any suture material preferred by the surgeon. If the distal tissue on the base of the proximally phalanx is tenuous, one can insert a small soft tissue anchor into the base of the proximal phalanx to allow for good approximation of the plantar plate (Fig. 6-41 A, B). The flexor tendons are allowed to return to their normal position and no deep closure is used in order to minimize excessive fibrosis and adhesions of the flexors (Fig. 6-42). The patient is kept non-weight bearing for approximately three weeks utilizing a low profile walking boot to eliminate ankle movement and movement of the tendons to the involved digit. Weight bearing is then allowed using the walking boot in order to eliminate the propulsive phase of gait for an additional three weeks. The use of a Darco™ digital splint is utilized by the patient at night to maintain the involved digit in the proper sagittal plane alignment once all bandaging has been removed for approximately one month.

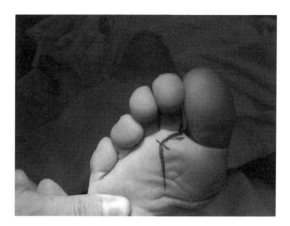

Figure 6-40: This photograph shows the planned plantar incision approach for a plantar plate repair.

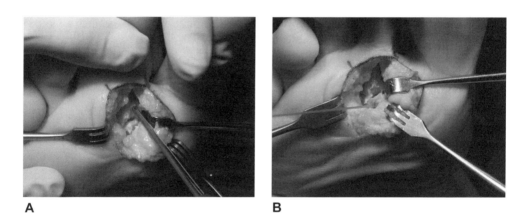

A   B

Figure 6-41: A: Intraoperative photograph showing a soft tissue anchor being inserted in the plantar aspect of the base of the proximal phalanx. **B:** Intraoperative photograph showing the plantar plate rupture being sutured together.

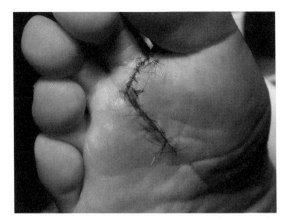

Figure 6-42: Clinical photograph of an incision closure following a primary repair of the plantar plate.

Inherent Complications:

In our experience the following are inherent complications of a flexor tendon transfer, plantar sulcus ellipse or plantar plate repair:

1. Chronic edema of the involved digit has been our most common complication following the flexor tendon transfer. This can usually be treated adequately with physical therapy and a steroid injection as described in Chapter 3 for a dactylitis.

2. Floating digit. Treatment for this condition depends upon the perceived etiology. If it is secondary to fibrosis and stiffness of the involved MTPJ, it may be treated by aggressive manipulation of the MTPJ and digit under local anesthesia followed by physical therapy and the use of a Darco™ digital splint at night and a Budin splint during the day. If it appears that the plantar skin at the sulcus of the digit is very redundant, and this was not addressed at the time of surgery, then an ellipse of this tissue has proven to be beneficial in allowing the digit to purchase the ground. If the FDB tendon was utilized for the transfer and it does not appear to have adequate strength, then one can consider another procedure using the FDL tendon under better physiological tension.

3. Stiffness of the involved digit. If this is the result of the chronic edema, then once the edema is resolved the stiffness will diminish. At times, stiffness of the involved MTPJ may be resolved with another dorsal soft tissue release.

4. Hyperextension of the distal aspect of the involved digit. When this occurs it is usually due to the loss of the FDL tendon to the distal phalanx. If this proves problematic, an arthrodesis of the DIPJ of the involved digit will need to be considered.

5. Fibrosis of the plantar sulcus scar. In some situations patients have complained of being able to feel a thickness where the plantar redundant skin had been ellipsed. An injection of an acetate steroid directly into the scar following a local anesthetic block can resolve this issue.

6. Soft tissue anchor irritation. In a few patients in where a soft tissue anchor was used, it backed out to a degree (Fig. 6-43 A, B) creating symptoms with ambulation. Using a plantar incision, the soft anchor can be removed and the flexor tendons sutured to the proximal phalanx.

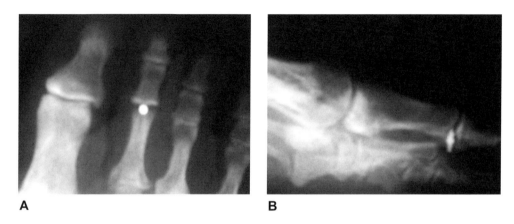

A   B

Figure 6-43: A: AP X-ray view five months following a PIPJ arthroplasty and FDL/FDB tendons transfer using the FASTak™ Arthrex anchor. The patient began complaining of pain along the plantar aspect of the digit with ambulation. The anchor can be seen to have migrated into the site of the arthroplasty. **B:** Lateral X-ray view showing the anchor having migrated distally and plantarly. The anchor was removed through a plantar incision and the FDL/FDB tendons sutured to the stump of the proximal phalanx.

Clinical Pearls:

The following are tips that we believe can assist the surgeon in providing a more predictable favorable outcome and preventing postoperative complications when attempting to correct a dislocated lesser MTPJ:

1. Identify the etiology(ies) for the dislocation.

2. Determine preoperatively the flexibility of the MTPJ by using the Kelikian Push-Up test.

3. Utilize a dorsal serpentine incision across the involved MTPJ.

4. Release the soft tissues around the MTPJ in a sequential fashion loading the forefoot after each maneuver.

5. Release both the medial and lateral capsular structures when attempting to re-balance the MTPJ on the transverse plane.

6. When possible, utilize a K-wire across the MTPJ to stabilize the digit when performing a flexor tendon transfer.

7. Evaluate for plantar skin redundancy at the sulcus of the involved digit after the digit has been brought into a corrected position and if found to be significant it should be excised.

8. Utilize a PIPJ open arthrotomy or arthrodesis with a flexor tendon transfer for the most effective results.

9. Utilize a dorsal approach for a flexor tendon transfer in which the tendon is split and sutured to each other on the dorsal surface of the phalanx to minimize the chance of digital vasculature embarrassment.

10. Use a low profile walking boot during the healing period to immobilize the ankle and minimize tendon action on the involved digit.

11. Utilize a Darco™ digital splint at night and a Budin splint during the day for one month after the bandages have been removed.

References:

Baravarian B. Essential Insights on Flexor Tendon Transfers. *Podiatry Today.* 20: 66-74, 2007.

Becerro de Bengoa, et al. Transfer of the Flexor Digitorum Brevis Tendon. *J Am Podiatry Assoc.* 98:27-35, 2008.

Blitz NM, Christensen JC, Ford LA. Plantar plate ruptures of the second metatarsophalangeal joint. *J Foot Ankle Surg* 41:138-141, 2002.

Blitz NM, Ford LA, Christensen JC. Plantar plate repair of the second metatarsophalangeal joint: Technique and Tips. *J Foot Ankle Surg* 43:266-270, 2004.

Boyer ML, DeOrio JK. Transfer of the flexor digitorum longus tendon for the correction of lesser-toe deformities. *Foot Ankle Int* 28:422-430, 2007.

Buxbaum FD. Surgical correction of the metatarsophalangeal joint dislocation and arthritic deformity: the partial head and plantar condylectomy. *J Foot Surg* 18:36-40, 1979.

Coughlin MJ. Subluxation and dislocation of the second metatarsophalangeal joint. *Orthop Clin North Am* 20: 535-551, 1989.

Coughlin MJ. Second metatarsophalangeal joint instability in the athlete. *Foot Ankle Int* 14:309-319, 1993.

Coughlin MJ. Lesser toe deformities. <u>Surgery of the Foot and Ankle</u> 8th edition, Coughlin, MJ, Mann RA, Saltzman CL, Eds., Elsevier, Philadelphia, Pa., 2007.

Deland JT et al. Anatomy of the plantar plate and its attachments in the lesser metatarsophalangeal joint. *Foot Ankle Int* 16: 480-486, 1995.

Ford LA, Collins KB, Christensen JC. Stabilization of the subluxed second metatarsophalangeal joint: flexor tendon transfer versus primary repair of the plantar plate. *J Foot Ankle Surg* 37:217-222, 1998.

Fortin PT, Myerson MS. Second metatarsophalangeal joint instability. *Foot Ankle Int* 16:306-313, 1995.

Gerbert, J. How to handle second MTPJ stress syndrome. *Podiatry Today* 18: 44-50, 2005.

Girdlestone GR. Physiotherapy for hand and foot. *J Chart Soc Physiother* 32:167-169, 1947.

Haddad SI et al. Results of flexor-to-extensor and extensor brevis tendon transfer for correction of the crossover second toe deformity. *Foot Ankle Int* 20:781-788, 1999.

Hofbauer MH, Shane-Reeves AM. Lesser digital surgery: Arthroplasty, arthrodesis and flexor tendon transfer. Master Techniques in Podiatric Surgery: The Foot and Ankle, Chang TJ Ed., Lippincott Williams & Wilkins, Philadelphia, Pa., 2005.

Kuwada GT, Dockery GL. Modification of the flexor tendon transfer procedure for the correction of flexible hammertoes. *J Foot Surg* 19:38-40, 1980.

Kuwada GT. A retrospective analysis of modification of the flexor tendon transfer for correction of hammertoe. *J Foot Surg* 27: 57 – 65, 1988.

Myerson MS, Jung HG. The role of toe flexor-to-extensor transfer in correcting metatarsophalangeal joint instability of the second toe. *Foot Ankle Int* 26:675-679, 2005.

Sgarlato TE. Tranplantation of the Flexor Digitorum Longus Muscle Tendon in Hammertoes. *J Am Podiatry Assoc* 60:383-388, 1970.

Taylor RG. The treatment of claw toes by multiple transfers of flexor into extensor tendons. *J Bone Joint Surg Br* 33B: 4: 539-542, 1951.

Yao L, Do HM, Cracchiolo A, Farahani K. Plantar plate of the foot: findings on conventional arthrography and MR imaging. *Am J Roentgenol* 163: 641-644, 1994.

Yao L, et al. Magnetic resonance imaging of plantar plate rupture. *Foot Ankle Int* 17: 33-36, 1996.

Yu GV et al. Predislocation syndrome: Progressive subluxation/dislocation of the lesser metatarsophalangeal joint. *J Am Podiatr Med Assoc* 92:182-199, 2002.

Lesser Metatarsal Osteotomies & Plantar Condylectomy 7

Joshua Gerbert, DPM, FACFAS

Introduction:

Numerous osteotomy procedures have been advocated for correction of pathologies associated with lesser metatarsals two, three, and four. These procedures involved various distal, mid-shaft and proximal osteotomies. After retrospective evaluation of the literature and our experiences with all of these procedures, we determined that the midshaft or proximal osteotomies were no more effective than the distal head procedures for isolated lesser metatarsal pathology and in many situations created a higher incidence of complications. In situations involving a metatarsus adductus in which multiple metatarsals require re-alignment, then a base procedure such as a Weil-type performed proximally or a crescentic may be indicated. These procedures for this pathology will be discussed in Chapter 12. Therefore this chapter will only discuss the osteotomies currently being performed by our department for isolated pathology of metatarsals two, three, or four. Correction of a brachymetatarsia will be covered in Chapter 12 even though there are situations in which the abnormally short metatarsal is secondary to a previous surgery or traumatic event. As with all procedures, the clinical evaluation to determine the specific pathology is extremely important in order to select the most effective osteotomy. The osteotomy procedures to be covered in this chapter are as follows:

1. Weil Osteotomy (modified Mau procedure)
2. Dorsal "V" Osteotomy of the metatarsal head

The utilization of a plantar condylectomy has been advocated for certain specific conditions for many decades. While osteotomy procedures have certainly replaced the need for plantar condylectomy in most situations, the procedure still has it uses.

Weil Osteotomy:

This metatarsal head procedure has becomes one of the most commonly performed osteotomies of lesser metatarsals two, three and four. It allows for significant shortening of the metatarsal while at the same time preserving the plantar grade position of the head (Fig. 7-1 A-C). This procedure will also allow for some transverse plane correction of the metatarsal head depending upon the width of the bone

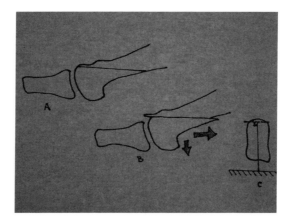

Figure 7-1: A: Sagittal view showing the long oblique osteotomy cut starting dorsal at the leading edge of the articular cartilage. **B:** Sagittal view showing the proximal displacement of the metatarsal head following the osteotomy cut. Note that as the capital fragment moves proximally it also moves slightly plantar to preserve weight bearing to the metatarsal head. One can also appreciate the dorsal overhang of bone that is created following the displacement of the capital fragment which is removed after the osteotomy site is fixated. **C:** This is a cross sectional view of the metatarsal head showing the proper position of the sagittal saw blade in making the osteotomy cut. It should be held perpendicular and parallel to the weight bearing surface.

involved. Lastly, because of the oblique design of the osteotomy, the use of a screw is a very effective means of fixation. Perhaps the biggest downside of this procedure is that with the shortening of the metatarsal of more than 2- 3 mm, the slip of the plantar fascia becomes slack as well as the flexor tendons which dramatically affect the windlass mechanism to the involved digit. The result is a floating digit in most cases. To counteract this problem, we have found it necessary to perform a flexor tendon transfer of some type (refer to Chapter 6) to the involved digit regardless of whether there is any digital deformity.

Clinical Indications:

1. Abnormally long metatarsal as compared to the adjacent metatarsals confirmed radiographically (Fig. 7-2). In some situations where one is performing a procedure on the first metatarsal in which shortening will occur and radiographically the second metatarsal is already relatively long, shortening of the second metatarsal should probably be considered in order to prevent an overload syndrome from developing.

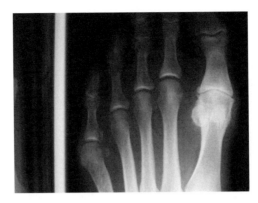

Figure 7-2: AP X-ray depicting an elongated second metatarsal relative to the first metatarsal and the third metatarsal.

2. Adequate width of the involved bone at the metatarsal head/neck area. This becomes critical when attempting to perform this procedure on the fourth metatarsal.

3. Lack of significant DJD of the involved MTPJ unless a lesser hemi MTPJ implant was to be used.

4. A dislocated MTPJ may be present along with MTPJ instability (positive modified Lachman's Test) (Fig. 7-3 A, B)

5. Transverse plane dislocation of the involved MTPJ in which the metatarsal head may be functionally adapted (Fig. 7-4 A, B).

6. A plantar hyperkeratotic lesion may be present under the involved metatarsal head.

7. Chronic MTPJ capsulitis secondary to a metatarsal overload/stress syndrome/metatarsalgia is usually present.

Surgical Procedure:

The following surgical description is the one that we perform at CSPM. Certainly other versions would be acceptable. A serpentine incision is made over the involved MTPJ extending as far distally on the digit to accommodate any digital procedure to be performed and as far proximally in order to perform the osteotomy without causing undue tension on the soft tissue structures (Fig. 7-5). Sharp and blunt dissection is performed down to the extensor expansion. Once this structure is identified, then depending upon the pathologies present it may be released in a sequential fashion (see Chapter 6). Again, depending upon the pathologies present, the extensor digitorum

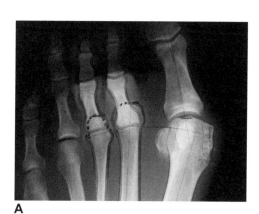
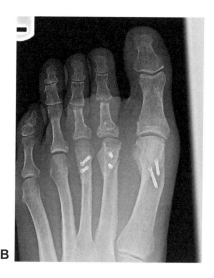

A   **B**

Figure 7-3: A: Preoperative AP X-ray view demonstrating significant dorsal dislocation of the second and third MTPJs. **B:** Postoperative AP X-ray view nine months status post Weil osteotomies of the second and third metatarsals along with digital procedures.

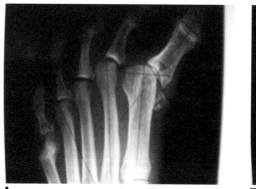
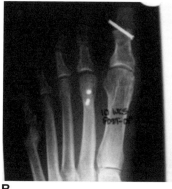
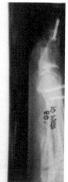

A   **B**

Figure 7-4: A: Preoperative radiograph showing a severe hallux varus with medial dislocations of the second and third digits. The second metatarsal is abnormally long. **B:** Postoperative radiograph at 10 weeks following a hallux IPJ fusion with FHL tendon transfer, arthroplasties of the second and third digits with flexor tendon transfers and a Weil osteotomy that both shortened the metatarsal as well as rotated the metatarsal head on the transverse plane in to better alignment.

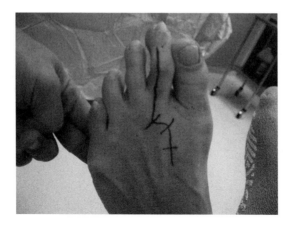

Figure 7-5: Preoperative clinical photograph showing planned serpentine incision extending from the digit over the involved MTPJ and proximally over the medial aspect of the metatarsal shaft. The "hash" marks are used to allow easier closure of the serpentine incision.

brevis may be severed. A dorsal linear capsulotomy is performed extending far enough proximally to adequately expose the dorsal surface of the metatarsal. If the MTPJ was dorsally dislocated then a transverse capsulotomy will also be performed. We have found that a number 125 MicroAire™ sagittal saw blade is very effective in performing the osteotomy. The osteotomy is started just at the most proximal portion of the dorsal edge of the cartilage of the metatarsal head and the blade is held as parallel to the weight bearing surface as possible making certain that the saw blade is as parallel to the weight bearing surface as possible (Fig. 7-6). Care should be taken to insure that the blade is not oriented at an angle on the frontal plane (Fig. 7-7). By holding the blade as parallel to the weight bearing surface as possible will insure an adequate oblique osteotomy in which two screws can be inserted (Fig. 7-8) and that when the head is moved proximally it remains parallel to the weight bearing surface. The metatarsal head is moved proximally to a point where the dorsal overhang of bone matches our predetermined shortening as seen on the preoperative template (Fig. 7-9 A, B). If the involved metatarsal head appears functionally adapted it can be moved on the transverse plane at this time in order to better re-align the digit (Fig. 7-4). We typically utilize the 2.0 cannulated OsteoMed™ screw. While one screw can in most cases create adequate fixation of the osteotomy, two screws will prevent any possible transverse plane rotation of the osteotomy fragment. The type of fixation to be used is best determined by the surgeon and the specific patient. Once the fixation has been competed, the dorsal overhang of bone is removed and the MTPJ is moved through its range of motion to make certain that there is no osseous impingement (Fig. 7-10 A, B).

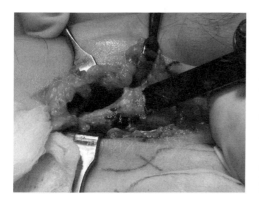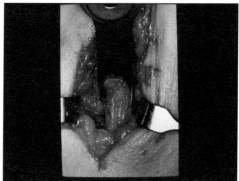

Figure 7-6: Intraoperative clinical photograph demonstrating the proper placement of the long sagittal saw blade beginning just proximal to the dorsal leading edge of the articular cartilage. Note that the saw blade is being held parallel to the weight bearing surface of the foot.

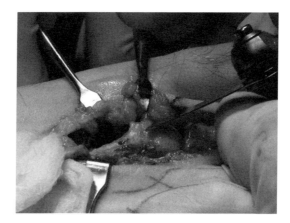

Figure 7-7: Intraoperative clinical photograph demonstrating the saw blade being held in an improper position relative to the weight bearing surface of the foot.

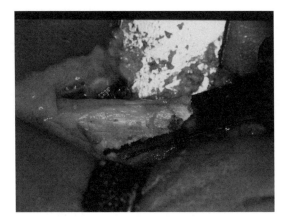

Figure 7-8: This clinical photograph demonstrates the long oblique cut being created by keeping the saw blade as parallel to the weight surface of the foot as possible.

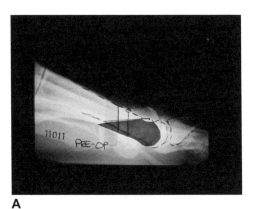
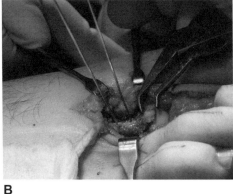

A   B

Figure 7-9: A: Preoperative X-ray with preoperative template showing the amount of shortening desired and the amount of dorsal overhang of bone that will be created. **B:** Intraoperative clinical photograph showing the use of calipers to check the amount of dorsal overhang as compared to the preoperative template. Temporary fixation for cannulated screws is shown.

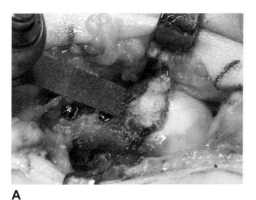 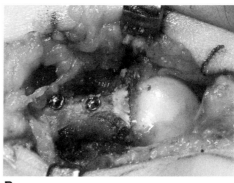

A   **B**

Figure 7-10: Clinical photographs: **A:** This intraoperative view demonstrates the sagittal saw blade in position to remove the amount of dorsal overhang of bone that was created following the shortening osteotomy and fixation. **B:** This intraoperative dorsal view shows the completed osteotomy fixated with two 2.0 cannulated OsteoMed® screws and the dorsal overhang of bone having been removed.

If one is not certain of the placement of the screws, the use of intraoperative fluoroscopy has proven to be beneficial (Fig. 7-11). 4.0 absorbable sutures are used to close the periosteum over the osteotomy site. Any digital procedure is then performed. As mentioned earlier, even if the involved digit has no deformity, a flexor tendon transfer is performed in order to help prevent a floating digit if the metatarsal is shortened more than 2-3 mm. The skin is re-approximated using several buried knot stitches of 5.0 absorbable material and 5.0 non-absorbable simple interrupted or horizontal mattress stitches. Appropriate bandages are applied making certain to splint the involved digit in a plantarflexed attitude. We prefer adding full strength Betadine® solution to the initial layer of bandages directly over the incision site to serve as a bactericidal agent and as a deterrent to the development of a hypertrophic scar. When the Betadine solution dries, it forms a "cast-like" firmness to the incision line which in our estimation lowers the incidence of hypertrophic scar formation.

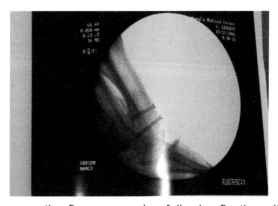

Figure 7-11: Intraoperative fluoroscopy view following fixation with two screws.

Postoperative Management:

The following is our protocol for the Weil osteotomy:

1. Elimination of the propulsive phase of gait for five to six weeks. We have found that the use of a low profile walking boot such as the Aircast™ (Fig. 7-12) has significantly reduced the patient's symptoms and pedal edema as compared to just a surgical shoe.

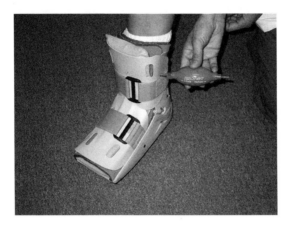

Figure 7-12: Clinical photograph of Aircast™ in which liner can be inflated or deflated to provide the best fit for the specific patient and to accommodate for increase or decrease in edema.

2. Utilization of a digital splint at night such as the Darco™ splint (Figs. 7-13A-B) for four to six weeks following suture removal to maintain the involved digit in a plantarflexed position.

3. X-ray evaluation either immediately following the procedure or within the initial week, again at the third week and again at the sixth or seventh week (Fig. 7-14 A-D).

4. Elimination of high impact activities for at least two months from the date of surgery.

5. Physical therapy as needed for residual edema or MTPJ stiffness.

6. Orthotic therapy as needed based upon any biomechanical pathologies that were present prior to surgery.

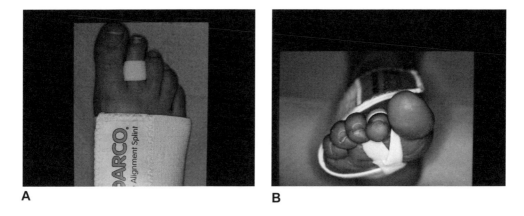

Figures 7-13: A, B: These photographs show how a Darco™ digital splint is used to maintain the second digit in proper transverse and sagittal plane alignment.

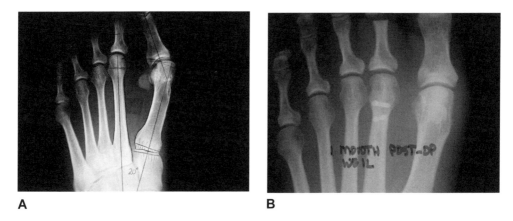

Figure 7-14: A: Preoperative X-ray view of patient with hypermobile first ray and second MTPJ stress syndrome. **B:** AP X-ray view one month post Weil osteotomy with two 2.0 OsteoMed™ screws.

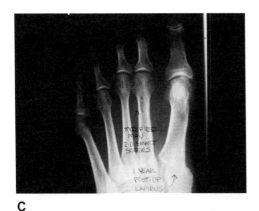
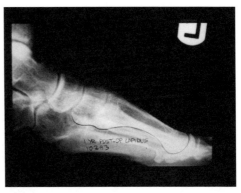

C   **D**

Figure 7-14: C: One year postoperative X-ray view following a first MCJ fusion and a Weil osteotomy of the second metatarsal in which polylactic screws were used for fixation. **D:** Lateral X-ray view at one year in which first and second rays are in good alignment on the sagittal plane.

Inherent Complications:

Over the years of performing the Weil osteotomy we have encountered the following complications.

1. Chronic edema. This can usually be treated adequately with physical therapy.

2. Floating digit which appeared in the majority of cases in which no digital procedure was performed. Treatment for this condition usually involves a digital procedure of at least a flexor tendon transfer along with the use of a Darco™ digital splint at night and a Budin splint during the day.

3. Transfer metatarsalgia/overload syndrome to the adjacent MTPJ when the metatarsal parabola was not maintained. In many cases this can be avoided by the use of a preoperative template to determine how much shortening should occur at the time of surgery. Once this problem occurs, it can be treated with either an orthotic device with accommodation to off load the involved metatarsal head or an osteotomy of the involved metatarsal head that is now bearing abnormal load (Fig. 7-15 A-C; Fig. 7-16 A-D).

4. Stress fracture of the surgical site area (Fig. 7-17 A-C) which seems to have occurred when the patient returned to the propulsive phase of gait and/or high impact activities too early. This can usually be treated with immobilization in an Aircast™ for a period of time, limiting physical activity, and having patient use more rigid sole shoe following the use of a walking boot. At times the use of an external bone stimulator to speed the rate of bone healing has proven to be very effective.

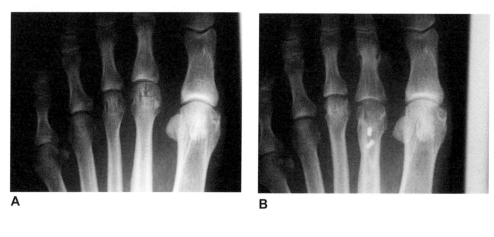

A   B

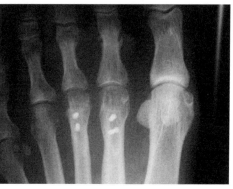

C

Figure 7-15: A: Preoperative AP X-ray showing an abnormally long second meta-tarsal relative to the first and third metatarsals. Patient had chronic second MTPJ stress syndrome. **B:** Postoperative AP X-ray view following a Weil osteotomy along with a flexor digitorum brevis tendon transfer on the proximal phalanx. Note that the third metatarsal now appears abnormally long as compared to the second and fourth metatarsals. One year following the initial Weil osteotomy on the second met-atarsal the patient began developing third MTPJ stress syndrome. **C:** Postoperative AP X-ray view following a Weil osteotomy on the third metatarsal to create a more normal parabola between 1, 2, and 3. This eliminated the patient's symptoms and no further forefoot problems developed.

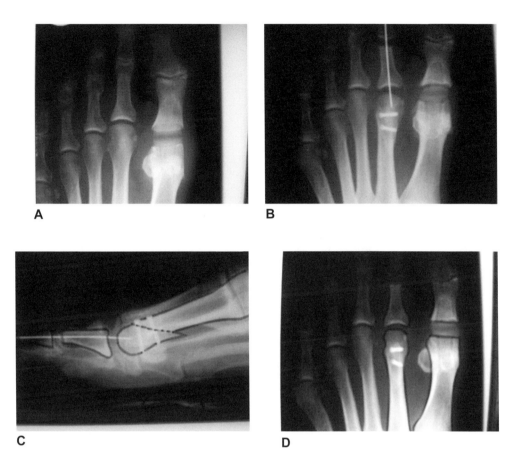

Figure 7-16: **A:** AP X-ray view following a total Silastic® hinge implant in the first MTPJ. Note that the second metatarsal appears abnormally long relative to the first metatarsal. The patient began developing a chronic second MTPJ stress syndrome one year following the implant procedure. **B:** AP X-ray view following a Weil oste-otomy on the second metatarsal which resolved the patient's forefoot symptoms. An arthroplasty of the PIPJ of the second digit along with a flexor digitorum brevis tendon transfer to the proximal phalanx was also performed. **C:** Lateral X-ray view showing Weil osteotomy with screw fixation and K-wire being used to stabilize digit. **D:** AP X-ray view at one year with relief of all symptoms.

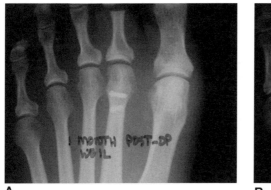

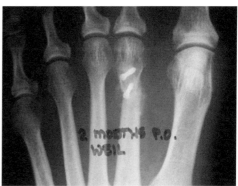

A   B

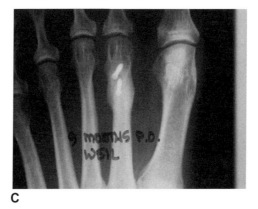

C

Figure 7-17: A: AP X-ray view one month postoperative Weil osteotomy. Patient had returned to her regular shoe gear and normal ambulation with minimal discomfort. **B:** AP X-ray view of the same patient two months postoperative Weil osteotomy. Patient related increase pain and edema at the surgical site for several weeks prior to having this X-ray taken which reveals a stress fracture. **C:** AP X-ray view of the same patient nine months post-op Weil osteotomy and seven and a half months post stress fracture of the second metatarsal. All symptoms have resolved.

Clinical Pearls:

The following are tips that we believe can assist the surgeon in providing a more predictable favorable outcome and preventing postoperative complications when performing the Weil osteotomy.

1. Make certain there is adequate width of the metatarsal neck area preoperatively.

2. Use a preoperative template to determine the amount of shortening necessary to maintain a normal metatarsal parabola.

3. Use a long enough sagittal saw blade and keep it as parallel to the weight bearing surface as possible in order to create a long oblique osteotomy.

4. Use intraoperative calipers to measure the amount of dorsal overhang created when the capital fragment is shortened and that it coincides with the measurements obtained by the preoperative template.

5. Perform a flexor tendon transfer on the involved digit to reduce the incidence of a floating toe syndrome regardless of whether there was associated digital pathology or a PIPJ fusion was performed.

6. Eliminate the propulsive phase of gait for at least five to six weeks to lower the incidence of a stress fracture.

7. Utilize a low profile walking boot such as an Aircast™ verus a surgical shoe to reduce postoperative symptoms and edema.

8. Take appropriate postoperative x-rays to access the healing of the osteotomy site.

9. Utilize a Darco™ digital splint at night for four to six weeks posteratively.

Dorsal "V" Osteotomy:

This metatarsal head procedure was very popular in the 1970s and 1980s; today it has largely been replaced by the Weil osteotomy. However, we believe it is still a useful procedure especially on the third and fourth metatarsals in certain situations. Initially this procedure was performed without fixation, allowing the metatarsal head to seek its own level postoperatively when the patient ambulated. This was made possible provided the suspensory ligaments were maintained from the epicondyle of the metatarsal head to the glenoid plate (Fig. 7-18 A-C). Today, when we perform this procedure we will usually fixate the capital fragment either by a K-wire that is being used to stabilize the involved digit or with an absorbable rod through the metatarsal head if no digital procedure was performed. A floating toe is usually not encountered to the extent as seen with the Weil procedure, provided one does not allow the metatarsal head to elevate to a significant level; typically, this only occurs when the suspensory ligaments have been severed. We have found that when using a 1 mm thick saw blade to create the osteotomy, with normal healing, the metatarsal will shorten approximately 2 to 3 mm.

Clinical Indications:

1. Minimally long metatarsal as compared to the adjacent metatarsals confirmed radiographically (Fig. 7-19).

2. Narrow width of the metatarsal neck does not contraindicate this procedure.

3. Lack of significant DJD of the involved MTPJ unless a lesser hemi MTPJ implant was to be used.

4. MTPJ instability (positive modified Lachman's Test) may be present; however, MTPJ dislocation is probably a contraindication.

5. A plantar hyperkeratotic lesion may be present under the involved metatarsal head.

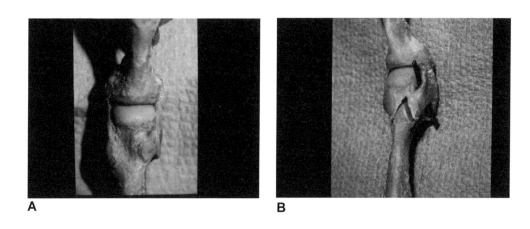

A   B

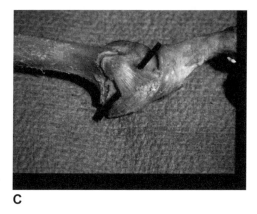

C

Figure 7-18: Clinical photographs: **A:** Dorsal view of a cadaver specimen demonstrating the MTPJ, the collateral ligaments extending from the epicondyle of the metatarsal head and the suspensory ligaments extending from the epicondyle to the glenoid plate. **B:** Dorsal/lateral view of a cadaver specimen following a dorsal "V" osteotomy in which one can see that the lateral suspensory ligament has remained intact going to the glenoid plate. **C:** Lateral view of a cadaver specimen following a dorsal "V" osteotomy in which the collateral ligament has been removed showing the intact lateral suspensory ligament extending from the epicondyle of the metatarsal head to the glenoid plate.

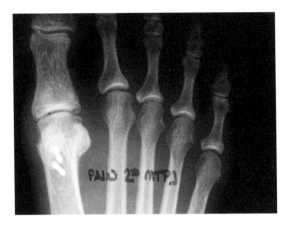

Figure 7-19: X-ray of patient who complains of second MTPJ stress syndrome nine months following a decompressional osteotomy of the first metatarsal to resolve a hallux limitus. The second metatarsal is now mildly elongated relative to the first metatarsal.

6. Chronic MTPJ capsulitis secondary to a metatarsal overload/stress syndrome/metatarsalgia is usually present.

7. Normal transverse plane articular position of the involved metatarsal head must be present.

8. Preventative procedure on a third metatarsal when a Weil osteotomy is being performed on the second and there is already a mild hyperkeratotic lesion sub third metatarsal head or a preventative procedure at times on the fourth when a Weil is performed on the third.

Surgical Procedure:

The following surgical description is the one that we perform at CSPM. Certainly other versions would be acceptable. A serpentine incision is made over the involved MTPJ, extending as far distally on the digit as needed to accommodate any digital procedure to be performed and as far proximally as needed in order to perform the osteotomy without causing undue tension on the soft tissue structures. The proximal portion of the incision is much less than required for the Weil procedure. Sharp and blunt dissection is performed down to the extensor expansion. Once this structure is identified, it may be released in a sequential fashion depending upon the pathologies present (see Chapter 6). Again, depending upon the pathologies present, the extensor digitorum brevis may be severed. A dorsal linear capsulotomy is performed extending just proximal to the metatarsal neck to allow exposure of the dorsal surface of the metatarsal. We attempt to preserve the suspensory ligaments and mark the "V" with a skin scribe (Fig. 7-20) with the apex located just distal to the epicondyles with its wings extending proximally preserving the epicondyles. This ensures that the suspensory ligaments remain attached from the metatarsal head to the glenoid plate, which is critical if one is not planning to fixate the osteotomy site. Once the cut has been made, the metatarsal is pushed slightly dorsally until one believes that the metatarsal is at its appropriate height. If a digital procedure is to be performed, then we will usually utilize a 0.045 K-wire through the digit, across the MTPJ and through the osteotomy site to stabilize the digital procedure as well as fixate the capital fragment. If no digital procedure was being performed and we wanted to fixate the capital fragment, we will use a 1.5 mm polylactic rod through the articular surface of the metatarsal head proximally into the osteotomy site (Fig. 7-21; Fig. 7-22). On the fourth metatarsal, we will often perform this procedure without any fixation and allow the metatarsal head to seek its own level when the patient ambulates. We have not encountered a transfer problem to the fifth metatarsal head. A 4.0 absorbable suture is used to close the periosteum over the osteotomy site. The skin is re-approximated using several buried knot stitches of 5.0 absorbable material and 5.0 non-absorbable simple interrupted or horizontal mattress stitches. Appropriate bandages are applied making certain to splint the involved digit in a plantarflexed attitude. Full strength Betadine solution to the initial layer of bandages directly over the incision site as discussed in the surgical discussion of the Weil procedure.

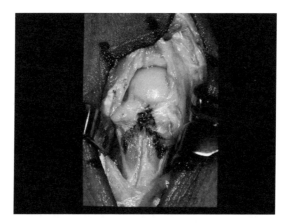

Figure 7-20: Intraoperative clinical photograph showing the planned osteotomy site marked on the metatarsal head in which the suspensory ligaments attached to the epicondyles are kept intact.

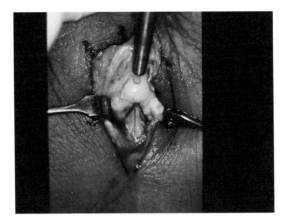

Figure 7-21: Intraoperative clinical photograph showing the insertion of a 1.5 mm polylactic rod through the metatarsal head into the shaft to fixate the osteotomy site once the metatarsal head was elevated to the position desired by the surgeon.

Postoperative Management:

The following is our protocol for the Dorsal "V" osteotomy:

1. Elimination of the propulsive phase of gait for five to six weeks. We have found that the use of a low profile walking boot such as the Aircast™ has significantly reduced the patient's symptoms and pedal edema as compared to just a surgical shoe.

2. Utilization of a digital splint at night such as the Darco™ splint for four to six weeks following suture removal to maintain the involved digit in a plantar-flexed position.

3. X-ray evaluation either immediately following the procedure or within the initial week, again at the third week and again at the sixth week (Fig. 7-23).

4. Elimination of high impact activities for at least two months from the date of surgery.

5. Physical therapy as needed for residual edema or MTPJ stiffness.

6. Orthotic therapy as needed based upon any biomechanical pathologies that were present prior to surgery.

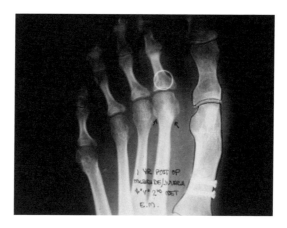

Figure 7-22: AP X-ray view at one year following a dorsal "V" osteotomy of the second metatarsal head in which a 1.5 mm PLA rod was utilized for fixation.

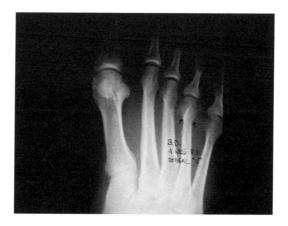

Figure 7-23: AP X-ray view at four weeks following a dorsal "V" osteotomy of the fourth metatarsal head in which no fixation was utilized and the patient allowed to ambulate in a surgical shoe. Note the absence of external callus formation.

Inherent Complications:

Over the years of performing the Dorsal "V" osteotomy, we have encountered the following complications.

   1.   Chronic edema. This can usually be treated adequately with physical therapy.

2. Floating digit when the metatarsal head was elevated to a significant degree. Unfortunately, this can only be treated by performing another osteotomy to lower the metatarsal head or a digital procedure in an attempt to re-establish digital toe purchase.

3. Transfer metatarsalgia/overload syndrome to the adjacent MTPJ when the metatarsal parabola. This usually occurs when there has been a delayed healing resulting in excessive bone absorption at the osteotomy site (Fig. 7-24 A-E). This can be treated with either orthotic devices with accommodation to off load the involved metatarsal head or an osteotomy of the metatarsal head which now is being over loaded.

4. Delayed and non-unions. These are usually the result of the patient returning to full high impact activities too early. This can be treated initially with the use of an external bone stimulator and/or further immobilization. If this does not resolve the problem, bone grafting surgery may be necessary (Fig. 7-25 A-E).

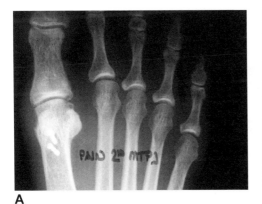

A

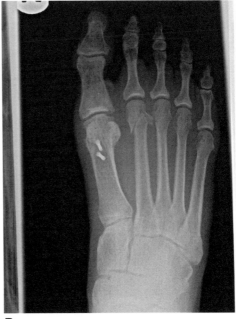

B

Figure 7-24: A: AP X-ray view nine months post-op decompressional osteotomy first metatarsal. Patient developed second MTPJ stress syndrome which was not responsive to conservative therapy. **B:** AP X-ray view three weeks postoperative dorsal "V" osteotomy second metatarsal head. Note that the lateral arm of the osteotomy fractured. The alignment of the second metatarsal head relative to the first appears good.

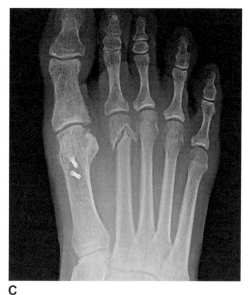

C

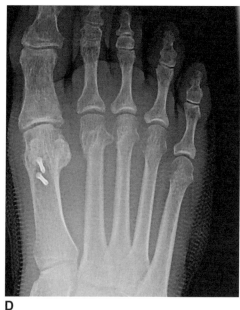

D

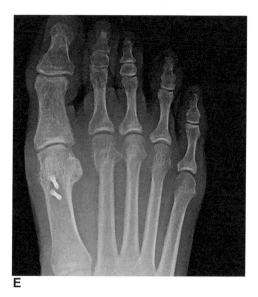

E

Figure 7-24: C: AP X-ray view six weeks postoperative showing increase re-sorption of bone at the osteotomy site. Note that the third metatarsal is now relatively longer as compared to the first and second metatarsals. **D:** AP X-ray view nine months following the second metatarsal osteotomy which has healed and symptoms related to this metatarsal resolved. The patient developed third MTPJ stress syndrome which did not respond to conservative therapies. A dorsal "V" osteotomy of the third metatarsal head was performed fixated with 1.5 mm PLA rod. **E:** AP X-ray view two months post-op third metatarsal osteotomy which appears to have resolved all symptoms and metatarsals 1, 2 and 3 are in good alignment.

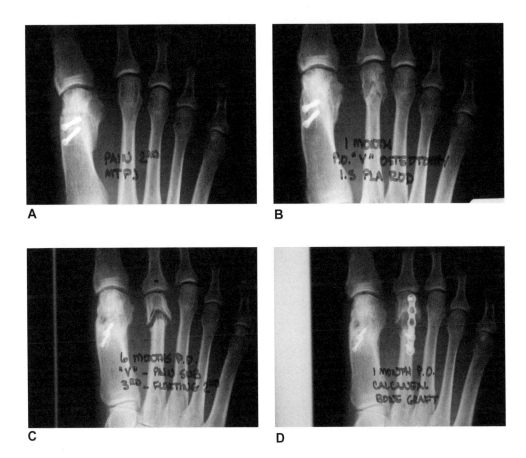

Figure 7-25: A: AP X-ray view 12 months postoperative decompressional osteotomy of the first metatarsal. The second metatarsal is now relatively longer as compared to the first metatarsal and the patient has developed second MTPJ stress syndrome. **B:** AP X-ray view one month postoperative dorsal "V" osteotomy of the second metatarsal head area in which a 1.5 mm PLA rod was used to fixate the capital fragment. The alignment appears good. **C:** AP X-ray view six months postoperative dorsal "V" osteotomy. The patient returned to high impact activities immediately following the previous photograph. The second metatarsal has shortened significantly and shows signs of delayed/non-union. The patient began developing third MTPJ stress syndrome. An external bone stimulator was used and custom orthotic devices fabricated to off-load the area. **D:** AP X-ray view nine months postoperative dorsal "V" osteotomy in which no further bone healing occurred and the symptoms sub third metatarsal head increased. A calcaneal autogenous bone graft with a mini-plate was used to lengthen the second metatarsal in an attempt to re-establish some weight bearing.

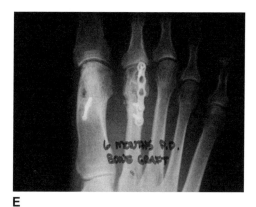

E

Figure 7-25: E: AP X-ray view six months following the bone grafting procedure which has now consolidated. The bone plate was later removed to allow better second MTPJ motion. The symptoms beneath the third metatarsal head resolved.

Clinical Pearls:

The following are tips that we believe can assist the surgeon in providing a more predictable favorable outcome and preventing postoperative complications when performing the Dorsal "V" osteotomy.

1. Utilize the procedure in only those cases where minimal shortening of the metatarsal is needed.

2. Do not utilize this procedure in the presence of a significant dorsal dislocation of the involved MTPJ.

3. Preserve the suspensory ligaments to the glenoid plate.

4. Fixate the osteotomy site on the second and third metatarsal heads.

5. Eliminate the propulsive phase of gait for at least five to six weeks to lower the incidence of external callus formation and increase osseous absorption resulting in increase metatarsal shortening especially in those cases where the osteotomy site is not fixated.

6. Take appropriate postoperative X-rays to access the healing of the osteotomy site.

7. Utilize a Darco™ digital splint for four to six weeks postoperatively to lower the incidence of a floating toe syndrome.

Plantar Condylectomy:

This metatarsal head procedure has been utilized for decades and while not used as commonly as the Weil or Dorsal "V," it still has its merits. It allows for elimination of a prominent plantar aspect of a metatarsal head while preserving the integrity of the MTPJ and the length of the metatarsal. Since this procedure is only an ostectomy, the postoperative management and expected disability is much less involved as compared to an osteotomy procedure.

Clinical Indications:

1. Plantar hyperkeratotic lesion is usually present under the involved metatarsal head.

2. Normal length of the metatarsal.

3. Lack of significant DJD of the MTPJ unless a lesser MTPJ implant was to be used or a partial metatarsal head resection was needed.

4. A dislocated MTPJ may be present along with MTPJ instability (positive modified Lachman's Test)

5. Plantar axial X-rays reveal a prominent metatarsal head (Fig. 7-26).

6. Intraoperative inspection of the plantar aspect of the metatarsal head reveals a prominent lateral plantar condyle.

7. Elderly patient in whom one believes performing a metatarsal osteotomy procedure would not be in the best interest of the patient.

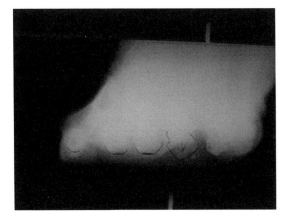

Figure 7-26: This is a preoperative plantar axial view demonstrating a prominent plantar condyle of the second metatarsal head.

Surgical Procedure:

A serpentine incision is made over the involved MTPJ extending as far distally on the digit as needed to accommodate any digital procedure to be performed and proximally to the metatarsal neck/shaft area. Sharp and blunt dissection is performed down to the extensor expansion. Once this structure is identified, it may be released in a sequential fashion depending upon the pathologies present. Again, depending upon the pathologies present, the extensor digitorum brevis may be severed. A dorsal linear capsulotomy is performed extending far enough proximally to adequately expose the dorsal surface of the metatarsal head and neck. If the MTPJ was dorsally dislocated, then a transverse capsulotomy will also be performed. Using a McGlamry® elevator, the metatarsal head is elevated dorsally exposing the plantar condyles. Maintaining the elevator in place, an appropriate width osteotome is used to remove the offending plantar condyles (Fig. 7-27 A, B). It should be noted that the fibular condyle is the most plantar prominent aspect of the metatarsal head; therefore the angulation to remove the condyle should be such to remove more bone from the lateral aspect as compared to the medial side (Fig. 7-28). Once the condyles have been cut with the osteotome, care is taken to apply pressure to the elevator and the osteotome to wedge the loose condyles distally into the MTPJ (Fig. 7-29 A-D). A small hand rasp or power burr can be used to smooth any rough edges on the plantar surface of the metatarsal head (Fig. 7-30). The area is flushed and the capsular structures closed in an appropriate fashion. Any digital procedure is then performed. The skin is re-approximated using several buried knot stitches of 5.0 absorbable material and 5.0 non-absorbable simple interrupted or horizontal mattress stitches. Appropriate

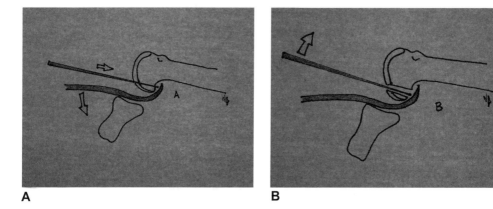

A   **B**

Figure 7-27: A: This drawing shows the McGlamry Elevator® in place and the osteotome cutting the plantar condyle. **B:** This drawing shows how one can use the osteotome to wedge the cut condyle against the elevator and remove it distally, thereby preventing this loose piece of bone from migrating proximally under the metatarsal.

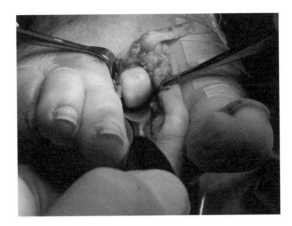

Figure 7-28: This is a frontal clinical photograph of the surgical site showing the exposed second metatarsal head. Note that the fibular condyle is the more prominent condyle.

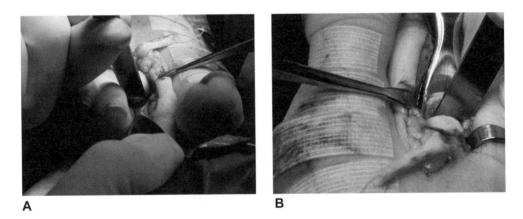

A   B

Figure 7-29: Clinical photographs: **A:** This photograph shows selecting a proper width osteotomeand angulating it to remove more bone from the lateral plantar aspect of the metatarsal head. **B:** Dorsal view following the cut by the osteotome in which the plantar cut portion of the metatarsal head is wedged between the elevator and the osteotome and pried distally.

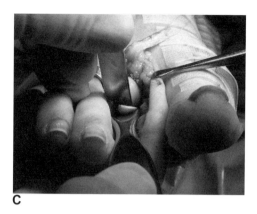
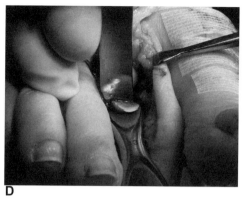

C   D

Figure 7-29: C: Frontal view in which the plantar cut portion of the metatarsal head is wedged between the elevator and the osteotome and pried distally. **D:** Frontal view in which the plantar cut portion of the metatarsal head has been pried distally and can easily be removed.

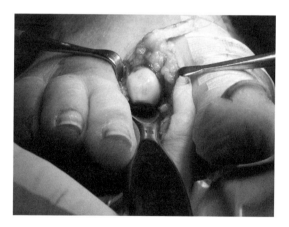

Figure 7-30: Clinical photograph from a frontal view showing the plantar surface of the second metatarsal head following removal of the plantar condyles.

bandages are applied making certain to splint the involved digit in a plantarflexed attitude. We prefer adding full strength Betadine solution to the initial layer of bandages directly over the incision site to serve as a bactericidal agent and as a deterrent to the development of a hypertrophic scar.

Postoperative Management:

The following is our protocol for a plantar condylectomy:

1. Immediate ambulation is permitted in a surgical shoe. At home the patient may ambulate just in the postoperative bandages with a propulsive gait provided a digital procedure performed at the same time does not dictate more restrictive ambulation.

2. Utilization of a digital splint at night such as the Darco™ splint for three to four weeks following suture removal in order to help maintain the involved digit in a plantarflexed position for better toe purchase.

3. Plantar axial X-ray evaluation as soon as feasible for the patient to take such an X-ray view in order to evaluate the surgical site.

4. Physical therapy as needed for residual edema or MTPJ stiffness.

5. Orthotic therapy as needed based upon any biomechanical pathologies that were present prior to surgery.

6. Return to regular shoes and activities as soon as the sutures are removed provided a digital procedure that may have been performed at the same time does not dictate other management and restrictions.

Inherent Complications:

Over the years of performing a plantar condylectomy we have encountered the following complications.

1. Chronic edema. This can usually be treated adequately with physical therapy.

2. Stiffness of the MTPJ. Treatment for this condition usually involves physical therapy and possibly an injection with a phosphated steroid.

3. Transfer metatarsalgia/overload syndrome to the adjacent MTPJ. This usually occurs when an excessive amount of the plantar aspect of the metatarsal head was removed. This can usually be treated with an orthotic device with accommodation to off load the involved metatarsal head.

4. Failure to remove the cut portion of the plantar condyles which creates chronic plantar pain. Treatment for this condition necessitates a surgery to remove the condyle portion.

Clinical Pearls:

The following are tips that we believe can assist the surgeon in providing a more predictable favorable outcome and preventing postoperative complications when performing a plantar condylectomy.

1. Make certain that the metatarsal is not abnormally long.

2. Use a McGlamry® elevator to elevate the metatarsal head into the surgical site to expose the plantar surface of the bone.

3. Maintain the elevator in place as the osteotome is used to remove the plantar condyles.

4. Remove more bone from the plantar lateral aspect of the metatarsal head since the fibular condyle is the more prominent structure.

5. Maintain the elevator in place and use the osteotome to wedge the cut plantar condyles against the metatarsal into the MTPJ in order to prevent accidental proximal migration of the condyles once cut.

6. Utillize a Darco™ digital splint at night for three to four weeks posteratively to assist with digital/MTPJ stability.

References

Beech I, Rees S, Tagoe M. A retrospective review of the Weil metatarsal osteotomy for lesser metatarsal deformities: an intermediate follow-up analysis. *J Foot Ankle Surg* 44:358-364, 2005.

Buxbaum FD. Surgical correction of the metatarsophalangeal joint dislocation and arthritic deformity: the partial head and plantar condylectomy. *J Foot Surg.* 18:36-40, 1979.

Downey MA, Dorothy WL. A radiographic technique to demonstrate the plantar aspect of the forefoot in stance. *J Am Podiatr Assoc.* 59, 1969.

Goforth PW, Overbeek TD, Odom RD, et al. Lesser-metatarsal medial displacement osteotomy for the treatment of digital plane deformities. *J. Am Podiatr Med Assoc.* 95:550-555, 2005.

Goforth PW, Karlin JM, DeValentine S, et al. Distal Metatarsal Osteotomy: A retrospective study. *J Amer Podiatr Assoc.* 74:402-405, 1984.

Grimes J, Coughlin M. Geometric analysis of the Weil osoteotomy. *Foot Ankle Int* 27:985-920, 2006.

Heller AG. Plantar condylectomy and some modifications for plantar keratoma. *J Am Podiatr Assoc* 53:347-348, 1963.

Hofstaetter SG, Hofstaetter JG, Petroutsas JA, et al. The Weil osteotomy: a seven-year follow up. *J Bone Joint Surg Br* 87:1507-1511, 2005.

Jex, CT, Wan CJ, Rundell S, et al. Analysis of three types of fixation of the Weil osteotomy. *J Foot Ankle Surg* 45:13-16, 2006.

Khalafi A, Landsman AS, Lautenschlager EP, Kelikian AS. Plantar forefoot pressure changes after second metatarsal neck osteotomy. *Foot Ankle Int* 26:550-555, 2005.

Lau JT, Stamatis ED, Parks, BG, Schon LC. Modifications of the Weil osteotomy have no effect on plantar pressure. *Clin Orthop Relat Res*: 421:194-198, 2004.

Lauf E, Weinraub GM. Asymetric "V" osteotomy: a predictable surgical approach for chronic central metatarsalgia. *J Foot Ankle Surg* 35:550-559, 1996.

McGlamry ED, Kitting RW, Butlin WE. Plantar condylectomy, Current Modifications in Technique. *J Amer Podiatr Assoc* 59:345-348, 1969.

Migues A, Slullitel G, Bilbao F, et al. Floating-toe deformity as a complication of the Weil osteotomy. *Foot Ankle Int*: 25:609-613, 2004.

Podskubka A, Stedy V, Kafunek M. Distal shortening osteotomy of the metatarsals using the Weil technique: surgical treatment of metatarsalgia and dislocation of the metatarsophalangeal joint. *Acta Chir Orthop Traumatol Cech* 69:79-84, 2002.

Pontious J, Lane GD, Moritz JC, Martin W. Lesser metatarsal V-osteotomy for chronic intractable plantar keratosis. Restrospective analysis of 40 procedures. *J Am Podiatr Med Assoc* 88: 323-331, 1998.

Trnka HJ, Gebhard C, Muhlbauer M, et al. The Weil osteotomy for treatment of dislocated lesser metatarsophlangeal joints: good outcome in 21 patients with 42 osteotomies. *Acta Orthop Scand* 73:190-194, 2002.

Vandeputte G, Dereymaeker G, Steenwerckx A, Peeraer L. The Weil osteotomy of the lesser metatarsals: a clinical and pedobarographic follow-up study. *Foot Ankle Int* 21:370-374, 2000.

Young DE, Hugar DW. Evaluation of the V-osteotomy as a procedure to alleviate the intractable plantar keratoma. *J Foot Surg* 19:187-189, 1980.

Tailor's Bunionette Deformity **8**

William M. Jenkin, DPM, FACFAS

Introduction:

This chapter will deal with the Tailor's Bunionette. A lateral prominence of the fifth metatarsal head is referred to as a Tailor's bunion or bunionette deformity. It is so named because historically it was associated as an occupational hazard of ancient tailors who sat cross legged upon the ground as they worked. It was believed that this chronic irritation produced the enlargement.

Etiologies:

The bunionette can be as a result of pathology at the level of the fifth metatarsal head, distal metatarsal shaft, proximal metatarsal base or a combination of levels.

- Enlargement of the metatarsal head/lateral condyle (Fig. 8-1).

- Bony exostosis.

- Excessive lateral deviation of the distal metatarsal shaft (Fig. 8-2).

- Excessive intermetatarsal angle IV making the lateral aspect of the fifth metatarsal head prominent (Fig. 8-3).

- Fifth digital adductus deformity causing retrograde force against the fifth metatarsal head, thereby increasing the fourth IMA (especially in the latter two presentations) (Fig. 8-4).

- Fifth ray hypermobility. Ground reactive forces upon the fifth metatarsal cause it to move about its own independent axis of motion creating maximal dorsiflexion in the sagittal plane, abduction in the transverse plane and eversion in the frontal plane. The end positional result makes the lateral condyle of the fifth metatarsal head more prominent and therefore subject to irritation from the interior of a shoe.

- Splay foot, or metatarsus latus, results when the patient presents with both abnormal IM angle I and IV which usually results in having symptoms both medially and laterally.

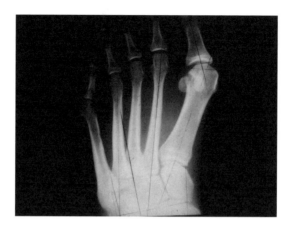

Figure 8-1: AP view radiograph demonstrating prominent lateral condyle.

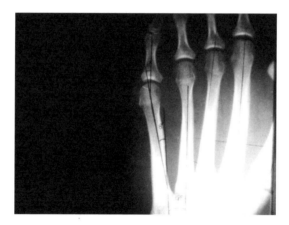

Figure 8-2: AP view radiograph demonstrating excessive lateral deviation angle.

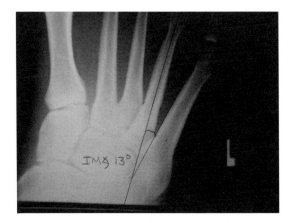

Figure 8-3: AP view radiograph demonstrating excessive IM angle.

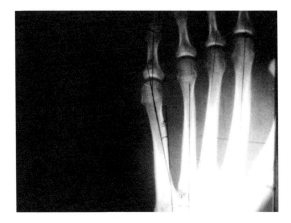

Figure 8-4: AP view radiograph demonstrating fifth digital adductus.

Signs and Symptoms:

Signs

- Laterally prominent fifth metatarsal head (Fig. 8-5).
- Erythema surrounding fifth metatarsal head.
- Edema lateral to fifth metatarsal head.
- Mechanically induced hyperkeratosis, lateral or lateral plantar to fifth metatarsal head (Fig. 8-6).

Symptoms

- Lateral metatarsalgia: Focal pain lateral or lateral/plantar to fifth metatarsal head.

Symptoms are secondary to mechanical irritation from footgear or ground reactive force creating a pressure point at the bunion site. The patient's complaint consists of lateral metatarsalgia or intermittent pain lateral to the fifth metatarsal head primarily occurring when weight bearing in shoes. The symptoms can be associated with an adventitious bursitis, nerve entrapment, mechanically induced hyperkeratosis lateral and sometimes plantar to fifth metatarsal head, or rarely arthrosis of the fifth MTPJ.

Clinical Evaluation:

During the non-weight bearing portion of the physical examination, have the patient describe where the point of maximum tenderness is located and then attempt to reproduce pain with palpation. Determine if the pain radiates indicating nerve involvement. Note the presence and location of any mechanically induced hyperkeratosis and, if present, determine if their location corresponds to the area of pain. With an acute onset of symptoms note signs of underlying inflammation which most often indicates the presence of a bursitis, but could also be associated with an infection or gout attack. Evaluate the integrity of the MTPJ to determine if pain is intra–articular or extra-articular. Determine if there is a significant fifth toe adductus or adductovarus deformity and if present whether the adductus is reducible, semi-reducible, or non-reducible in the transverse plane at the fifth MTPJ level. Determine the fifth metatarsal position as well as the forefoot to rearfoot and rearfoot to leg relationships to see if there is a forefoot varus or valgus deformity contributing to the problem at the fifth metatarsal level. Evaluate for fifth ray hypermobility, the ability to "lock" the midtarsal joint, and for the presence of an ankle equinus as described in Chapter 1.

During the weight bearing portion of the examination while the patient stands in the relaxed calcaneal stance position (RCSP, determine if the deformity increases. Then place the foot in the neutral calcaneal stance position (NCSP) to determine if the deformity significantly reduces making the lateral aspect of the fifth metatarsal head less prominent. If this occurs, custom functional foot orthotics holding the foot in the "corrected" position may be helpful in the long term management.

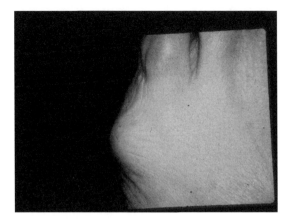

Figure 8-5: Clinical photograph of Bunionette deformity.

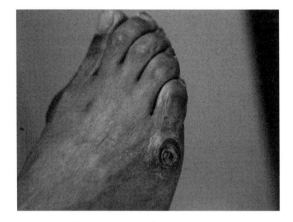

Figure 8-6: Clinical photograph demonstrating mechanically induced hyperkeratosis lateral to Bunionette deformity.

Finally, classify the foot type into rectus (straight forefoot), pronated (abducted forefoot), supinated (adducted forefoot), or splay foot. Evaluate footgear to determine fit and areas of internal pressure points by observing wear pattern inside shoe along its lateral side. Assure that the "last" of the shoe corresponds to the shape of the foot (foot type). The "last" is determined by mentally bisecting the rear portion of the shoe and comparing it to the bisection of the fore part of the shoe. A straight "last" shoe is for a rectus foot. An in-flared "last" shoe is for an adducted type foot and an out-flared "last" shoe is for an abducted forefoot. (Fig. 8-7) Finally, evaluate the shod foot to assure that the widest part of the shoe corresponds to the widest part of the foot. The shoe itself can cause irritation to the fifth metatarsal head in several ways: (1) When wearing an in-flared "last" shoe on a foot type with abducted forefoot, the fifth metatarsal head will become a pressure point and (2) if the shoe is short (improper heel to ball length) the first and fifth metatarsal heads will be pinched by the interior of the shoe.

X–Ray Evaluation:

Radiographic evaluation further defines the level and extent of pathology and confirms the findings of the clinical examination. Lesion markers can be placed at area of maximum tenderness and over areas of mechanically induced hyperkeratosis in order to more accurately correlate clinical symptoms/signs with the underlying osseous pathology. The views we routinely take are an anterior-posterior (AP) and lateral.

AP and lateral views are obtained of the foot while positioned in the angle and base of gait. X-ray projections taken of both feet at the same time will provide inaccurate information. The following should be evaluated on the AP view:

- Hypertrophy of the fifth metatarsal head.
- Prominent lateral condyle or a lateral exostosis of fifth metatarsal head (Fig. 8-1).
- Abnormally high lateral deviation angle (Fig. 8-2).
- Abnormally high intermetatarsal angle IV (Fig. 8-3).
- Fifth toe adductus or adductovarus deformity. (Fig. 8-4).
- Location of lesion marker.
- Arthritic changes within fifth MTPJ.
- Splay Foot Type (metatarsus latus).
- Width of the metatarsal neck.

Because of a bowed appearance of the fifth metatarsal in the transverse plane occurring just distal to its base, obtaining a true bisection of the entire fifth metatarsal is not always possible. Therefore, a radiographic reference line is established by placing a tangential line paralleling and next to the medial proximal cortical margin of the base of the fifth metatarsal. The inter-metatarsal angle is determined by comparing the bisection of the fourth metatarsal to this reference line. (Fig. 8-8 A, B). If the angle is abnormally increased, the pathology is mostly at the metatarsal base. The normal IM angle IV has been reported between 6.5 to eight degrees depending upon author.

If the bowing occurs more distally one will encounter an abnormal lateral deviation angle. The lateral deviation angle of the fifth metatarsal is determined by bisecting the head and neck of the fifth metatarsal and comparing it in relationship to

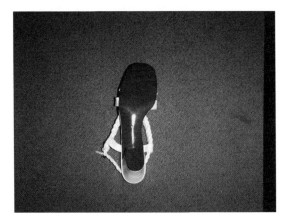

Figure 8-7: Photograph of an in-flare shoe "last" design.

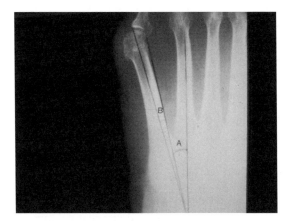

Figure 8-8: AP radiographic view demonstrating placement of fifth metatarsal reference line along medial proximal shaft. **A:** Angle A is the intermetatarsal angle IV determined by comparing bisection of fourth metatarsal to reference line. **B:** Angle B is the lateral deviation angle determined by comparing bisection of head and neck of fifth metatarsal to reference line.

the reference line along the medial cortical margin of the base of the fifth metatarsal (Fig. 8-8 B). The lateral deviation angle has even greater variability and ranges from 2.6 to 4.8 degrees and has been reported as high as eight degrees.

In any event these measurements correlated with the clinical findings help to determine the level of the deformity in order to choose an appropriate procedure.

The width of the metatarsal neck is important as it determines the limit of translocation of the capital fragment during the performance of a distal osteotomy. An exceptionally thin neck will dictate a shaft or base procedure.

On the lateral view one should note the following:

- Fifth metatarsal declination
- Prominent plantar condyle
- Arthritic changes of the fifth metatarsal head

Conservative Therapies:

In the acute presentation, symptomatic measures are employed to reduce inflammation and pain. Once the possibility of an infectious process has been eliminated, the following can be instituted:

- NSAIDs for inflammatory conditions.
- Steroid injection for an acute bursitis/neuritis.
- Pressure off pads.
- Shoe gear modification to reduce pressure.
- Patient education regarding proper footgear (shoe "last" selection, etc).
- Physical therapy measures to relieve inflammation.
- Custom functional foot orthotics to control fifth ray hypermobility and abnormal pronation.

Surgical Procedures:

Surgical intervention is indicated when there is a poor response to conservative therapy or where there are no reasonable conservative therapies for that specific patient. Procedure selection is determined by the extent and level of pathology, the patient's medical status, age and ambulatory status. Distal procedures performed upon the metatarsal head and distal shaft are less disabling and allow for immediate weight bearing postoperatively. Proximal procedures performed in the proximal metatarsal diaphysis or metatarsal base create more disability since weight bearing has to be avoided or carefully guarded post operatively.

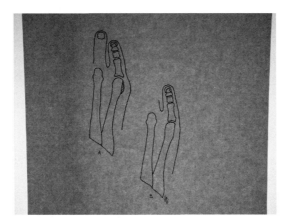

Figure 8-9: Diagram demonstrating lateral condylectomy.

Lateral Condylectomy:

The lateral condylectomy involves resecting the lateral condyle of the fifth metatarsal head or any prominent lateral exostosis (Fig. 8-9). It may be performed as an isolated procedure or as an adjunctive procedure in combination with other procedures.

Indications:

- Enlarged fifth metatarsal head lateral condyle or lateral exostosis

Contraindications:

- High intermetatarsal angle IV
- High lateral deviation angle
- Arthritic fifth MTPJ

Surgical Technique:

A curvilinear incision is placed dorsal laterally centered over the fifth MTPJ measuring 3 cm in length (Fig. 8-10 A). The incision is deepened by sharp and blunt dissection to the capsule. The capsule is exposed dorsally and laterally and a dorsal linear or lateral "T" shaped capsulotomy is performed (Fig. 8-10 B). The joint is entered, and the lateral suspensory and collateral ligaments are released exposing the lateral condyle and metatarsal head. The fifth toe is adducted while an ostectomy is performed resecting the lateral condyle even with or parallel to the distal lateral metatarsal shaft (Fig. 8-10 C). The ostectomy is angled or biased in the frontal plane such that slightly more bone is taken dorsally than plantarly. This helps to insure that the prominence is eliminated dorsally but also leaves the plantar condyles intact for articulation with the flexor plate. The fifth toe is held in a corrected position while the lateral capsule is evaluated for redundancy. Any redundant capsule is excised and capsulorrhaphy is performed as the fifth toe is properly aligned. The skin incision is approximated and closed and sterile dressing is applied.

Post Operative Management:

Patient is allowed to ambulate in a post operative healing shoe as tolerated. Bathing restrictions are in place until the sutures are removed. Patient may return to a regular shoe as tolerated usually at two weeks once the sutures are removed. The fifth toe is splinted into abductus as needed for several weeks post operatively. X-rays are taken within one week post operatively and prior to any planned activity change (Fig. 8-10 D). Physical therapy is rarely needed following this procedure.

Inherent Complications:

- Fifth digital adductus deformity post operatively causing irritation to fourth toe. Most often this is not a problem. Splinting the toe post operatively into an abducted position for several weeks can minimize or prevent this problem. If this becomes problematic, it is usually a result of not correcting an underlying osseous pathology. Surgical revision is indicated which should involve performing an appropriate osteotomy either at the metatarsal distally or at the base as well as reefing up on the lateral capsule.

Horizontal "V" Osteotomy (Mini–Austin, Chevron):

The horizontal "V" osteotomy is performed in the fifth metatarsal head extending into the neck of the metatarsal. The apex of the "V" is distally and the arms extend proximally at various lengths and angles to each other depending upon choice of fixation or surgeon's preference. It is performed in conjunction with a lateral condylectomy (Fig. 8-11 A, B). It primarily reduces the lateral deviation angle by creating a relative reduction when transposing the metatarsal head and neck medially. Its performance should be guided by fabrication of preoperative templates.

Indications:

- High lateral deviation angle.
- Adequate width of the metatarsal neck to allow for capital fragment medial transposition.
- Adequate bone stock within metatarsal neck area.

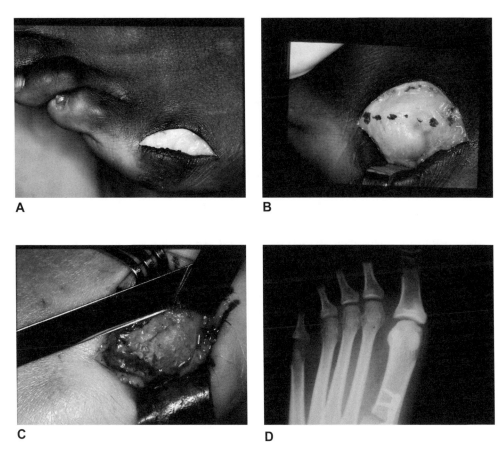

Figure 8-10: A: Clinical photograph of skin incision placement for lateral condylectomy. **B:** Clinical photograph of dorsal lateral linear capsulotomy. **C:** Clinical photograph of resection of lateral condyle. **D:** Postoperative X-ray demonstration lateral condylectomy.

Contraindications:

- High IM angle
- Open epiphysis of the fifth metatarsal neck
- Arthritic fifth MTPJ
- Excessively narrow/thin metatarsal neck

Surgical Technique:

The skin incision is made as above but is approximately 5 cm in length. A lateral condylectomy is performed as previously described except a wider exposure of the surgical neck of the metatarsal is obtained. An osteoperiosteal tunnel is made dorsally just proximal to the joint from lateral to medial under the EDL tendon which will serve as an exit point for the dorsal arm of the osteotomy. The osteotomy design is then transcribed onto the cancellous bone of the met head (Fig. 8-12 A). Each arm exits proximal to the joint capsule dorsally and plantarly. A 0.45 K-wire can be inserted at the apex of the design through the metatarsal head from lateral to medial to serve as an axis guide for the bone cut. This temporary guide pin is cut leaving enough wire to serve as a guide (3 cm). Utilizing an osteotomy guide attachment (Fig. 8-12 B) a "V" or "L" designed osteotomy is performed horizontally from lateral to medial penetrating both cortices (Fig. 8-12 B, C). The guide wire is removed and the capital fragment is then transposed medially up to two-thirds the width of the metatarsal and impacted into the metatarsal shaft (Fig. 8-12 D). The osteotomy site is temporarily fixated by driving a 0.45 K-wire through the metatarsal head from distal to proximal. The osteotomy can be fixated in a variety of methods based upon the surgeon's preference. We utilize one of the following: (1) A 1.5 mm. absorbable rod which is retrograded from distal to proximal through the metatarsal head into the metatarsal shaft (Fig. 8-13 A, B). (2) A 2.0 mm cannulated screw inserted from dorsal to plantar. The surgeon can either design the osteotomy with a long dorsal arm or a long plantar arm (Fig. 8-11 A, B). The temporary fixation is removed. The proximal lateral overhanging metatarsal shaft is then resected even with the medially translocated metatarsal head (Fig. 8-13 C). Capsular closure and skin closure are performed as described above.

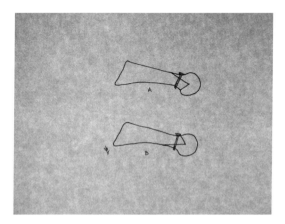

Figure 8-11: A: Diagram demonstrating horizontal "V" osteotomy utilizing a long dorsal arm with screw fixation from distal to proximal. **B:** Long plantar arm with screw from distal to proximal.

Post Operative Management:

Apropulsive, guarded weight-bearing is allowed in a surgical shoe with a rigid sole or in a prefabricated walker with a rocker sole. Bathing restrictions are in place until the sutures are removed at 10 to 14 days. X-rays are taken within the first week post operatively and again at three and six weeks to access healing prior to any planned activity change. Patient may usually return to regular shoes and a propulsive gait at two to three weeks post operatively depending upon the fixation utilized and the X-ray results. High impact activities are usually allowed at eight weeks. Physical therapy is rarely needed following this procedure.

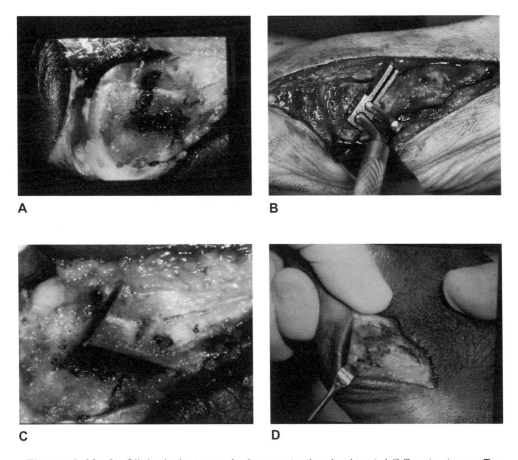

Figure 8-12: A: Clinical photograph demonstrating horizontal "V" osteotomy. **B:** Clinical photograph demonstrating osteotomy guide in place. **C:** Clinical photograph of horizontal V osteotomy completed and capital fragment transposed medially. **D:** Clinical photograph of capital fragment osteotomy site being impacted.

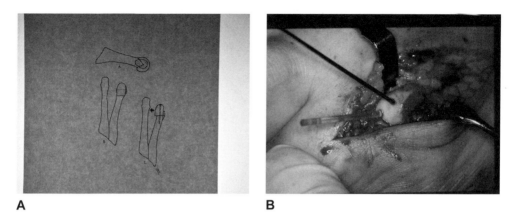

A   B

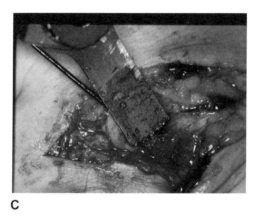

C

Figure 8-13: A: Diagram of horizontal "V" osteotomy being fixated with an intramedullary resorbable rod. **B:** Clinical photograph demonstrating temporary K-wire fixation for fixation of osteotomy with 1.5 mm absorbable rod. **C:** Clinical photograph demonstrating resection of lateral overhang of distal fifth metatarsal after translocation of capital fragment.

Inherent Complications:

- Delayed union with chronic edema requiring further immobilization and use of an external bone stimulator.

- Osteotomy site fracture requiring further immobilization.

- Dislocation of osteotomy site secondary to fixation failure requiring further surgical intervention as needed.

- Under correction of the deformity which may or may not require further surgical intervention.

Juvara -Type Diaphyseal Osteotomy:

This osteotomy design is performed within the base and proximal diaphysis of the fifth metatarsal with its length being at least twice the width of the metatarsal shaft to allow for screw fixation. It is a wedge shaped osteotomy with the apex proximal-laterally and the base distal-medially leaving the lateral cortex intact. Preoperative templates are constructed to determine the size wedge of bone to be removed to achieve the necessary IM reduction. When the wedge of bone is removed the osteotomy is closed and fixated reducing the distance between the fourth metatarsal and fifth metatarsal (Fig. 8-14 A, B).

Indications:

- High IM angle which can not be reduced by a more distal procedure
- Open fifth metatarsal epiphysis may be present
- Adequate width of the metatarsal shaft in area of proposed osteotomy

Contraindications:

- Patient who can not remain non-weight bearing
- Severe osteoporosis
- Narrow shafted fifth metatarsal
- Arthritic fifth MTPJ

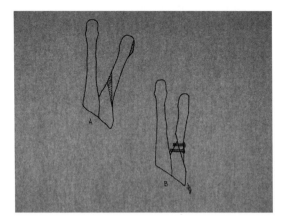

Figure 8-14: A: Diagram demonstrating Juvara diaphyseal osteotomy. **B:** Diagram demonstrating two screw fixation.

Surgical Technique:

The skin incision is placed dorsal laterally along the fifth metatarsal shaft extending proximally to the base of the fifth metatarsal measuring 8 cm in length. A lateral condylectomy is performed as previously described. The amount of condyle bone resection and its angulation to the shaft is guided by the preoperative templates. The incision is deepened proximally exposing the metatarsal base and shaft. A linear incision is made in the periosteum which is lifted off the shaft. A 0.45 K-wire is inserted from dorsal to plantar at the lateral apex of the proposed wedge site just medial to the lateral cortex. This will act as an aid to keeping the lateral cortex intact as well as serve as a guide to performing the osteotomy. The K-wire is then cut leaving enough length to accommodate application of the osteotomy guide. The arms of the osteotomy and the desired sized wedge are then marked on the bone with a sterile scribe. An osteotomy guide is then placed upon the K-wire and an oblique wedge shaped osteotomy is made leaving the lateral cortex intact (Fig. 8-15 A-D). The wedge of bone is then removed, and the osteotomy is reduced (Fig. 8-15 E) and fixated with two 2.0 mm cannulated screws (Fig. 8-15 F). After a copious lavage, the periosteum is closed with a 4-0 absorbable suture and the skin margins are approximated and closed using suture material and technique of the surgeon's preference. Sterile bandages are applied.

Postoperative Management:

The patient is either placed in a non-weight BK cast or posterior splint for six weeks. In selected cases with a compliant patient one can utilized guarded weight bearing in a prefabricated walker in which the sole area has been modified in such a fashion as to off weight or float the fifth metatarsal (Fig. 8-16 A, B). Post operative base line X-rays are taken within the first week, and serial X-rays are taken at the third week and the fifth to seventh week in order to evaluate healing and allow activity change. Sutures are normally removed at the second week. Return to a propulsive gait will depend upon the X-ray findings but will not occur before six weeks. High impact activities can be resumed at three months. Physical therapy is utilized as necessary but only after osseous healing has occurred.

Inherent Complications:

- Delayed union with chronic edema (External Bone Stimulator).
- Osteotomy site fracture secondary to premature weight bearing requiring further immobilization.
- Dislocation of osteotomy site secondary to fixation failure usually necessitating surgical intervention as needed.
- Non – union treated with a bone stimulator and additional surgery as needed often requiring a bone graft and absolute non weight bearing for healing to occur.
- Under-correction of the deformity, requiring revisional surgery as needed.

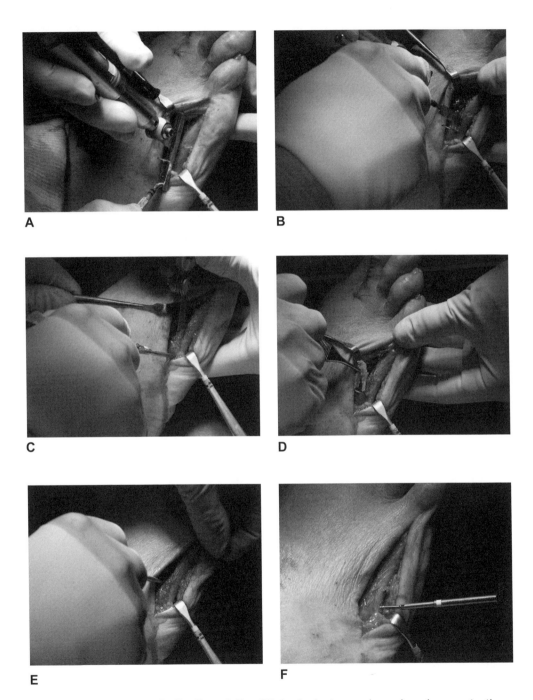

Figure 8-15: A, B, C, D, E and **F:** Clinical photograph series demonstrating performance of diaphyseal osteotomy.

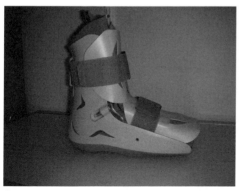
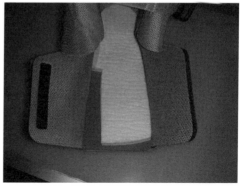

A   **B**

Figure 8-16: A. Clinical photograph demonstrating prefabricated BK cast. **B.** Clinical photograph showing cast modification with one-quarter inch adhesive back felt with a cut out to off load the fifth ray from the cuboid distally in order to allow guarded weight bearing.

Base Wedge Osteotomy:

This osteotomy is also performed in the base of the fifth metatarsal by placing a short transverse wedge osteotomy at the diaphyseal metaphyseal junction leaving the lateral cortex intact (Fig. 8-17 A, B). The amount of wedge removed is calculated using preoperative templates.

Indications:

- High IM angle with a normal or narrow metatarsal neck/shaft
- Open epiphysis of fifth metatarsal may be present (Fig. 8-18)

Contraindications:

- Inability for patient to be NWB postoperatively (ambulatory challenged)
- Severe osteoporosis
- Arthritic fifth MTPJ

Surgical Technique:

The surgical procedure is performed as described previously for the Juvara except that a shorter transverse osteotomy is performed at the diaphyseal metaphyseal junction leaving the lateral cortex intact. The design of the osteotomy does not allow for screw fixation. Fixation can be obtained with either a staple or a mini bone plate placed dorsally, or a monofilament stainless steel wire, or a diagonal K-wire (Fig. 8-19).

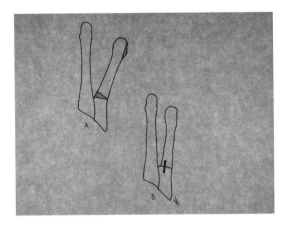

Figure 8-17: A: Diagram demonstrating placement of adductory base wedge osteotomy at base of the fifth metatarsal. **B:** Diagram of result with fixation in place.

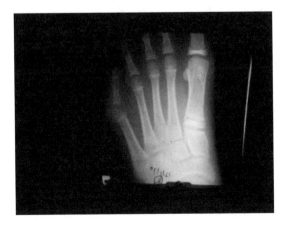

Figure 8-18: AP X-ray view demonstrating open epiphysis fifth metatarsal neck associated with a bunionette deformity secondary to a high IM angle IV.

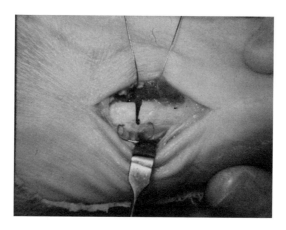

Figure 8-19: Clinical photograph demonstrating placement of 28 g double stranded monofilament wire fixation of fifth metatarsal base wedge osteotomy.

Postoperative Management:

This procedure requires absolute non weight bearing using crutches in either a BK cast, prefabricated walking boot or a posterior splint for six weeks as if managing a Jones fracture. Serial X-rays are taken within the first week, again at the third week to access osseous healing and at the sixth week to determine whether weight bearing can be instituted (Fig. 8-20). Weight bearing should not be allowed until bony trabeculation is seen across the osteotomy site and when clinical evaluation reveals no motion or pain at the osteotomy site when stressed. Physical therapy is utilized as needed but only after osseous healing has occurred.

Inherent Complications:

The same as listed for the Juvara osteotomy with a potentially greater chance of a non- union due to placement of the osteotomy at the diaphyseal metaphyseal junction.

Fifth Metatarsal Head Resection:

In rare situations complete resection of the fifth metatarsal head is performed at the anatomic neck (Fig. 8-21 A, B). The procedure eliminates any lateral or plantar prominence of the fifth metatarsal head; thereby, neutralizing any pressure points, eliminates the fifth MTPJ, and shortens the fifth metatarsal. It does not require fixation, does not rely on bone healing, and creates minimal disability. It is a joint destructive, end stage procedure reserved for the geriatric, medically compromised or ambulatory challenged patient population.

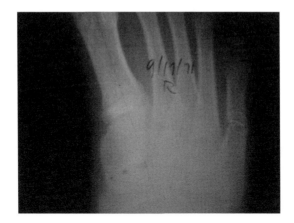

Figure 8-20: Postoperative AP X-ray of a base wedge osteotomy fixated with double stranded 28 g monofilament wire.

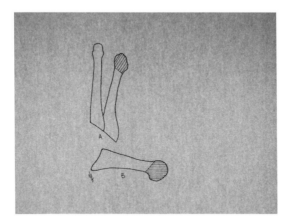

Figure 8-21: A: Diagram demonstrating fifth metatarsal head resection orientation in the transverse plane. **B:** Demonstration of the resection design in the sagittal plane so as to prevent post surgical pressure points.

Indications:

- IPK sub or lateral fifth metatarsal head (elderly patient)
- Chronic pressure ulceration
- Arthritic fifth MTPJ
- Osteoporosis (severe)
- Medically compromised patient
- Ambulatory challenged patient

Contraindications:

- Younger, active patients
- Ability to salvage the fifth MTPJ

Surgical Technique:

The fifth MTPJ is approached as described above for the lateral condylectomy utilizing a skin incision measuring four cm in length. A linear capsulotomy is performed and the joint is disarticulated. The fifth metatarsal head is resected at its anatomic neck. The osteotomy cut is oriented in the transverse plane from distal medial to proximal lateral and in the sagittal plane distal dorsal to proximal plantar to prevent potential pressure points from developing. A 0.45 or 0.62 inch K-wire can be retrograded through the fifth toe crossing the void created by the resection and ending within the fifth metatarsal to support the soft tissue as fibrosis occurs in place of the resected metatarsal head. This helps to minimize proximal recession of the fifth digit (Fig. 8-22 A, B). The capsule is closed. The skin margins are approximated and sutured closed. Sterile bandages are applied.

Postoperative Management:

Immediate weight bearing in a post operative shoe is allowed. If a K-wire was utilized then the patient needs to ambulate in a surgical shoe for two to three weeks to eliminate the propulsive phase of gait and to prevent bending of the K-wire. The wire is usually removed at two to three weeks at which time the patient can begin a propulsive gait and a return to regular shoes. If no K-wire was used then a surgical shoe is used to accommodate the bandages; however, at home the patient may ambulate without the shoe and can return to regular shoes at two weeks when the sutures are removed. Bathing is restricted until the sutures and K-wire are removed. The patient is usually seen at the first week post operatively to change the bandage and again at two weeks to remove sutures. X-rays are taken at the first week to serve as a baseline for future reference. Physical therapy is rarely required for this procedure.

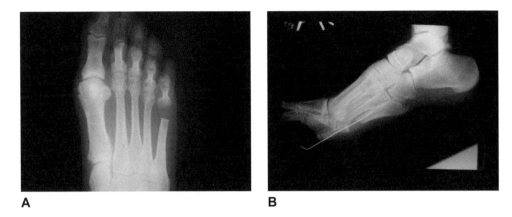

A　　　　　　　　　　　　　**B**

Figure 8-22: A: Postoperative AP X-ray view with 0.45 inch K-wire in place. **B:** Lateral X-ray view.

Inherent Complications:

Most of the complications are due to the volume loss created by the removal of the entire metatarsal head resulting in fifth toe instability and possible load transfer to the fourth metatarsal. Fifth toe instability is often treated by surgical syndactylism of the fifth to fourth toes. The reader is referred to Chapter 3.

- Flail/floppy toe (refer to section on syndactylism).
- Proximal recession of fifth toe (refer to section on syndactylism).
- Transfer metatarsalgia requiring treatment with an accommodative foot orthotic.

Clinical Pearls:

- Identify level of pathology within the fifth metatarsal.
- Select procedure based upon level of pathology.
- Consider patients ambulatory status and ability to be non weight bearing when planning a shaft or base osteotomy.
- Utilize preoperative templates for planning osteotomy procedures as well as determining the amount of bone resection from the lateral aspect of the metatarsal head (condylectomy).
- Utilize an osteotomy guide when performing a wedge osteotomy.

- Adequately protect shaft and base osteotomy procedures post op for six to seven weeks.

- Obtain serial X-rays to evaluate healing of osteotomy site and prior to activity change.

References:

Boyer ML, DeOrio JK. Bunionette deformity correction with distal chevron osteotomy and single absorbable pin fixation. *Foot Ankle Int* 24:834 -837, 2003.

Castle JE, Cohen AH, Docks G. Fifth metatarsal distal oblique wedge osteotomy utilizing cortical screw fixation. *J Foot Surg* 31:478-485, 1992.

Catanzarariti AR. Oblique Osteotomy of the fifth met: A five year review. *J Foot Surg*: 27:316-320, 1988.

Coughlin MJ. Treatment of Bunionette deformity with longitudinal diaphyseal osteotomy with distal soft tissue repair. *Foot Ankle* 11:195-203, 1991.

Fallat LM, Buckholtz JL. An analysis of the tailor's bunion by radiographic and anatomic display. *J Am Podiatry Assoc* 70:597-603, 1980.

Fallat LM. Pathology of the fifth ray, including the tailor's bunion deformity. *Clin Podiatr Med Surg* 7:689-715, 1990.

Gerbert J, Sgarlato TE, Subotnick SI. Preliminary study of a closing wedge osteotomy of the fifth met for correction of a tailor's bunion deformity. *J Am Podiatry Assoc* 62:212-218, 1972.

McKeever DC. Excision of the fifth metatarsal head. *Clin Orthop* 13:321-1322, 1959.

Schoenhaus H, Rotman S, Meshon AL. A review of normal intermetatarsal angles. *J Am Podiatry Assoc* 70:597-603, 1980.

Thul JR. Neuromas associated with tailor's bunion. *J Foot Surg* 24:342-344, 1985.

Throckmorton JK, Bradlee N. Transverse "V" sliding osteotomy: A new surgical procedure for the correction of tailor's bunion deformity. *J Foot Surg* 18:117-121, 1978.

Inter-Metatarsal Neuritis or Neuroma

9

Joshua Gerbert, DPM, FACFAS
William M. Jenkin, DPM, FACFAS

Introduction:

Inter-metatarsal neuritis and neuroma are fairly common entities which often prove to be difficult to diagnosis due to lack of clinical signs and/or radiographic pathology. This chapter will discuss the clinical evaluation, conservative therapy, surgical techniques, postoperative management and inherent risks to each procedure. This chapter will also discuss the management of a symptomatic amputation neuroma which can occur as the result of excision of the inter-metatarsal nerve.

Clinical Evaluation and Diagnostic Tests:

The following are important aspects of the clinical evaluation to enable the surgeon to differentiate a neuritis from an actual neuroma from adjacent MTPJ pathology.

Patient's description of the location of the symptoms: The third interspace is the most common location for an inter-metatarsal nerve entrapment with resultant neuritis or neuroma. While this pathology can also occur in the other inter-metatarsal spaces, one should always be hesitant to make the diagnosis of nerve pathology in one of these other interspaces before ruling out all other possible etiologies.

Patient's description of symptoms: Typically the symptoms are episodic and include a burning-type pain with ambulation exacerbated with increase pressure to the ball of the foot, paresthesias distally into the involved digit(s) and pain relief with non-weight bearing. Symptoms that occur predominantly with toe-off and have only been present for a short period of time are usually indicative of a transverse metatarsal ligament nerve entrapment resulting in neuritis, while those that occur with any form of weight bearing and have been present for more than one year are usually indicative of a neuroma.

- **Direct palpation of the involved interspace:** (Fig. 9-1 A, B) Pain associated with neuritis or a neuroma secondary to a transverse metatarsal ligament nerve entrapment will become evident with direct dorsal-plantar palpation.

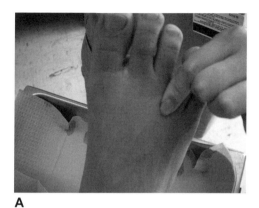
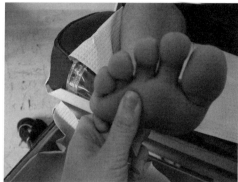

A   **B**

Figure 9-1: A: Clinical photograph demonstrating the palpation of the involved interspace from dorsal to plantar. **B:** Clinical photograph demonstrating the plantar palpation if the involved interspace in which one is attempting to compress the nerve against the transverse metatarsal ligament.

- **Lateral-Medial Squeeze Test:** (Fig. 9-2) Pain that is produced within the involved interspace by squeezing the lateral and medial aspects of the forefoot is usually indicative of a bursitis or MTPJ effusion. This maneuver cannot indicate a neuroma since the nerve lies beneath the transverse metatarsal ligament and cannot be compressed between the metatarsal heads when they are squeezed together.

- **Mulder's Click:** (Fig. 9-3 A, B) Pain/clicking sensation produced by applying pressure to the involved interspace from dorsal/plantar and dragging your finger distally while squeezing the foot from medial to lateral. This is usually indicative of perineural fibrosis resulting in a neuroma and not an entrapment neuritis. This maneuver when positive is due to bringing the enlarged portion of the perineural fibrosis or neuroma over the distal aspect of the transverse metatarsal ligament.

- **Separation of the involved digits:** Noticeable separation of the involved digits in stance may be indicative of a soft tissue mass such as a neuroma in the involved interspace or adjacent lesser MTPJ instability pathology.

- **Direct palpation of the adjacent MTPJs and/or range of motion:** Failure to reproduce any symptoms with direct pressure to the adjacent MTPJ and/or range of motion is usually indicative of no MTPJ pathology.

- **X-ray evaluation:** Standard anterior-posterior X-rays of the forefoot will demonstrate most lesser MTPJ pathologies and should be taken. Failure to notice any apparent osseous pathology would not automatically rule out

MTPJ pathology or rule in an entrapment neuritis or neuroma. Very often a pre-dislocation syndrome may create symptoms similar to those encountered with an inter-metatarsal neuritis or neuroma; however, usually the symptoms are in the second MTPJ/second interspace.

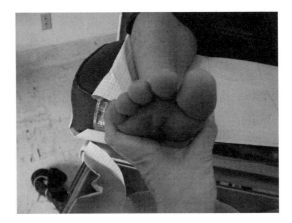

Figure 9-2: Clinical photograph showing the medial-lateral squeeze test.

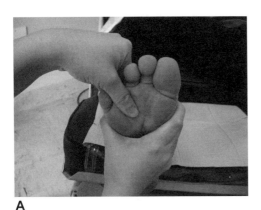
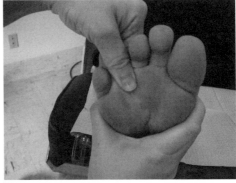

A   B

Figure 9-3: A-B: These two photographs demonstrate the performance of the Mulder's test in which one is attempting to move the nerve under the transverse metatarsal ligament and to feel for a "click" which would be indicative of an enlargement of the nerve. As the enlarged portion of the nerve moves distally from under the transverse metatarsal ligament the sensation will be noticed.

- **MRI and Ultrasonography:** These imaging modalities can help to confirm the presence of a neuroma once it reaches a certain size (transverse diameter greater than 3-5 mm) but are not helpful in diagnosing an entrapment neuritis. The MRI is especially useful in evaluating for other pathology which may cause forefoot pain especially in the second distal intermetatarsal space. Both the MRI and ultrasound are helpful in evaluating for neuromata in multiple interspaces. In all cases the result of the imaging modalities must be correlated with clinical findings.

- **Diagnostic Injection:** The use of an intra-articular injection of a local anesthetic with or without contrast dye into an adjacent MTPJ that eliminates the patients symptoms with ambulation will in most cases rule out an inter-metatarsal nerve entrapment or neuroma. If the symptoms are not eliminated then an injection of the local anesthetic should be performed into the involved interspace. Elimination of symptoms following this injection will usually be indicative of inter-metatarsal nerve pathology of some type. At times injecting several interspaces at different times may be necessary to isolate the involved interspace.

Conservative Therapies:

In most situations, the most we obtain from conservative therapy is a reduction in the symptoms; however, since these therapies are benign and usually easy for the patient, they are worth pursuing initially. The following are the therapies that we utilize.

- **Functional foot orthoses:** These devices are indicated in the patient who exhibits excessive abnormal pronation with flexor stabilization. The devices help to stabilize the MTPJs and improve muscle function.

- **Injection therapy:** This is usually effective in those situations where a bursa is suspected in the involved interspace. It may also be effective in reducing the symptoms associated with neuritis but not a neuroma.

- **Digital pad:** At times, the use of a small digital pad to separate the involved toes has proven to be beneficial (Fig. 9-4).

- **Accommodative foot orthotic:** The use of an accommodative orthotic device with a metatarsal cookie placed under the third and/or fourth metatarsal head to help elevate the involved metatarsal heads and metatarsal ligament may take pressure off the involved nerve.

- **Physical therapy:** This only proves beneficial in reducing the inflammation in the involved area and usually does not provide any long term relief.

- **Shoe gear modification:** Wearing any form of shoe gear that reduces the flexing of the involved digits at propulsion such as a rocker bottom soled shoe or a shoe with a more rigid toe box may be effective in those cases of nerve entrapment resulting in neuritis versus a neuroma.

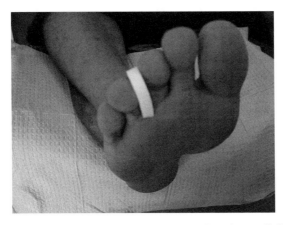

Figure 9-4: Clinical photograph showing the use of an inter-digital pad to slightly separate the involved digits.

Surgical Procedures:

Regardless of the procedure to be performed, decompression of the nerve or surgical excision of the nerve, the patient should be adequately informed of the problems associated with performing surgery on a nerve. When choosing to perform a decompressional procedure through a minimal incisional approach, the patient needs to be informed that the surgeon cannot visualize the nerve; therefore, if there is a neuroma present, the minimal decompressional technique will be not be effective and the symptoms will continue requiring an additional open procedure.

Surgical Decompression or Neurolysis:

This procedure can be utilized in those cases where the surgeon believes the symptoms are secondary to a nerve entrapment involving the transverse metatarsal ligament. There are several different surgical procedures that have been advocated for decompressing the involved interspace when one believes the etiology of the problem is secondary to nerve irritation from the transverse metatarsal ligament and/or the mooring ligament (Fig. 9-5 A, B). These procedures can be divided into minimal incisional decompressional procedures or an open surgical neurolysis.

Minimal Surgical Decompression:

One technique involves the use of endoscopy through small incisions and the other involves also a small web incision and the use of specialized instrumentation known at the OsteoMed KobyGard System™. The Surgery Department at the California School of Podiatric Medicine utilizes this latter technique to decompress the involved

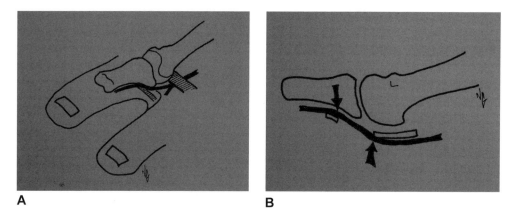

A   **B**

Figure 9-5: A: Drawing depicting the inter-metatarsal nerve as it comes under the transverse metatarsal ligament at the level of the metatarsal head/neck area and continues distally into the involved digit crossing over the mooring ligament that extends from the flexor tendon sheath at the base of one digit to another. **B:** Drawing from a side view of an MTPJ depicting the two locations where the inter-metatarsal nerve may become irritated or entrapped. The arrow from plantar is pointing to the distal aspect of the transverse metatarsal ligament and the arrow from dorsal is pointing to the proximal aspect of the mooring ligament.

interspace. We are not aware of any definitive research that has demonstrated one technique more effective than another.

This procedure is not performed with a tourniquet; however the use of one is certainly not contraindicated. The KobyGard System™ utilizes a series of instruments shown in Figure 9-6. The surgical technique involves making a small vertical incision in the involved web space (Fig. 9-7). We advocate making a line with a marking pen on the dorsal surface of the involved interspace to indicate the actual angle of the interspace. By making this line the surgeon can then better direct the instrumentation in the correct direction avoiding trauma to the adjacent metatarsals (Fig. 9-8). The next step is to introduce a mosquito and create a small plane on the plantar aspect of the transverse metatarsal ligament (Fig. 9-9). The tissue locator is then use to create a plane over the dorsal and plantar aspects of the transverse metatarsal ligament (Fig. 9-10). When the tissue locator is on the plantar surface of the ligament, the surgeon should turn the locator into a vertical position and then attempt to move it dorsally into the interspace. If the locator is in the correct position, one will not be able to move the locator in a vertical direction. The locator is then removed and the ligament separator is inserted which encompasses the transverse metatarsal ligament (Fig. 9-11A, B). Many of us will skip this step and go directly to the insertion of the Isogard Flex Tip™ (Fig. 9-12). Once again this instrument is inserted to encompass the transverse

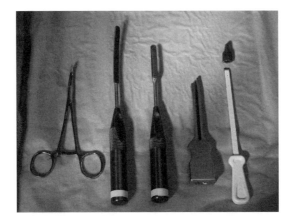

Figure 9-6: Clinical photograph showing the instruments used when performing a minimal incision nerve entrapment release with the KobyGard™ system. From left to right: a mosquito, a tissue locator, a ligament separator, the cannulated Isogard Flex Tip Instrument™ and the Isogard™ single-use blade.

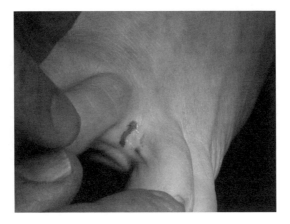

Figure 9-7: Intraoperative photograph showing the placement of the small vertical incision to be performed to release the ligaments.

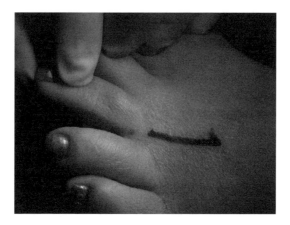

Figure 9-8: Intraoperative photograph shows the line drawn on the dorsal surface of the foot along the actual angle of the involved interspace.

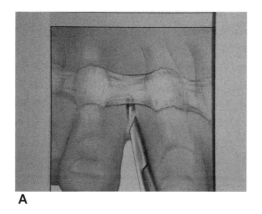

A

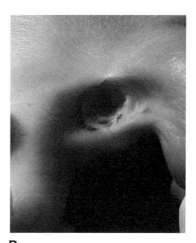

B

Figure 9-9: A: This drawing, from the informational material provided by OsteoMed Corporation with their permission, depicts the use of a mosquito through the vertical incision to create a blunt separation of adipose tissue in order to insert the various instruments to be used in performing this procedure. **B:** Intraoperative photograph showing the vertical incision having been opened after using the mosquito.

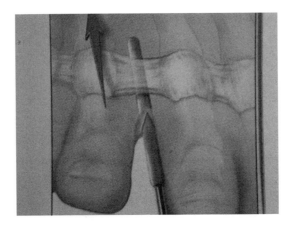

Figure 9-10: This drawing from the informational material provided by OsteoMed Corporation with their permission depicts the tissue locator being inserted to create a plane under the transverse metatarsal ligament. One can rotate the locator 90 degrees and attempt to move it dorsal to plantar which is not possible due to the integrity of the transverse metatarsal ligament. Once this is accomplished it is removed and re-introduced to create a plane over the dorsal aspect of the ligament.

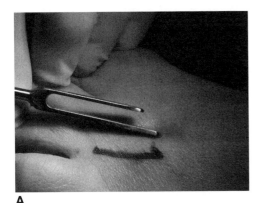

A

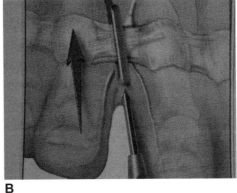

B

Figure 9-11: A: This intraoperative photograph shows the ligament separator being held along the dorsal aspect of foot prior to be inserted. **B:** This drawing, from the informational material provided by OsteoMed Corporation with their permission, depicts the ligament separator inserted to encompass the transverse metatarsal ligament.

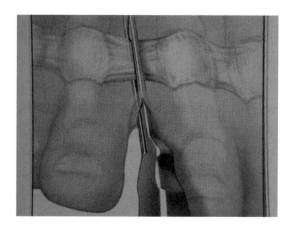

Figure 9-12: This drawing from the informational material provided by OsteoMed Corporation with their permission depicts the Isogard Flex Tip cannulated instrument being inserted to encompass the transverse metatarsal ligament.

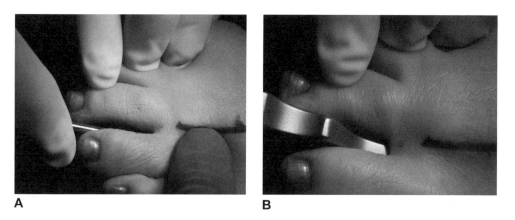

A   B

Figure 9-13: A: Intraoperative photograph showing the Isogard instrument being rotated toward the third digit so that the surgeon can feel the elevation of the fourth metatarsal head. If the instrument has encompassed the transverse metatarsal ligament then as it is rotated it will cause the metatarsal head to either dorsiflex or plantarflex. **B:** The instrument is now rotated toward the fourth digit thereby elevating the third metatarsal head.

metatarsal ligament. Once in position, the surgeon can check to make certain the ligament has been encompassed by turning either the ligament locator or Isogard clockwise which will cause one metatarsal head to move dorsally and then by turning the instrument counter clockwise will cause the adjacent metatarsal head to move dorsally (Fig. 9-13 A, B). Once the surgeon believes the Isogard is in the correct position, the specialized knife blade is inserted into the cannulated portion of the Isogard and the transverse metatarsal ligament which had been encompassed is severed (Fig. 9-14 A, B). The tissue locator is then re-inserted and moved vertically in the interspace to make certain that no further aspect of the ligament remains intact. If the tissue locator cannot move freely dorsally and plantarly, then the Isogard is re-inserted and the remaining portion of the ligament is cut. The small vertical incision in the web space can usually be closed with several skin sutures. A small bandage is applied and the patient is allowed to ambulate with a propulsive gait. The sutures are normally removed at one week and the patient is allowed to return to their regular foot gear and activities.

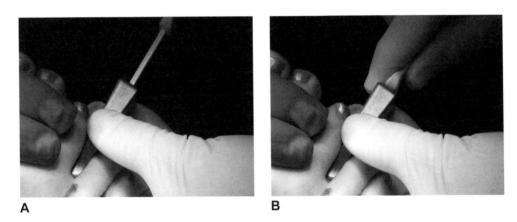

A   B

Figure 9-14: A: In this intraoperative photo, the Isogard instrument had been placed to encompass the transverse metatarsal ligament and the Isogard blade is being inserted into the cannulated portion of the Isogard. **B:** This photograph shows the blade fully inserted. As the blade is inserted the surgeon can feel the resistance as the transverse metatarsal ligament is severed.

Inherent Risks:

- **Hematoma**. This has been the most common complication with this procedure which creates interspace induration and soreness. It usually resolves by itself with time and at times has necessitated an interspace injection with a steroid and/or physical therapy.

- **Neuritis**. Contusion of the involved nerve can occur with repeated and forcible introduction of the specialized instrumentation. The symptoms will usually resolve with time; however the use of an NSAID and/or interspace injection of a steroid will be hasten the recovery.

- **Continued Pre-operative Symptoms**. This will occur if the underlying pathology was not an entrapment neuritis but rather a neuroma. An additional surgery to remove the neuroma will need to be performed. Unfortunately, it is not always easy to distinguish an entrapment neuritis from an actual neuroma.

Dorsal "Open Technique" for a Neurolysis:

The utilization of a pneumatic ankle cuff for hemostasis depends upon the surgeon's preference. The skin incision is placed dorsally to the involved interspace extending distally from the web space proximally for 4-5 cm. It is deepened by sharp and blunt dissection. If a bursa is noted at the level between the adjacent MTPJs, it is excised. The deep transverse metatarsal ligament is then located. Using a curved mosquito clamp, it is inserted under the ligament and the jaws are opened allowing one to incise the ligament from inferior to superior. If a neuroma existed, it will now be quite visible and need to be removed; however, based upon the preoperative evaluation and the impression that the pathology was an entrapment neuritis, the nerve will appear normal. It will lie in the adipose tissue beneath the ligament. Once it is identified the nerve is followed distally past its division into the digital proper branches. A vessel loop can be placed around the nerve and used to apply mild traction which assists in the neurolysis (Fig. 9-15). The nerve is further inspected for areas of

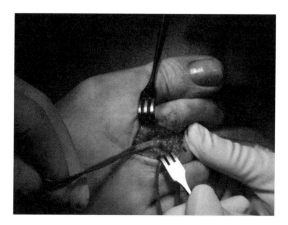

Figure 9-15: This photograph demonstrates the use of a vessel loop, which is a small elastic rubber band used to retract blood vessels without tension, being used to retract the inter-metatarsal nerve to aid in its dissection.

entrapment such as the mooring ligament located at the level of the web space. The nerve is bathed with a phosphated steroid to minimize inflammation and postoperative fibrous adhesions. The intermetatarsal ligament is not reattached. The skin and superficial tissues are closed based upon the surgeon's preference. In cases where postoperative bleeding may be of concern, a small drain such as a Porex TLS™ (Fig. 9-16 A-C) can be used for a few hours following the procedure. A small compressive bandage is applied and the patient is allowed to ambulate with a propulsive gait. A surgical shoe is used to accommodate the postoperative bandages. The patient is seen one week postoperatively to change the bandages and again at two weeks to have the sutures removed. At that time the patient can return to regular activities and normal footgear.

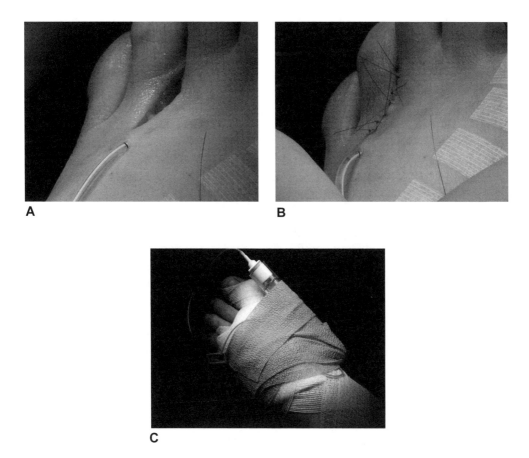

A

B

C

Figure 9-16: Clinical photographs: **A:** TLS drain shown exiting proximal to the incision site. **B:** TLS drain following skin closure. **C:** TLS drain system incorporated in the outer layer of the bandages.

Inherent Risks:

- Hematoma. This has been the most common complication with this procedure which creates interspace induration and soreness. It usually resolves by itself with time and at times has necessitated an interspace injection with a steroid and/or physical therapy. The use of a small drain for several hours following the surgery can minimize this complication.

- Neuritis. Contusion of the involved nerve can occur with repeated manipulation of the nerve. The symptoms will usually resolve with time; however the use of an NSAID and/or interspace injection of a steroid will be hasten the recovery.

Dorsal Linear Incision Approach for Neuroma Excision:

We usually utilize a dorsal approach for exploration and excision of a neuroma provided no prior surgery had been performed in that involved interspace; however, this is really a surgeon's preference and there is no research that has shown that a linear dorsal approach is more effective than a transverse or linear plantar approach. Also the utilization of a tourniquet for this procedure is at the discretion of the surgeon. We normally use an ankle tourniquet inflated to 275 mm Hg.

A 5 cm incision is made extending from the web space proximally, staying between the adjacent metatarsal shafts. Using sharp and blunt dissection, any superficial veins are identified and coagulated. Dissection is carried deeper to the transverse metatarsal ligament which is then incised. At this time, with pressure from the distal/plantar surface of the web space, the neuroma should become very visible. Care should be taken to attempt to dissect only the nerve itself. Once the neuroma is identified, the most proximal trunk of the nerve is severed as far proximal as possible, which should appear normal. By severing the proximal portion of the nerve initially, the neuroma can be manipulated without producing painful stimulation to the patient that even under any form of anesthesia can produce an unfavorable reaction. The dissection is continued, trying to identify the digital nerve trunks which are then severed as they enter the two involved digits (Fig. 9-17 A-D). The interspace is inspected for any aberrant nerve that could be involved in the pathology. If the surgeon believes that a hematoma formation in the interspace is probable, then the use of a small drain system is advised. The drain is normally removed prior to the patient being discharged from the hospital or surgery center. Rarely do we utilize any deep closure. Depending upon the surgeon's preference, several buried knot sutures could be employed and then skin closure. The neuroma specimen is sent to pathology for analysis.

A compressive type bandage will assist in creating hemostasis and minimizing a hematoma formation. The patient is allowed to ambulate with a propulsive gait; however a surgical shoe is needed just to accommodate the bandages. The patient is normally seen at one week for a bandage change and then at the second week to remove the sutures. At that time the patient is allowed to return to regular shoe gear and normal activities.

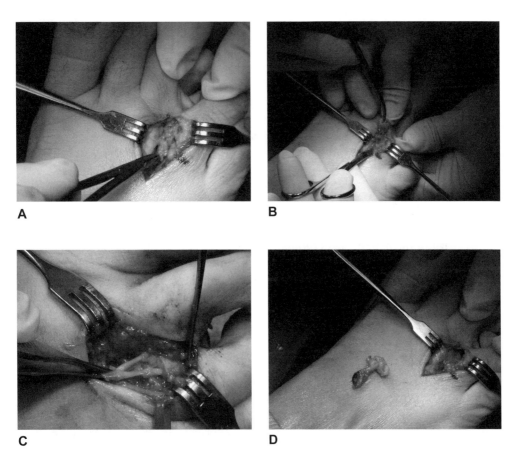

Figure 9-17: A: Clinical photograph showing the nerve being grasped after its most proximal portion has been severed. **B:** Clinical photograph showing the nerve being dissected distally into the digital branches. **C:** Clinical photograph clearly revealing the digital branches being dissected. **D:** Clinical photograph showing the neuroma following excision.

Inherent Risks:

- Hematoma. This has been one of the most common complications, creating interspace induration and soreness for several months postoperatively. It usually resolves by itself with time and at times has necessitated an interspace injection with a steroid and/or physical therapy.

- Neuritis. Inflammation of the proximal aspect of the severed neuroma may be present for four to six weeks following surgery. The symptoms will usually resolve with time; however the use of an NSAID and/or interspace injection of a steroid will be hasten the recovery if the symptoms are present.

- Chronic Inflammation. This usually occurs as the result of aggressive dissection. Very often this problem is difficult to distinguish from a hematoma. Treatment usually involves NSAIDs, physical therapy and possibly an injection of a phosphated steroid.

- Regrowth of the nerve. This problem does not occur with any frequency but nerve tissue can regenerate. At times one is able to determine that this has occurred without symptoms being present when testing the sensation of the involved digits. Normally following a resection of a neuroma, the medial plantar skin of one digit and the lateral plantar skin of the adjacent digit will be permanently numb. At times, regrowth of the nerve will result in normal sensation in the involved digits and neurological pain in the interspace; in these cases, if NSAIDs and physical therapy are not beneficial, additional surgery may be required.

- Amputation Stump Neuroma. This complication probably occurs in one percent of the patients undergoing neuroma surgery. It can be differentiated from symptomatic regrowth of the nerve by checking the sensation pattern on the involved digits; this will demonstrate numbness of the areas that would be expected following a nerve resection. Treatment for this condition is discussed later in this chapter.

Plantar Transverse Incision Approach for Neuroma Excision:

We usually utilize a plantar transverse approach for exploration and excision of a neuroma when a there are recurring symptoms after a dorsal incision to excise a neuroma but an amputation stump neuroma has been ruled out. However, this surgical approach can certainly be used as the initial approach to excise a neuroma or to perform a neurolysis. Once again the utilization of a tourniquet for this procedure is at the discretion of the surgeon; however we find the tourniquet to be beneficial in performing the dissection. An ankle tourniquet is used and it is inflated to 275 mm Hg.

The incision is marked out using a marking pen and is centered approximately half way between the metatarsal heads and the sulcus on the plantar aspect of the foot (Fig. 9-18). Sharp and blunt dissection is used to reach the level of the inter-metatarsal ligament of the involved interspace. The neuroma is located below the inter-metatarsal ligament which may or may not be incised. Once again an attempt is made to severe the most proximal aspect of the nerve lesion at a level that appears normal and as far proximal as possible. Once this has been performed, the neuroma is dissected distally severing the digital nerve trunks as they enter each involved digit. The interspace is inspected for any aberrant nerve that could be involved in the pathology. If the surgeon believes that a hematoma formation in the interspace is probable, then the use of a small drain system is advised. The drain is inserted so that it exits the dorsal aspect of the interspace proximally and is normally removed prior to the patient being discharged from the hospital or surgery center. The wound is usually closed with several buried knot sutures and then a skin closure of the surgeon's preference. The neuroma is sent to pathology for analysis.

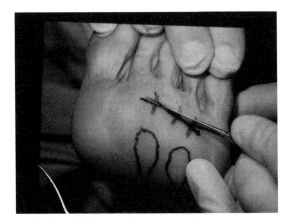

Figure 9-18: Clinical photograph showing the location for a transverse incision to be used to explore an interspace for a neuroma. It is located midway between the sulcus of the digits and the metatarsal heads.

A compressive type bandage will assist in creating hemostasis and minimizing a hematoma formation. The patient is allowed to ambulate using a surgical shoe in order to maintain an apropulsive gait. The patient is normally seen at one week for a bandage change and then weekly until the sutures are removed. For a plantar incision, the sutures may need to be kept in place for three weeks and during this time the patient should be kept in the surgical shoe to prevent a propulsive gait. Once the sutures are removed, the patient is allowed to return to regular shoe gear and normal activities.

Inherent Risks:

- Hematoma. This has been one of the most common complications, which creates interspace induration and soreness for several months postoperatively. It usually resolves by itself with time and at times has necessitated an interspace injection with a steroid and/or physical therapy.

- Neuritis. Inflammation of the proximal aspect of the severed neuroma may be present for four to six weeks following surgery. The symptoms will usually resolve with time; however the use of an NSAID and/or interspace injection of a steroid will hasten the recovery if the symptoms are present.

- Chronic Inflammation. This usually occurs as the result of aggressive dissection. Very often this problem is difficult to distinguish from a hematoma formation. Treatment usually involves NSAIDs, physical therapy and possibly an injection of a phosphated steroid.

- Regrowth of the nerve. This problem does not occur with any frequency, but nerve tissue can regenerate. At times, one is able to determine that this has occurred without symptoms being present when testing the sensation of the involved digits. Normally following a resection of a neuroma, the medial plantar skin of one digit and the lateral plantar skin of the adjacent digit will be permanently numb. At times, regrowth of the nerve will result in normal sensation in the involved digits and neurological pain in the interspace; in these cases, if NSAIDs and physical therapy are not beneficial, additional surgery may be required.

- Amputation Stump Neuroma. This complication probably occurs in one percent of the patients undergoing neuroma surgery. It can be differentiated from symptomatic re-growth of the nerve by checking the sensation pattern on the involved digits; this will demonstrate numbness of the areas that would be expected following a nerve resection. Treatment for this condition is discussed later in this chapter.

Amputation Neuroma:

The symptoms usually begin four to six weeks following the neurectomy. This is the time it normally takes to form an amputation neuroma. The symptoms are not as they were pre-operatively. Instead, the patient complains of a deep ache in the forefoot occurring with weight bearing, often at rest, and even at night. The pain is not foot gear related and is present with bare footed walking. Symptoms can be reproduced with deep palpation in the distal interspace where the neurectomy was performed. Anesthesia of the involved digits is present as expected due to the previous neurectomy.

Conservative treatment consists of diagnostic anesthetic blocks to identify the exact location of the source of pain. This is often followed by a series of steroid injections in an attempt to eliminate fibrous adhesions. Topical capsaicin can be utilized as well as physical therapy modalities to help desensitize the area. Any pressure placed on the area of the neurectomy will increase symptoms and should be avoided (i.e. metatarsal pads, etc.) Sclerosing agents such as three percent ethyl alcohol have been advocated, but if used should be used with extreme caution to prevent the development of tissue necrosis. If the symptoms are not resolved after a course of conservative therapy then surgical intervention will be necessary.

Neurectomy with Nerve Implantation:

The approach is from the plantar aspect of the forefoot. Prior to the procedure while the patient is alert the point of maximum tenderness is marked on the sole of the foot. Following anesthesia, two one quarter inch 27 g needles are inserted from dorsally exiting plantarly in the involved interspace. One is placed distally and the other mid-shaft. This will assist in the plantar incision placement (Fig. 9-19 A-C).

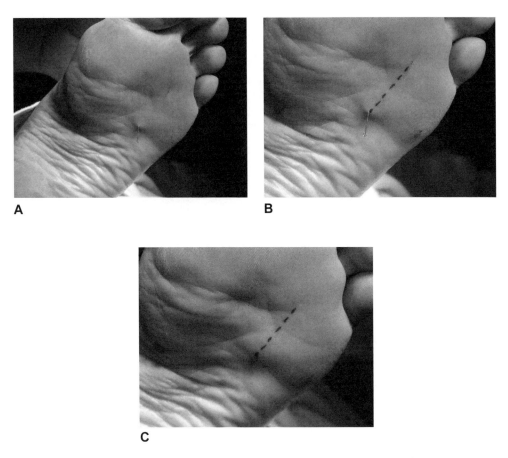

Figure 9-19: Clinical photographs: **A:** Plantar aspect of the foot in which two needles have been inserted from the dorsal aspect of the foot in the third interspace exiting the plantar skin. **B:** Marking pen used to draw a line connecting the two needles. **C:** Needles have been removed leaving the line for the proposed skin incision in the correct angle relative to the third interspace.

If only one interspace is to be inspected, then a linear incision connecting the two needles is made on the plantar skin. If multiple interspaces are going to be explored, a "Z" type incision is made (Fig. 9-20). The incision is deepened to the level of the plantar aponeurosis. A linear incision is made in the plantar fascia; the common digital nerve will be located immediately below the fascia. Once identified, the nerve is followed distally to the level of the amputation neuroma and fibrous adhesions. The distal nerve is dissected free and an epineural incision is made circumscribing the nerve. The epineurium is peeled proximally 1 cm and folded back upon itself. A fresh

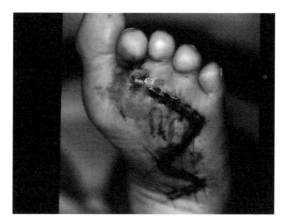

Figure 9-20: This photograph shows the closure of plantar "Z" incision which was utilized to explore several interspaces for a nerve entrapment.

neurectomy is then performed, resecting the amputation neuroma, which is sent to pathology for microscopic diagnostic confirmation. The epineural sleeve is then unfolded and an epineural plasty is performed with a 6-0 PROLENE suture placed through the epineurium in a purse string fashion. A small hole is then created in one of the intrinsic muscles in the area and the epineural sleeve along with the nerve ending is sutured into the muscle with the 6-0 PROLENE suture. It is imperative that the nerve is not placed on any tension whatsoever when implanting the nerve into the muscle. The fascial layer is closed with absorbable sutures to prevent muscle herniation and the skin margin is approximated and closed based upon the surgeon's preference. Care should be taken to make certain that this incision is not closed under tension.

A compressive dressing is applied. The patient is managed non-weight bearing on the operated foot for three weeks at which time the sutures are removed. Bathing restrictions are in place until the sutures are removed. The patient may return to regular footgear and activities as tolerated at one month postoperatively.

Inherent Risks:

- Hematoma. This has been one of the most common complications, creating interspace induration and soreness for several months postoperatively. It usually resolves by itself with time and at times has necessitated an interspace injection with a steroid and/or physical therapy. The use of a small drain for several hours after surgery minimizes this complication.

- Neuritis. Inflammation of the proximal aspect of the severed neuroma may be present for four to six weeks following surgery. The symptoms will usually resolve with time; however the use of an NSAID and/or interspace injection of a steroid will be hasten the recovery if the symptoms are present.

- Chronic Inflammation. This usually occurs as the result of aggressive dissection. Very often this problem is difficult to distinguish from that of a hematoma formation. Treatment usually involves NSAIDs, physical therapy and possibly an injection of a phosphated steroid.

- Continued Amputation Neuroma Symptoms. This problem does not occur with any frequency, but nerve tissue can regenerate and/or the implantation of the nerve into muscle is not always effective. If a course of NSAIDS and injection therapy with a steroid does not resolve the symptoms, the patient should be referred to a specialist who performs microscopic peripheral nerve surgery.

Clinical Pearls:

The following are tips that we believe can assist the surgeon in providing a more predictable favorable outcome and preventing postoperative complications when performing a nerve decompression procedure or an exploration with neuroma excision.

- Perform a diagnostic nerve block in the involved interspace to determine if symptoms are due to nerve pathology versus intra-articular MTPJ pathology.

- Take a detailed history to determine what creates the symptoms, the character of the symptoms and how long the symptoms have been present. Neurological symptoms that area associated only with propulsion, wearing higher heel shoes and has only been present for less than one year is more likely to be secondary to an entrapment versus a true neuroma.

- A positive Mulder's Click is indicative of a neuroma versus an entrapment neuritis.

- If symptoms and physical examination are inconclusive in distinguishing an entrapment neuritis from a neuroma, then an open exploration should be performed.

- When performing an open exploration with possible nerve excision and one anticipates increased bleeding within the interspace, then the use of a small drain system for a short period of time will significantly reduce the chances of a significant hematoma formation.

- When performing a minimal incision nerve entrapment release, make certain that the angle of the interspace is clearly appreciated which can be accomplished by drawing a line along the dorsal aspect of the involved interspace.

- Following a minimal incision nerve entrapment release, make certain that one can easily move an instrument in the sagittal plane within the involved interspace to indicate that the entire transverse metatarsal ligament has been severed.

- Blunt dissection should be used as much as possible during an open exploration with possible nerve excision to prevent unnecessary tissue damage.

- With a dorsal approach, the transverse metatarsal ligament should be severed prior to determining whether the inter-metatarsal nerve should be removed.

- When removing the inter-metatarsal nerve, the proximal portion of the nerve should be severed initially with a sharp scalpel or scissors as far proximal as possible; then the remaining portion of the nerve should be dissected distally.

- When performing a plantar linear incisional approach for an amputation neuroma, the utilization of two straight needles inserted from dorsal to plantar will enable the surgeon to better create an incision that is within the involved interspace.

- Any nerve specimen removed should be sent to pathology.

References:

Barrett S, Pignetti TT. Endoscopic decompression for intermetatarsal nerve entrapment – the EDIN technique. Preliminary study with cadaveric specimens and early clinical results. *J Foot Ankle Surg* 33:503-506. 1994.

Beskin JL, Baxter DE. Recurrent pain following interdigital neurectomy – a plantar approach. *Foot Ankle* 9:34-39, 1988.

Coughlin MJ, Pinsonneault T. Operative treatment of interdigital neuroma. A long-term follow-up study. *J Bone Joint Surg Am* 84:1276-1277, 2002.

Dellon AL, Mackinnon SE. Treatment of the painful neuroma by neuroma resection and muscle implantation. *Plast Reconstr Surg* 77:427-436, 1986.

Dellon AL. Treatment of Morton's neuroma as a nerve compression: The role of neurolysis. *J Am Podiatr Med Assoc* 82:399-402, 1992.

Diebold PF, Delagoutte JP. True neurolysis in the treatment of Morton's neuroma. *Acta Artgop Belg* 55:467-471, 1989.

Downey MS: Surgical treatment of peripheral nerve entrapment syndromes. Musculoskeletal Disorders of the Lower Extremities. Oloff LM, Ed. WB Saunders, Philadelphia, Pa., 1994.

Fannuci E, Masala S, Fabino S, et al. Treatment of intermetatarsal Morton's neuroma with alcohol injection under US guide: 10 month follow-up. *Eur Radiol* 14:514-518, 2004.

Gauthier G. Thomas Morton's disease: a nerve entrapment syndrome - A new surgical technique. *Clin Orthop* 142:90-92, 1979.

Goldstein SA, Sturim HS. Intraosseous nerve transposition for treatment of painful neuromas. *J Hand Surg* 10A:270-274, 1985.

Kankanala G, Jain AS. The operational characteristics of ultrasonography for the diagnosis of plantar intermetatarsal neuroma. *J Foot Ankle Surg* 46:213-217, 2007.

Mackinnon SE, Dellon AL, Hudson AR, Hunter DA. Alteration of neuroma formation by manipulation of its microenvironment. *Plast Reconstr Surg* 76:345-352, 1985.

Mulder JD. The causative mechanism in Morton's metatarsalgia. *J Bone Joint Surg Br* 33:94-95, 1951.

Kenzora JE. Symptomatic incisional neuromas on the dorsum of the foot. *Foot Ankle* 5:2, 1984.

Shapiro SL. Endoscopic decompression of the intermetatarsal nerve for Morton's neuroma. *Foot Ankle Clin* 9:297-304, 2004.

Sharp RJ, Wade CM, Hennessy MS, Saxby TS. The role of MRI and ultrasound imaging in Morton's neuroma and the effects of size of lesion on symptoms. *J Bone Joint Surg (Br)* 85-B:999-1005, 2003.

Wolfort SF, Dellon AL. Treatment of recurrent neuroma of the interdigital nerve by implantation of the proximal nerve into muscle in the arch of the foot. *J Foot Ankle Surg* 40: 404-410, 2001.

Management of the Arthritic Forefoot

10

William M. Jenkin, DPM, FACFAS

Introduction:

The prototype for the arthritic forefoot is the patient with rheumatoid arthritis (RA) with the entire forefoot deranged and deformed. The forefoot pathology consists of dorsally dislocated MTPJs with plantarly prominent metatarsal heads, metatarsalgia, digital deformities in the form of hammertoes, claw toes, hallux malleus, hallux abductus with or without metatarsus primus adductus or hallux rigidus, metatarsus elevatus, and a Tailor's Bunionette deformity (Fig. 10-1 A-D).

The goal of treatment is to minimize discomfort, eliminate deformity and the resultant pressure induced pathology (bursitis, callus, corns, ulceration) while providing an easier foot to "shoe" and a more stable foot for ambulation.

Approach to Forefoot Surgery in the Arthritic Patient:

The rheumatoid patient can present with little to no forefoot deformity but still have joint pain or, as is often the case, with forefoot deformity but without joint pain. In the latter presentation, the complaint is either a wound healing problem or pain from the pressure-induced consequences of the deformity itself. The arthrosis may involve a single MTPJ or multiple MTPJs with or without digital deformity.

In the past, it was more or less accepted that the surgical approach to the rheumatoid forefoot was to perform joint destructive procedures, as it was assumed that the disease would eventually progress to the end-stage rheumatoid forefoot deformity.

Today, however, disease-modifying anti-rheumatic drugs (DMARDs) are changing the approach to surgery, since they are very successful at controlling inflammation and therefore limiting joint destruction, pain and deformity. In the past, if more than one dislocated or arthritic MTPJ was involved, all of the metatarsal heads were resected even if there was little to no erosive destruction of the remaining metatarsal heads. Today, as long as the erosive changes within the MTPJ are not too significant, joint salvage procedures are being performed initially. One technique is the use of shortening osteotomies of metatarsals 2, 3, and at times 4 to surgically address the dislocated MTPJ by creating soft tissue laxity, decompression of the joint, and relocation of the digit(s).

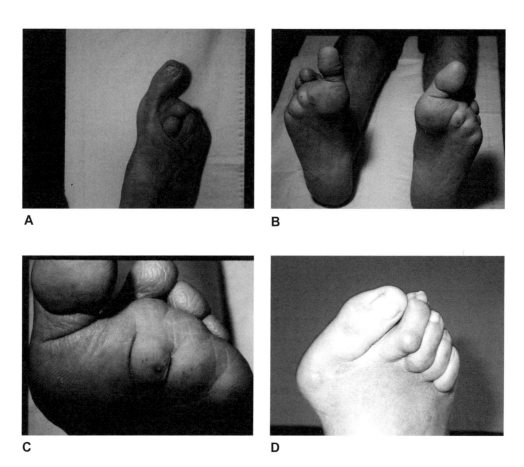

A   B

C   D

Figure 10-1: Clinical photograph of an "arthritic forefoot." **A:** Dorsal view demonstrating dislocated 2-5 MTPJs and hallux malleus. **B:** Plantar view demonstrating prominent metatarsal heads. **C:** Close up plantar view demonstrating mechanically induced hyperkeratosis under prominent metatarsal head. **D:** Dorsal view of an "arthritic forefoot" of a different patient demonstrating hallux abductus deformity with hammertoes and lateral deviation of the digits.

Forefoot surgery should always be considered in context with other joints in the lower extremity and at times the upper extremity as well. Since the forefoot is often the painful area, it is the first to be operated upon. However, if the rearfoot is involved and equally as painful, then operating upon the rearfoot should be performed first. Simultaneous surgery upon the rearfoot and forefoot should be approached with caution because of the risk of extensive edema, vascular compromise and wound healing issues.

In most instances, if there is a bilateral forefoot deformity, it is best to operate upon one foot at a time. In this way, the patient will have one limb to bear load as the other heals. This is especially important should a postoperative complication result.

A candidate for forefoot surgery may also be contemplating hip or knee surgery, in which case it is better to treat the foot first. If the feet are not treated first, once the hip or knee pain has been relieved by the arthroplasty, the metatarsalgia will worsen as the patent tries to increase mobility. This will interfere with the rehabilitation of the hip or knee surgery.

Perioperative Medical Considerations:

Perioperative management of the arthritic may be relatively straightforward or extremely complicated, depending upon the disease as well as its extent and activity. In complex multisystem disorders such as RA or systemic lupus erythematosus (SLE), surgical risk may be greatly increased, particularly when the disease is active or when major organ system change has occurred.

Management of these patients requires special knowledge and/or consideration of the following factors:

- **Glucocorticoid Supplemental Therapy for Patients Stressed by Surgery:**

    Patients who are taking or have taken glucocorticoids within the past 12 months are at risk for adrenal insufficiency when stressed by surgery. If the dose was greater than 5 mg prednisone a day, empiric supplementation is recommended to prevent adrenal insufficiency. Patients undergoing major procedures are treated with 50 to 100 mg hydrocortisone intravenously or intramuscularly prior to surgery and postoperatively every six hours for several days, tapering the dose by 50 percent per day to maintenance level over three to five days. For patients undergoing minor surgical procedures, the patient may not need coverage or prednisone can be increased to 15 mg per day for several days prior to surgery and returned to the baseline level immediately following the procedure.

- **Disease-Modifying Anti-rheumatic Drugs (DMARDs):**

    Many patients will be taking DMARDs. Even though these are immunosuppressive drugs and potentially can increase the risk of postoperative wound complications and infection, it is not routinely recommended to stop these medications, as doing so would risk a flare up of the rheumatoid process. However, this decision must be tempered by the risk of problems with wound healing. In some cases, performing the surgery a short time before administration of the immunosuppressive drug may help to minimize postoperative complications with wound healing and infection. Some have advocated stopping the immunosuppressive drug perioperatively and instead using steroids. If planning to stop tumor necrosis factor (TNF) alpha inhibitors, they should be discontinued two to three weeks before the surgery. Should an active infection develop, these medications will be discontinued in consultation with rheumatology and infectious disease specialists.

- **Bleeding concerns:**

    To minimize excessive bleeding and hematoma formation, aspirin should be discontinued 10 to 12 days before surgery because of its irreversible effect on platelet aggregation. Other NSAIDs should be discontinued for a period equal to five times their half-life (h) prior to surgery: ibuprofen, h=2 hrs. = 10 hrs.; naproxen, h = 12 hrs. = 60 hrs.; sulindac, h=16 hrs. = 80 hrs.; piroxicam, h=50 hrs. = 250 hrs.

NOTE: the COX-2 NSAIDs such as celecoxib have no effect on the platelets.

Anesthesia Concerns:

Upper airway

- Difficult intubation due to arthritis of the cricoarytenoid joints leading to fixed narrowing of the vocal cords. Signs/symptoms include hoarseness, laryngeal pain, dysphagia and inspiratory stridor.

- Cervical Spine Disease. Atlantoaxial joint subluxation/dislocation potential is always present. If suspected, lateral X-ray view of the neck in flexion and extension may be obtained. A distance greater than 4 mm between the arch of C 1 and the odontoid process represents asymptomatic cervical spine disease. In this case, orthopedic consultation prior to surgery is well advised. In selected cases, a cervical collar is prescribed to help stabilize the neck but most importantly to serve as a reminder to staff not to hyperextend the neck.

Dry Eyes (keratoconjunctivitis sicca)

- Sjogren's syndrome is found in seven percent of those who have RA. Symptoms include dry eyes, dry mouth (xerostomia), and connective tissue disease resulting in dry skin and lung involvement.

- Knowing the diagnosis before surgery is important because complications that may arise as a result of excessive dryness of the eyes, nose and mouth can be easily prevented (corneal abrasions, visual loss, choking aspiration).

- If known from history, alert the anesthesia department prior to surgery.

- Inquire about dry mouth, eyes and difficulty in swallowing.

Postoperative Management Concerns:

- The functional capacity of the upper extremity must be taken into consideration when determining the appropriate postoperative ambulatory assistive device for the patient. For example, the patient's upper extremity may make the patient incapable of using crutches. The ambulatory assistive device decision should be made prior to any surgical intervention (Fig. 10-2).

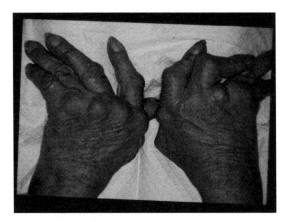

Figure 10-2: Clinical photograph of the hand of an arthritic patient whose functional capacity is compromised to the point of not being able to use crutches postoperatively.

Clinical and Radiographic Evaluation:

Clinical evaluation is centered on defining the extent of the deformity and determining how many joints and to what extent each is involved. The reader is referred to Chapter 1 for further discussion of the evaluation of metatarsalgia.

Weight bearing AP, lateral, and plantar axial views are obtained. The AP view is evaluated to identify which joints are involved, degree of subluxation or dislocation, erosive changes and amount of joint destruction, phalangeal base hypertrophy, digital deformity, metatarsal length, inter-metatarsal angles, hallux position and overall bone stock. The lateral view is observed for metatarsus elevatus, MTPJ contractures and dislocations. The plantar axial view is evaluated for erosive changes on the plantar metatarsal heads. The AP and lateral X-ray views are also utilized in preoperative planning (Fig. 10-3 A, B).

Conservative Therapies:

Extra depth or custom shoes with rocker soles and semi-rigid or accommodative insoles are the mainstay to the non-surgical treatment of the patient with an arthritic forefoot. Conservative therapy consists mostly of palliative measures which are repeated as needed consisting of the following:

- Lesion reduction.
- Pressure off pads.
- Footgear modification.
- Mono articular injection therapy with a steroid.

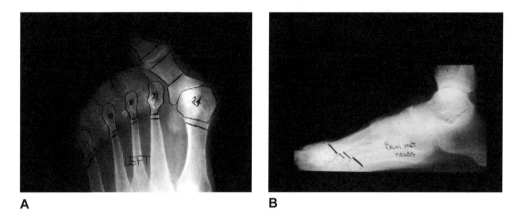

A   **B**

Figure 10-3: A: AP X-ray view of arthritic forefoot demonstrating dislocated 2-5 MTPJs and hallux abductus. Note preoperative planning orientation of resection osteotomy designs on each metatarsal. **B:** Lateral X-ray view of arthritic forefoot.

Definitive treatment involves surgical intervention. Surgery is indicated after a therapeutic trial of one or more of the above measures. However, in certain cases such as a history of prior ulceration due to fixed contractures and dislocations, surgery should be considered as the initial treatment.

Surgical Procedures:

Pan Metatarsal Head Resection (PMHR)

The PMHR involves resection of metatarsal heads 1, 2, 3, 4 and 5. It is a joint destructive procedure. It eliminates the prominent metatarsal heads as well as the inflamed MTPJ (Fig. 10-4). It is used in severe end-stage foot deformities which involve joint pain, erosive arthritis, dislocated MTPJs, digital deformities and plantarly prominent metatarsal heads, and is often associated with a hallux valgus or with a hallux rigidus.

By removing the metatarsal head soft tissue, laxity is created, allowing the digits to better align with the forefoot. Adjunctive procedures such as digital arthrodesis or arthroplasty of the PIPJ are performed as needed. Hammertoe or claw toe deformity of toes 1, 2, 3, and 4 are treated with fusion of the PIPJ, as this seems to provide better long term results as far as alignment than an arthroplasty. As always, if the fifth toe is involved, an arthroplasty is performed to create laxity and eliminate pressure points.

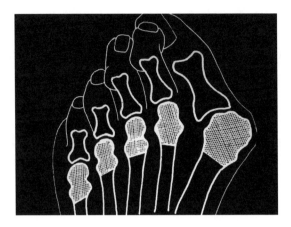

Figure 10-4: Diagram of transverse view of PMHR demonstrating level of metatarsal head resections.

PMHR is utilized in other patient populations that present with a severe deformed forefoot such as the diabetic patient with forefoot deformity and chronic plantar ulcerations and the post traumatic deformed foot, which also includes what is known as the "surgically failed foot" or the foot that is iatrogenically deformed by previous surgical failures. It should be noted that the arthritic and diabetic populations accept the long term results of the procedure better than the post traumatic population, probably because the latter group has normal pain sensation, is more active and has higher expectations.

Indications:

- Arthritic forefoot derangement with significant DJD.
- Diabetic with forefoot ulcerations and forefoot derangement.
- Post traumatic forefoot derangement with severe DJD.
- Prior foot surgery creating the "surgically failed foot."
- Dislocation/subluxation of the majority of MTPJs in the elderly patient.
- Digital mal-alignment.
- Plantar fat pad atrophy/displacement may be present.
- ROM pain with DJD of more than three MTPJs.
- Pressure points with mechanically induced hyperkeratosis (MIH) may be present.
- Greater than two metatarsal head resections from previous surgery.
- Failure of conservative care.

Contraindications:

- When lesser non-destructive procedures could be utilized.
- When an isolated partial metatarsal head resection could be effective.
- Younger, more active patient.

Incisional Approaches:

Dorsal and plantar incisional approaches to the forefoot are utilized. Dorsal linear skin incisions vary in number from three, four or five incisions (Fig. 10-5 A, B, C).

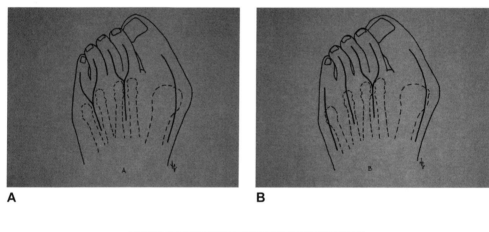

A   **B**

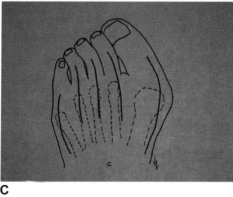

C

Figure 10-5: Diagram demonstrating various dorsal linear incisional approaches: **A:** Three incisional. Note the distal extension of the linear incision onto two adjacent digits in a "pitch fork" configuration. This "pitch fork" incision can be converted to a "V" to "Y" skin plasty if dorsal skin contracture is present. **B:** Four incisional approach. **C:** Five incisional approach.

The fewer the incisions, the longer each must be in order to mobilize the tissue without creating surgical retraction trauma. The incision should be chosen based upon the pathology being addressed. We recommend that the first MTPJ have its own dedicated dorsal incision. This is especially true if an adjunctive fusion of the first MTPJ is to be performed. A plantar transverse elliptical incision is recommended when the digits are dorsally dislocated with anteriorly displaced plantar fat pads, plantarly prominent metatarsal heads, tylomas, or scaring from previously healed ulcerations. Dedicated dorsal incisions are made in the digits to be surgically corrected and over the fifth MTPJ if there is a significant Tailor's Bunionette deformity.

Dorsal Linear Approach:

Utilizing a skin scribe, the incisions are drawn with the goal of avoiding vascular compromise by keeping the tissue islands created between each incision as wide as possible. In the five incisional approach, each is placed over the distal metatarsal shaft, MTPJ, and onto the digit as needed. The first dorsal incision is placed medial to the EHL tendon. The fifth dorsal linear incision is placed more lateral to the EDL tendon and is several centimeters longer to gain better access to the fifth metatarsal shaft. Dissection is continued to the extensor expansion. The expansion is freed as needed exposing the EDL tendon. A transverse EDL tenotomy is performed at the joint level exposing the MTPJ. A linear incision is made into the dorsal capsule onto the metatarsal shaft which is freed to expose the anatomic neck of the metatarsal. The joint is disarticulated and the metatarsal head is prepared to be delivered into the surgical wound (Fig. 10-6). All of the metatarsal heads are exposed in a similar manner.

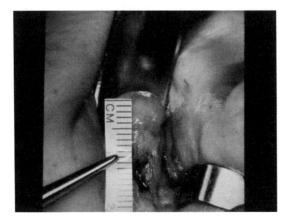

Figure 10-6: Intraoperative photograph demonstrating dorsal view of isolated metatarsal head to be resected. Note the use of a McGlamry elevator to help deliver the metatarsal head into the surgical wound.

At this time, starting with the second metatarsal, all of the metatarsal heads are resected at their anatomic neck; the amount of the resection must be calculated from the preoperative AP X-ray, with the goal of creating a good postoperative metatarsal parabola. The goal of the resection is to remove enough of the metatarsal so as to eliminate pressure points and create soft tissue laxity in order to align the digits upon the forefoot, while at the same time attempting to leave as much metatarsal length as needed to provide a forefoot platform for stability (longer lever arm). To avoid postoperative pressure points, the metatarsal is cut at an angle in the sagittal plane resecting more bone plantarly, as the cut is made from dorsal distal to plantar proximal (Fig. 10-3 B). In the transverse plane, the second metatarsal is left the longest and is resected at its anatomic neck perpendicular to the long axis. The third, fourth, and fifth metatarsals are each cut on a bias at their anatomic neck, each shorter by 3 mm angled from distal medial to proximal lateral. The first metatarsal head is cut at an angle from distal lateral to proximal medial (Fig.10-3 A). Once all of the metatarsal heads are resected, the surgeon should confirm that the metatarsal heads form an appropriate parabola, where 2 is the longest followed by 1 and 3, then 4, and lastly 5 (Fig. 10-7 A, B, C).

Digital procedures are performed as needed. Arthroplasty of the PIPJ of the fifth toe is performed to create laxity and eliminate pressure points. It is recommended that PIPJ arthrodesis be attempted on digits 1, 2, 3, and 4 to provide better long time digital stability. Phalangeal base resection, especially of the fifth proximal phalanx, is performed if it is hypertrophic but not as a routine.

Stabilization of the digits is provided by 0.045 or 0.062 inch K-wires inserted into each digit which had an adjunctive procedure except perhaps the fifth toe. The K-wires are antegraded out the end of the toe and then retrograded back into the metatarsal extending to the tarsal bones. Tenodesis of the EDL tendons to the metatarsal is accomplished by placing the end of the tendon from dorsal to plantar over the resected end of the metatarsal as the K-wire is retrograded proximally into the metatarsal shaft. This will neutralize their effect on the toes by preventing a recurrent contracture. A layered closure is performed. If significant dead space is anticipated, a drain is placed. The skin is closed with interrupted sutures of 4-0 PROLENE. Sterile dressings are applied. The patient is placed in a postoperative shoe or prefabricated BK – rocker sole walker with the inner sole accommodated for K-wires by placing a quarter inch adhesive felt from heel to ball of foot to prevent bending of the wires as the patient ambulates.

Plantar Transverse Elliptical approach:

The incision is marked out on the plantar forefoot directly under the MTPJs. The elliptical incision will remove the callous tissue and will help in assisting relocation of the digits and the anteriorly displaced plantar fat pad. The elliptical incision is placed directly below the prominent metatarsal heads (Fig. 10-8 A, B, C). The incision is deepened to the plantar plate or metatarsal head. The entire wedge of tissue is then

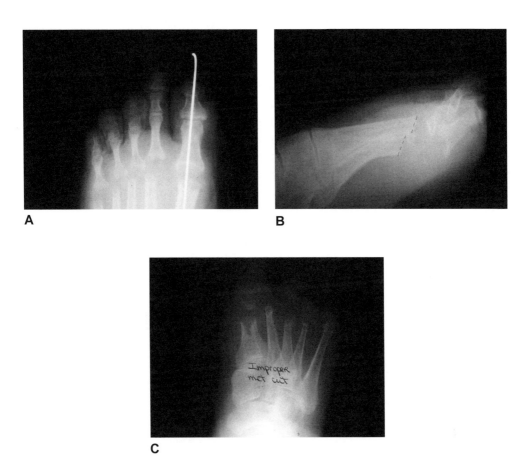

Figure 10-7: Intraoperative X-rays: **A:** AP view demonstrating resected metatarsal heads 1 – 5 creating a normal metatarsal "parabola" with digits in excellent alignment and with a K-wire in the first MTPJ exiting the end of the hallux. **B:** Lateral view demonstrating resected metatarsal heads with the osteotomy cut obliquely angled in the sagittal plane from dorsal to plantar with no bone spicules noted. **C:** AP view of another surgical case demonstrating an improper resection of the metatarsal heads leaving the second and especially the fifth too long calling for immediate revision.

dissected and removed. Most often the flexor plate and flexor tendons will have been dislocated to one side of the joint. In any event, the joint is entered and disarticulated. The digits are dorsally dislocated upon the head of the metatarsal exposing the metatarsal head and neck (Fig. 10-8 D). In this way the resection of metatarsal heads 2, 3, 4 and sometimes 5 can be performed as described from dorsal to plantar. A dorsal dedicated incision is made for the first MTPJ, and it is either resected or fused. Once the metatarsal heads are resected, digital procedures are performed as needed. K-wires are inserted as described and the plantar tissue is approximated and closed utilizing 4-0 Prolene retention sutures with simple interrupted sutures (Fig. 10-8 E). Sutures are left in place and removed at three weeks in most cases (Fig. 10-8 F, G, H). The use of a postoperative shoe or walking boot as described above is utilized.

A dedicated dorsal linear incision for the fifth MTPJ is sometimes indicated (Fig. 10-9).

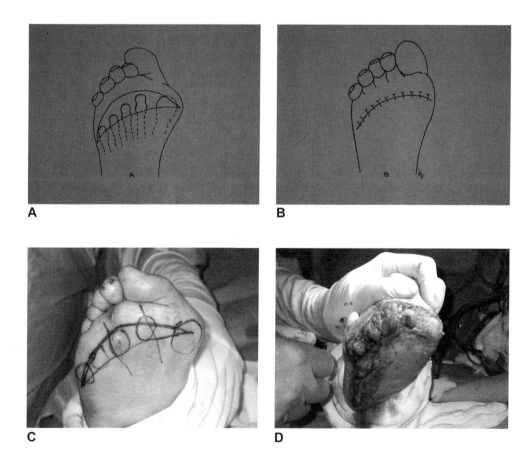

A

B

C

D

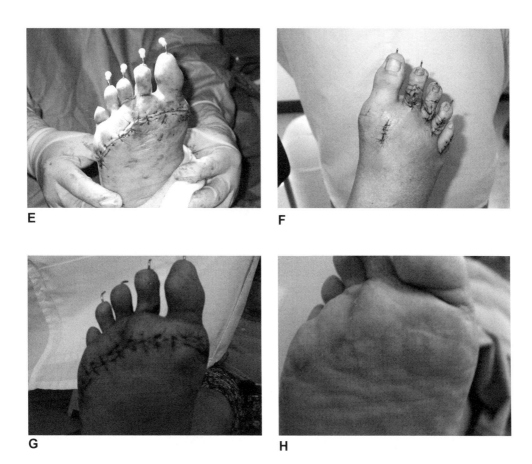

Figure 10-8: **A:** Diagram of placement and appearance of a plantar transverse elliptical incision to expose the metatarsal heads when associated with dorsally dislocated digits. **B:** Diagram of closure of plantar transverse elliptical incision. Note the relocation of the digits. **C:** Intraoperative photograph demonstrating design and placement of the plantar elliptical incision incorporating scaring from a previously infected plantar callus. **D:** Intraoperative photograph demonstrating exposure of all the metatarsal heads from the plantar approach prior to metatarsal head resection. **E:** Intraoperative photograph demonstrating closure of plantar ellipse and with K-wires in toes. **F:** Postoperative photograph of dorsal view of foot demonstrating linear incisions in the digits with sutures and K-wires in place at three weeks. **G:** Clinical photograph of plantar view of foot demonstrating the plantar ellipse at three weeks post operatively. **H:** Clinical photograph of plantar view of foot demonstrating healed incision four months post operatively.

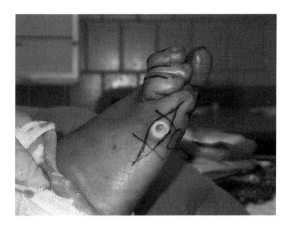

Figure 10-9: Clinical photograph demonstrating dedicated dorsal linear elliptical incision incorporating skin ulceration centered over the fifth MTPJ.

Keller Resectional Arthroplasty Combined with Lesser MHR:

Resection of the base of the proximal phalanx of the hallux in association with resection of the heads of the lesser metatarsals creates more weight transfer to the central metatarsals than when the first metatarsal head resection is performed in conjunction with lesser MHR. It eliminates all of the intrinsic muscle insertions to the hallux. It also leaves the first metatarsal longer than the second. It is associated with a high incidence of recurring digital deformity and transfer central metatarsalgia and is not recommended.

Hallux Proximal Phalangeal Base Resection Combined with a PMHR:

Resection of the base of the proximal phalanx of the hallux in association with a PMHR is indicated in the patient with severe osteoporosis and in certain situations such as: an excessively long hallux, subluxation/dislocation of the first MTPJ, an extremely high hallux abductus angle or a large metatarsus primus adductus. This patient population would have difficulty healing an osteotomy or accepting internal fixation. The primary goal here is not to provide stability but to eliminate pain and pressure points, while allowing for shoeing (Fig. 10-10 A, B, C).

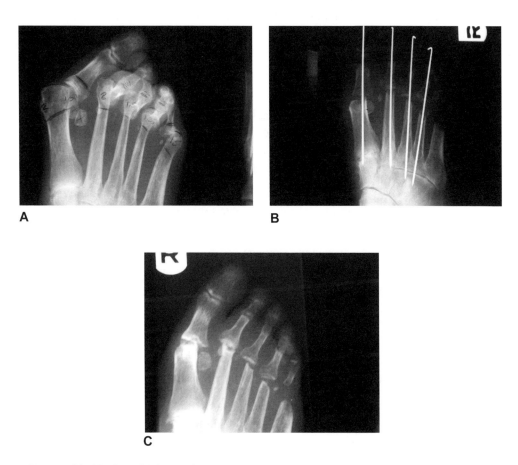

Figure 10-10: A: AP X-ray view demonstrating arthritic forefoot with dislocation of 1 – 5 MTPJs, metatarsus primus adductus, hallux abductus, and an excessively long hallux. **B:** Immediate postoperative AP X-ray view demonstrating a PMHR combined with resection of the base of the excessively long proximal phalanx of the hallux. **C:** Postoperative AP X-ray view of above at eight months demonstrating excellent digital alignment.

First MTPJ Resectional Arthroplasty with Total Joint Implant Combined with Lesser MHR:

On occasion, a first MTPJ implant arthroplasty has been performed in combination with lesser metatarsal head resections. Although providing some transverse plane stability of the hallux, the implant creates most of the same problems as mentioned above regarding the Keller resectional arthroplasty. Furthermore, most candidates for a PMHR do not have good bone stock to receive a first MTPJ joint implant. In addition, at times the implant has to be removed because it cannot withstand the ground reactive forces being placed upon it and either dislodges or causes stress fractures of the adjacent bone. Therefore, in our opinion, it is a procedure with very little indication.

Postoperative Management:

Postoperative management is individualized based upon the overall condition of the patient and the procedure(s) performed. Most often the procedure is performed on a come and go basis. Patients are admitted to the hospital for at least one day if bilateral procedures have been performed, if drains have been used, for pain management, or if the patient is medically compromised and needs closer monitoring.

- Guarded weight bearing in a prefabricated walking boot or rigid postoperative shoe is allowed for six weeks.

- Other ambulatory assistance devices are employed as needed (wheelchair, crutches, Canadian crutches).

- X-rays are taken at one week to access the alignment of the digits and K-wires.

- Sutures are removed at three weeks.

- Bathing restrictions are in place until K-wires are removed.

- Physical therapy is utilized as needed once the K-wires have been removed.

Inherent Complications of PMHR:

- Recurring digital deformity and mal-alignment. If hallux valgus occurs and is problematic, it can be treated with a revisional arthrodesis of the first MTPJ. Digital mal-alignment can be treated with PIPJ arthrodesis or a revisional arthrodesis if a fusion was initially performed.

- Transfer metatarsalgia and pressure points. Revisional surgery may become necessary to remove prominent bone if it is the etiology of the pressure point. If instability of the first ray is the cause of the transfer metatarsalgia, revisional arthrodesis of the first MTPJ is indicated providing the patient is a viable candidate.

- Chronic forefoot edema. This is more common with dorsal incisions. It can be managed with physical therapy and compression bandages.

- Postoperative shortening and widening of the foot. It is addressed by shoe gear modification or custom shoes.

- Apropulsive gait. This is also a predictable known side effect of the procedure and needs to be discussed with the patient preoperatively. The use of shoe gear modification will often assist the patient with this problem.

Arthrodesis First MTPJ Combined with Lesser MHR:

Fusion of the first MTPJ in association with resection of the heads of the lesser metatarsals creates stability of the first ray. It helps maintain alignment of the hallux and lesser toes preventing recurrent lateral digital mal-alignment and subsequent metatarsalgia (Fig. 10-11 A, B). Prior to fusing the first MTPJ, the metatarsal should be shortened to the level of the resected second metatarsal, so that the fusion will occur at this level preventing the first ray from being excessively longer than the lesser rays (Fig. 10-12 A, B). The presence of a significant metatarsus primus adductus or metatarsus elevatus will dictate an additional procedure to correct these pathologies. These additional procedures will probably necessitate being non-weight bearing post operatively for six to eight weeks.

The fusion of the first MTPJ should be accomplished with fixation which does not have to cross the IPJ of the hallux. Arthritic degeneration of the hallux IPJ is more frequent in patients in whom threaded Steinmann pins were used for fixation of the first MTPJ and were inserted longitudinally penetrating the IP joint (Fig. 10-12 A).

Postoperative retrospective studies have demonstrated that overall patient satisfaction is no greater for the first MTPJ fusion combined with lesser MHR than with a PMHR wherein all the metatarsal heads are resected even though it does provide more stability and prevention of recurring deformity initially.

Postoperative Management:

- Management is as for PMHR except that guarded weight bearing utilizing crutches for six to eight weeks is instituted. A prefabricated cast with a rocker sole in which the inner sole is modified to off weight the first ray is utilized.

- X- rays are taken at one week, three weeks and six weeks to access the healing of the fusion site.

- The use of a shoe with a rocker sole may be more comfortable for the patient than any other type of foot gear once the fusion site has healed (Fig. 10-13 A, B).

Inherent Complications:

- Non- union: Revisional arthrodesis of the first MTPJ with a bone graft can be considered or the fusion could be converted to a metatarsal head resection.

- Arthritis of the DIPJ: Fusion or arthroplasty of the DIPJ can be performed. The reader is referred to Chapter 2.

- Pressure points: If the pressure point is due to a mal-position of the fusion site then a revisional arthrodesis is indicated or the fusion can be converted to a metatarsal head resection.

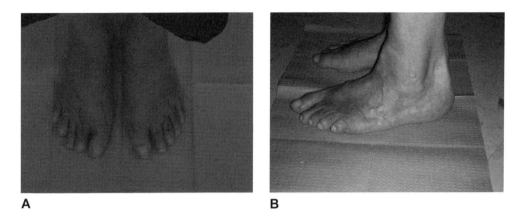

A   B

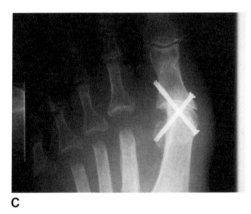

C

Figure 10-11: A: Postoperative weight bearing photograph of a stable, well-aligned forefoot status post first MTPJ fusion with lesser MHR performed bilaterally one foot at a time. **B:** Clinical photograph of the above foot from the side. The patient walks in shoe with a rocker sole.**C:** Postoperative AP X-ray view demonstrating first MTPJ fusion with lesser MHR and arthrodesis of the PIPJ of toes 2, 3, 4 and an arthroplasty of the fifth toe PIPJ at eight months.

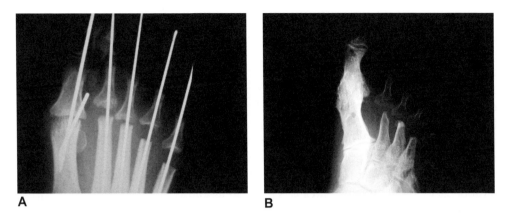

A   B

Figure 10-12: A: AP X-ray view demonstrating fusion site of first MTPJ at the same level as the resected distal end of the second metatarsal. **B:** AP X-ray view demonstrating excessively long first ray post fusion of the first MTPJ with lesser MHR.

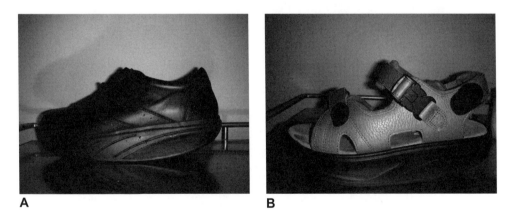

A   B

Figure 10-13: A: Shoe with rocker sole. **B:** Sandal with rocker sole.

Isolated Partial Metatarsal Head Resection(s) (Resectional Arthroplasty)

Resectional arthroplasty of the lesser MTPJs 2, 3, and 4, involves a 4 - 6 mm resection of the distal metatarsal head (Fig. 10-14 A). By not removing the entire metatarsal head, less MTPJ instability is created than with a complete metatarsal head resection resulting in a more stable forefoot and digit. It is utilized most often when there is an isolated arthrosis involving a single subluxed or dislocated MTPJ which demonstrates erosive articular changes. The procedure eliminates the joint, shortens the metatarsal, creates laxity, and decompression of the joint. A plantar condylectomy is performed as needed to eliminate plantar pressure (Fig. 10-14 B, C, D, E). No fixation is required except for placement of a temporary 0.045 or 0.062 inch K-wire as an arthrofibrosis is formed at the involved MTPJ. The procedure allows for immediate postoperative weight bearing. It causes minimal disability and is well accepted by the geriatric population. With minor modification in technique, the procedure can be utilized with implant arthroplasty of the isolated central MTPJ (see Chapter 5) providing the bone stock is adequate.

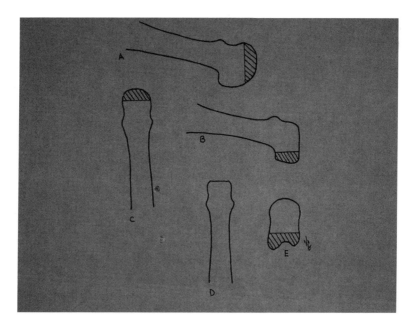

Figure 10-14: A: Diagram demonstrating partial metatarsal head resection orientation and appearance in the sagittal plane. **B:** Sagittal plane diagram demonstrating resected distal metatarsal head and planned plantar condylectomy. **C, D:** Transverse plane diagram demonstrating amount and orientation of the planned partial resection of the distal metatarsal head. **E:** Frontal plane diagram of a metatarsal head demonstrating plantar condyles with fibular condyle extending the farthest plantarly.

In situations where there is a need to shorten the metatarsal due to chronic MTPJ dislocation with no erosive changes but with significant osteoporetic bone in the elderly patient, a partial metatarsal head resection may be favored over a Weil shortening osteotomy (Fig. 10-15 A, B, C).

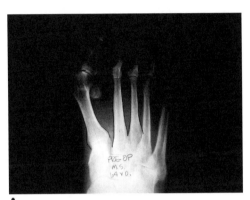

A

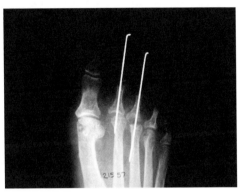

B

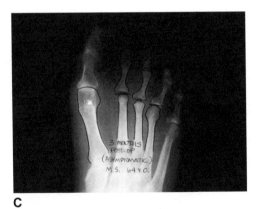

C

Figure 10-15: A: AP X-ray view demonstrating dislocated second and third MTPJs. **B:** Immediate postoperative AP X-ray view demonstrating partial metatarsal head resection of the second and third relocation of the joint and arthrodesis of the PIPJ of toes 2, and 3. **C:** AP X-ray view demonstrating partial metatarsal head resections of two and three metatarsals, three months postoperatively.

Indications:

- Isolated MTPJ derangement with DJD.
- Erosive arthritis with or without chronic MTPJ dislocation.
- Freiberg's infraction.
- IPK may be present.
- Elongated metatarsal may be present.
- Plantarflexed metatarsal may be present.
- Prominent plantar condyle may be present.
- Osteoporosis may be present.
- Geriatric apropulsive population.

Contraindications:

- Younger/active patient.
- Joint preservation procedure is possible.
- Multiple joint involvement. Usually if more than two MTPJs are involved a PMHR is indicated (Fig. 10-16 A, B).

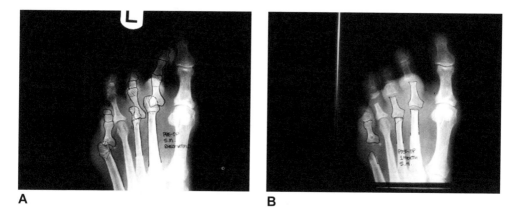

A

B

Figure 10-16: A: AP X-ray view demonstrating dislocated second, third and fifth MTPJ. **B:** Postoperative AP view demonstrating resected second, third and fifth metatarsal heads with a resultant long fourth ray. The fourth metatarsal head was eventually resected.

Surgical Procedure:

The MTPJ is approached as previously described in chapters 5, 6 and 7. The joint is entered and disarticulated. The metatarsal head is delivered into view and a partial resection is performed by removing the distal 4 – 6 mms of metatarsal head (Fig. 10-17 A). A plantar condylectomy is performed as needed (Fig. 10-17 B). An adjunctive flexor transfer or PIPJ fusion is recommended to help prevent a floating toe postoperatively. Temporary K-wire stabilization across the MTPJ is critical (Fig. 10-18) unless an adjunctive lesser MTPJ implant procedure has been performed to help stabilize the isolated MTPJ. The reader is referred to Chapter 5 for a complete discussion on central MTPJ implant arthroplasty.

Post Operative Management:

- Guarded weight bearing as described for PMHR for three weeks or until K-wire removal.
- Bathing restriction until K-wire is removed.
- X-rays are taken at one week to evaluate MTPJ alignment.
- K-wire removal at three weeks.
- Digital splinting in mild plantar flexion for several months.

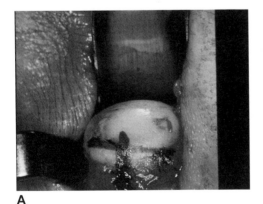
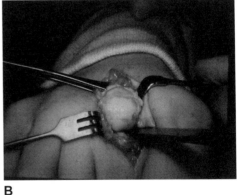

A   **B**

Figure 10-17: A: Intraoperative photograph of metatarsal head exposed and marked for the performance of a partial head resection. **B:** Intraoperative photograph of a frontal plane view of a metatarsal head prepared for a plantar condylectomy.

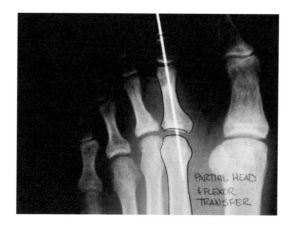

Figure 10-18: Postoperative AP X-ray view demonstrating partial second metatarsal head resection with K-wire in place.

Inherent Complications:

- Floating toe: This can be managed with a flexor tendon transfer of the involved toe.

- Transfer metatarsalgia: This can be managed with an accommodative orthotic device.

Joint Preservation Shortening Osteotomy(ies)

Multiple Weil metatarsal shortening osteotomies can be performed to treat central metatarsalgia involving MTPJs 2, 3 and 4 if the pain is primarily from the deformity and not from intra articular pathology (see Chapter 7).

Indications:

- Elongated metatarsal 2, 3 and 4.

- Subluxed or dorsally dislocated MTPJ without erosive arthritis of metatarsal head.

- Subluxed or dislocated MTPJ without erosive arthritis or hypertrophy of the base of the proximal phalanx.

Contraindications:

- Erosive arthritis/severe DJD of the MTPJ.

- Severe osteoporosis.

- First ray instability unless an adjunctive fusion of the first MTPJ and/or metatarsal cuneiform joint is performed.

Clinical Pearls:

- When performing a PMHR the patient should be informed that foot will be shorter and most often wider, requiring custom shoes or shoes that are a size or two smaller postoperatively.

- When performing PMHR, neutralize the effect of the extensor tendons on the toes in order to prevent recurrent dorsal contracture by tenodesing the EDL tendons into their respective metatarsals.

- Always have a dedicated dorsal incision when approaching the first MTPJ.

- Perform an arthrodesis of the first MTPJ when the patient's activity level would benefit from a more stable forefoot.

- When fusing the MTPJ shorten the first metatarsal to the length of the second resected metatarsal prior to fusing.

- To lessen the chance of Hallux IPJ arthritis, do not cross the joint with pins or wires when fusing the first MTPJ.

- In cases of osteoporosis place the stabilizing 0.062 inch K-wires so that they extend proximally to the tarsal bones so as to engage as much bone – pin contact as possible (Fig. 10-10 B).

References:

Bitzan P, Giurea A, Wanivenhaus A. Plantar pressure distribution after resection of the metatarsal heads in rheumatoid arthritis. *Foot Ankle* 18:391-397, 1997.

Bolland BJRF, Sauve PS, Taylor GR. Rheumatoid forefoot reconstruction: first metatarsophalangeal joint fusion combined with Weil's metatarsal osteotomies of the lesser rays. *J Foot Ankle Surg* 47:80-88, 2008.

Coughlin MJ. Rheumatoid forefoot reconstruction: A long-term follow-up study. *J Bone Joint Surg Am* 82: 322-341, 2000.

Current Rheumatology Diagnosis and Treatment Second Edition. Imboden J, Hellmann D, Stone J, Eds., McGraw-Hill Co., Inc. New York, NY, 2007.

Dereymaeker G, Mulier T, Stuer P, Peeraer L, Fabry G: Pedodynograhic measurements after forefoot reconstruction in rheumatoid arthritis patients. Foot Ankle 18:270-276, 1997.

Grondal L, Bronstgrom E, Wretenberg P, Stark A. Arthrodesis versus Mayo resection: the management of the first metatarsophalangeal joint in reconstruction of the rheumatoid forefoot. *J Bone Joint Surg* 88-B: 914-919, 2006.

Hanyu T, Yamazaki H, Murasawa A, Tohyama C. Arthroplasty for rheumatoid forefoot deformities by a shortening oblique osteotomy. *Clin Orthop Relat Res* 338:131-138, 1997.

James D, Young A, Kulinsakaya E, et al. Orthopaedic intervention in early rheumatoid arthritis: occurrence and predictive factors in an inception cohort of 1064 patients followed for 5 years. *Rheumatology* 43:369-376, 2004.

Mulcahy D, Daniels TR, Lau JT, Boyle E, Bogoch E. Rheumatoid forefoot deformity: a comparison study of 2 functional methods of reconstruction. *J Rheumatol* 30:1440-1450, 2003.

Nassar J, Cracchiolo III A. Complications in surgery of the foot and ankle in patients with rheumatoid arthritis. *Clin Orthop* 391:140-142, 2001.

Saltrick KR, Alter SA, Catanzariti A. Pan metatarsal head resection: Retrospective analysis and literature review. *Journal of Foot Surgery* 28:340-345, 1989.

Yu GV, Shook J. Arthrodesis of the first metatarsophalangeal joint: current recommendations. *J Am Podiatr Med Assoc* 84:266- 271, 1994.

Woodburn J, Barker S, Helliwell PS. A randomized controlled trial of foot orthoses in rheumatoid arthritis. *J Rheumatol* 29:1377- 1383, 2002.

Vahvanen V, Piirainen H, Kettunen P. Resection arthroplasty of the metatarsophalangeal joints in rheumatoid arthritis. A follow-up study of 100 patients. *Scand J Rheumatol* 9:257-265, 1980.

Foot Amputations

11

Albert E. Burns, DPM, FACFAS

Introduction:

There are approximately twenty-one million people with diabetes mellitus in the United States, and greater than 60 percent of all the lower extremity amputations are performed on patients with diabetes. Minor external trauma is the leading pivotal event for amputation in high risk patients with diabetes, so treatment of the diabetic foot will, therefore, require the foot and ankle surgeon to inevitably face the need for amputation of part or all of the foot. In the past, amputations were considered a failure of treatment, but an amputation can mark the beginning of a comprehensive rehabilitation process. The primary goal of amputation surgery is to salvage the greatest amount of functional limb that will heal, so any pedal amputation attempts to maintain as much forefoot length as possible to improve biomechanical function. Partial foot amputations should be regarded as a limb salvage step, avoiding higher and more disabling procedures, since the more proximal the amputation level, the greater the increase in energy expenditure to ambulate. Whatever the level of amputation, however, the goals are the same:

- Create a distal stump that can be easily accommodated by a shoe insert, orthotic device, modified shoe, or prosthesis.

- Create a distal stump that is durable and unlikely to break down.

- Create a distal stump that will not cause muscle or other dynamic imbalance.

Additionally there are advantages of partial foot ablations such as preservation of end-weight bearing, normal proprioception, and limited disruption of body image. The amputations to be discussed in this chapter are:

- Digital amputations
- Ray resections – single and multiple
- Transmetatarsal amputation

Generic Indications:

Although individual indications and criteria will be listed for each of the amputations to be discussed, there are generalized criteria for all lower extremity ablations. They are:

- Diabetic infections: The neuropathic foot is easily traumatized, resulting in non-healing ulcers and/or soft tissue infections and wet gangrene with progression to acute and ultimately chronic osteomyelitis.

- Ischemia: The dysvascular limb secondary to diabetes or peripheral vascular disease can result in tissue necrosis and ultimately dry gangrene.

- Trauma: Traumatic amputations and crush injuries can result in non-viable tissue of the foot.

- Congenital deformities: Symptomatic and even asymptomatic deformities such as polydactyly and macrodactyly are indications for ablation.

- Tumors: Malignant tumors that require wide ablation or even large, aggressively invasive benign tumors are indication for ablation.

- Cold-induced injuries: Frostbite with the development of painful or non-viable tissue is indication for ablation.

- Burns: Burn injury resulting in non-viable tissue are indication for ablation.

General Amputation Principles:

Each amputation discussed in this chapter will have the specific technique described, but for all amputations there are principles in common. There is obviously no absolute consensus on many of the technique considerations, but attempt will be made to present what the alternative approaches are, culminating with a description of the method preferred by the CSPM surgical faculty and why.

1. The Guillotine amputation - At this point in time of the evolution of amputations, the overall consensus is that the guillotine amputation is a procedure that has its greatest application as a preliminary debriding operation to remove an infecting source as would be encountered in an acute diabetic infection. It is part of the initial incision and drainage that is performed to remove the source of infection and is left open and treated with appropriate wound care and antibiotics. Once the infection is cleared, a formal primary amputation at the appropriate level should be performed. There is the possibility that in a localized infection such as wet gangrene of a digit, the guillotine and primary amputation could be one and the same and done in one procedure.

2. Hemostasis – Studies have shown that no complications have been ascribed to the use of tourniquets at any level except above the knee amputations, and the CSPM surgery department faculty advocates the use of a tourniquet in all

cases except where there is a specific contraindication such as the patient who has had revascularization surgery. The CSPM surgery department faculty also does not advocate dropping the cuff before closure. The lumen of any vessel that requires ligation is visible and all other vessels are coagulated with a bovie or adequately compressed with an appropriate compression dressing. It is felt that this method best avoids the development of a hematoma, which could lead to pressure on adjacent tissues sufficient to cause death of the tissue and act as an excellent culture medium for bacteria. Specific to transmetatarsal amputations, the patient should be typed and crossed for a minimum of 2U of packed red blood cells in anticipation of intraoperative bleeding.

3. Level of amputation – The decision on the appropriate level of amputation is based on the extent of the forefoot infection, the presence of osteomyelitis and a sufficient vascular supply necessary for healing. That decision relies on the clinical exam which assesses the quality of the tissue, the extent of the infection, the amount of vascularity and the patient's nutritional, immune, and ambulatory status. The use of vasoconstrictors such as nicotine or caffeine should be actively discouraged. Serum albumin levels below 3.0 g/dL, protein levels greater than 6 g/dL, and a lymphocyte count below 1500/mm^3 would indicate the inability to heal a wound. Pulses either audible with Doppler or easily palpated in the diabetic patient have little predictive value in determining wound healing capability. Ankle brachial index and pulse volume wave forms are not useful in the diabetic patient. Transcutaneous oxygen pressure measurements (TcPO2) greater than 30 mm/Hg have been touted as predictive of wound healing capability, but no preoperative hemoglobin levels, distal blood pressures, or forefoot transcutaneous oximetry have provided a standard, reliable test to predict wound healing. Even angiographic findings of blood flow to the foot have been reported to not be predictive of wound healing success and cannot be used to determine the level of amputation, except in cases of more proximal arterial occlusions in the region of the thigh or pelvis. Ultimately the level of amputation in patients with vascular insufficiency is determined by clinical criteria, such as peripheral pulses, skin color and temperature.

4. Tissue handling techniques – All skin incisions should be full thickness, without dissection by layers, using sharp elevation from bone to preserve the circulation to the skin flaps. Skin edges should be handled with gentle manipulation and should not be crushed. The soft tissue envelope in forefoot amputations is formed of skin, subcutaneous tissue and fascia alone, unlike more proximal amputations, where muscle tissue forms an integral part of the soft tissue envelope. There should be no tension on the flaps with closure, and the skin should never directly adhere to bone. Nerves should be sharply transected under tension to allow for nerve retraction to avoid the development of stump neuromas. Tendons should also be transected under tension

and allowed to retract. Bone cuts should be made with a power saw, because bone cutting forceps crush remaining bone ends which increase the risk of delayed healing and wound failure. The bone ends should be properly contoured to remove all sharp edges to prevent damage of the soft tissues when compressed between the bone and the outside environment.

5.   Closure – Prior to closure the wound should have high pressure lavage with 2-6 liters depending on the degree of remaining contamination. Deep cultures are taken after the lavage. There is no absolute consensus on leaving the wound open and doing delayed primary closure later versus primary closure; the CSPM surgery department faculty advocates primary closure unless there is a reason not to do so. There is a higher healing rate with closure than with open wounds that are allowed to heal by granulation. The worst case for primary closure is the wound will become purulent and be opened and treated the same as an open wound from the beginning. The CSPM surgery department faculty does not advocate the use of drains in any foot amputation, unless there is a significant dead space that could result in a hematoma. If a drain is used, it should not exit out through the incision because of the increased risk of infection, but rather through a separate stab incision proximal to the surgical site. No deep closure is accomplished with absorbable sutures, and if there is a perceived need for deep closure, it is accomplished with retention sutures. A compression dressing is applied, and the weight bearing status is determined by the procedure performed. If the amputation was in part or in toto for osteomyelitis, it is assumed that all of the infected bone was resected and the antibiotics are continued for two weeks postoperatively to treat the soft tissue infection. Suture removal is no sooner than three weeks for all foot amputations.

Digital Amputations:

There are three levels of digital amputations:

1.   Terminal Syme's
2.   Partial digital amputation
3.   Digital disarticulation

The terminal Syme's has been described to address onychopathology, chronic paronychia, chronic ulceration of the tip of the digit and osteomyelitis of the tip of the distal phalanx. The CSPM surgery department faculty views a simple matricectomy as more appropriate for pathology of the nail plate, so there is rare indication for this procedure.

The partial digital amputation is the primary procedure utilized for problems localized to the digit. It preserves the base of the proximal phalanx which preserves the attachments of the intrinsics, allowing the remaining digit to act as a buttress to the adjacent digits and preventing future migration of the neighboring toes. For the second toe this would help preclude the development of hallux abductovalgus. Additionally, the intact phalangeal base prevents exposure of the cartilage of the metatarsal head which is avascular and prone to infection. The partial digital amputation is performed with either a medial and lateral flap (Fig. 11-1) or a dorsal and plantar flap. The medial and lateral flap has the advantage of preserving more of the area in which the digital arteries run; in addition, gravity allows any drainage to pass plantarly through the incision. It also allows for easy extension of the incision in the central digits if the infection needs to be explored more proximally. A dorsal and plantar flap would allow a hematoma to accumulate over the plantar flap, but has the advantage of putting more durable skin in a weight bearing position. Practically, either method works well; the CSPM surgical faculty prefers to use medial and lateral flaps on the central digits and dorsal and plantar flaps on the hallux and fifth digit (Fig. 11-2). On the hallux and the fifth digit this incision can be easily extended proximally if necessary and it allows for contouring on the medial and lateral sides of the foot. If the hallux and an additional digit are involved, we advocate doing a transmetatarsal amputation. If multiple lesser digits are involved we advocate transmetatarsal amputation of the lesser digits with preservation of the hallux. We do not advocate the utilization of digital disarticulation procedures, and if the base of the proximal phalanx cannot be preserved, instead advocate a partial ray resection. This provides both a better functional and cosmetic result.

Indications:

Terminal Syme's

1. Severe deformity of the distal digit

2. Traumatic avulsion of the tip of the digit

3. Chronic ulceration of the tip of the digit

4. Tumor of the distal half of the distal phalanx

Partial digital amputation

1. Osteomyelitis of the proximal, intermediate, or distal phalanx

2. Wet gangrene of the distal half of the digit

3. Dry gangrene of the distal half of the digit

4. Recurring ulcers on the tip or dorsum of the digit

5. Necrotic ulceration of the distal one half of the digit

6. Tumor of the distal one half of the digit

7. Polydactyly whether symptomatic or asymptomatic

8. Macrodactyly

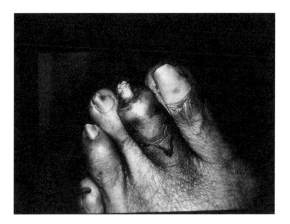

Figure 11-1: Clinical photograph of a partial digital amputation of the second digit illustrating the use of medial and lateral flap technique.

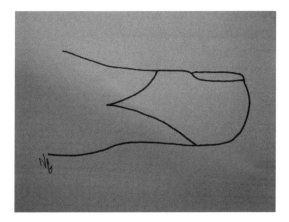

Figure 11-2: The drawing illustrates on the hallux the dorsal and plantar flap technique used in partial digital amputation of the hallux and fifth digit.

Surgical Procedure:

Terminal Syme's – The procedure utilizes two converging, semielliptical incisions (Fig. 11-3). The first is transverse proximal to the nail matrix but distal to the distal interphalangeal joint (the interphalangeal joint of the hallux). The second is below the ungualabia and courses distal then back proximal connecting the two ends of the first incision. Both incisions are carried from skin to bone and there is no dissection by layers. The dorsal nail bed is sharply dissected off of the distal phalanx. A bone cut is made through the distal phalanx perpendicular to the weight bearing surface with a small power oscillating saw. Enough bone is removed to allow for closure of the distal flap but making sure that the attachment of the extensor tendon is intact. The surgical site is irrigated with one liter of high pressure lavage, and the wound is reapproximated with 3-0 or 4-0 monofilament simple interrupted suture. If the digit was amputated for an infection or osteomyelitis, a gram stain and culture and sensitivity of the deep tissue is taken after the lavage. The flap is modified as necessary prior to closure. A compression dressing is applied.

Partial digital amputation – The incision is drawn out using a skin scribe, using either medial and lateral, or dorsal and plantar flaps. The incisions are carried from skin to bone with no dissection by layers (Fig. 11-4). The flexor and extensor tendons are divided in line with the skin incision. The distal part of the digit is grasped with a traumatic clamp and the distal soft tissue is dissected off of the proximal phalanx to the proximal interphalangeal joint of the lesser digits or the interphalangeal joint of the hallux and is disarticulated at that level (Fig. 11-5). The proximal phalanx is resected with a small oscillating power saw perpendicular to the weight bearing surface leaving at least one centimeter of the base of the proximal phalanx. The surgical site is irrigated with one liter of high pressure lavage, and the wound is reapproximated with 3-0 or 4-0 monofilament simple interrupted suture (Fig. 11-6). If the digit was amputated for an infection or osteomyelitis, a gram stain and culture and sensitivity of the deep tissue is taken after the lavage. The flap is modified as necessary prior to closure. A compression dressing is applied.

Postoperative Management:

1. Immediate postoperative X-rays (Fig. 11-7, 11-8).

2. Patient is ambulatory in a postoperative shoe to eliminate the propulsive phase of gait.

3. Antibiotics are continued for two weeks, if the amputation was for an infection or osteomyelitis. It is assumed that if osteomyelitis was present that all of the bone infection was removed and that the treatment is for the soft tissue infection. Since most patients are immunocompromised (e.g. diabetic), coverage is broad spectrum to cover both the gram positive and gram negative organisms.

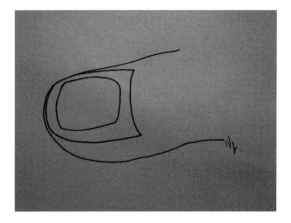

Figure 11-3: Drawing illustrating Terminal Syme's amputation utilizing a transverse incision proximal to the nail matrix connected to a second incision below the ungual-abia and courses distal and back proximal connecting the two ends of the first incision.

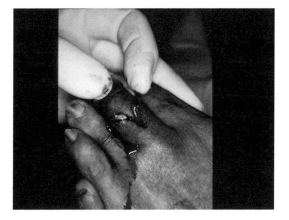

Figure 11-4: A clinical photograph of a partial digital amputation. The incision is made skin to bone with no dissection by layers, dividing the extensor and flexor tendons in line with the skin incision.

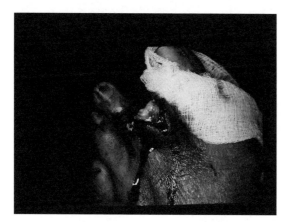

Figure 11-5: A clinical photograph of a partial digital amputation with disarticulation at the proximal interphalangeal. The proximal phalanx is then resected with a small power saw leaving one centimeter of the base of the proximal phalanx.

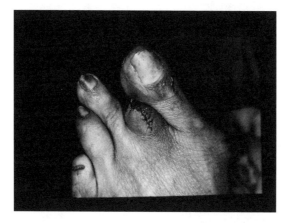

Figure 11-6: Clinical photograph showing closure of partial digital amputation.

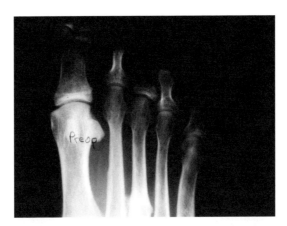

Figure 11-7: An X-ray of a partial digital amputation. Preserving the base of the proximal phalanx preserves the attachments of the intrinsic muscles and allows the remaining digit to act as an abutment to the adjacent digits, thus preventing drift of these digits.

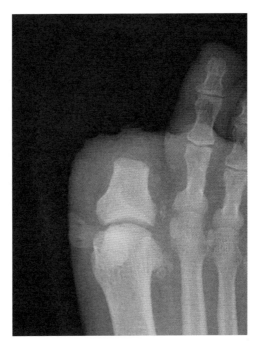

Figure 11-8: An X-ray of a partial digital amputation of the hallux. This preserves the attachments of the intrinsic muscles and, therefore, the function of the great toe.

4. The patient returns to the clinic in one week for a dressing change to evaluate for purulence of the wound. If the wound is purulent, the sutures are removed, the wound irrigated, and the patient started on daily dressing changes. The culture and sensitivity is used to determine the continuance or change in antibiotics.

5. Suture removal is at three weeks if the wound does not become purulent.

6. After suture removal the patient can be progressed to normal shoes and requires no filler, orthotic, or prosthesis. If the patient has neuropathy or vascular insufficiency, they should have routine palliative care and be well educated on proper foot care.

Inherent complications:

1. Stump neuroma – entrapment of the nerves in the incisional scar is unusual in digital amputations, but may require a more proximal amputation.

2. Wound dehiscence – this can be particularly problematic if the proper digital arteries are compromised and may require a more proximal amputation.

3. Further spread of the infection – this will require further incision and drainage, proximal exploration and more proximal amputation.

4. Structural deformities – deviated digits, digital contractures, and hallux abductovalgus can develop that can result in irritation, ulceration, and infection that may require further amputation.

5. Stump ulceration – this could progress to infection and may require further amputation.

Clinical pearls:

1. Do not dissect by layers and do not undermine the skin in order to preserve all possible blood supply.

2. Make sure that flaps are long enough or that adequate bone has been removed so that the flaps are not closed under tension.

3. Dissection should be done sharply and not bluntly to avoid crushing the tissues.

4. Do not use deep absorbable sutures that would cause more trauma to the tissues by causing an increased inflammatory reaction and or acting as a nidus for infection.

5. Use a compression dressing in order to prevent hematoma and edema which may compromise results.

Ray Resections:

Ray resections are generally utilized for problems previously discussed that cannot be managed with a partial digital amputation. Single lesser ray amputations provide an excellent functional and cosmetic result that does not require the use of shoe fillers, orthotics, or prosthetics. However, an isolated first ray amputation will have a serious debilitating effect on stance and gait because an intact medial column is essential for proper foot function. Multiple ray resections should be avoided because of the risk of subsequent transfer lesion development, but there are exceptions. If two or more of the lesser rays are involved, it is best to remove all of the lesser rays, and leave the hallux intact, since this provides both a better functional and cosmetic result. This is preferable to a transmetatarsal amputation. The removal of multiple lesser rays is acceptable if it involves just the fourth and fifth rays (Fig. 11-9 A-C). The removal of the lateral column can be adequately compensated for by a good pedorthic fitting. Care must be taken in this instance to try and preserve the base of the fifth metatarsal in order to preserve the insertion of the peroneus brevis, or the unopposed pull of the posterior tibial tendon will result in the foot being pulled into a severe varus position. If the debridement of an acute infection resulted in the detachment of the peroneus brevis, it cannot be reattached at that time, but would be anchored into the cuboid in a second operation after the infection had been cleared. If the first ray and any additional single lesser ray are involved, then it is best to proceed with a transmetatarsal amputation. With a first ray amputation, caution should be taken to maintain the attachment of the anterior tibial tendon in order to obviate valgus deformity of the foot. Most ray resections are partial, with the metatarsal bone resections performed in the middle one-third of the metatarsal.

Indications:

1. Recurrent ulceration under a metatarsal head.
2. Recurrent ulceration medial to the first metatarsal head or lateral to the fifth metatarsal head.
3. Ischemic digit or dry gangrene of a digit that is not amenable to a partial digit amputation.
4. Wet gangrene of a digit that is not amenable to a partial digit amputation.
5. Osteomyelitis of the digit and/or the distal aspect of the corresponding metatarsal.
6. Polydactyly with partial or complete duplication of the corresponding metatarsal.
7. Macrodactyly with involvement of the distal corresponding metatarsal.
8. Tumor of the digit or distal aspect of the involved metatarsal.

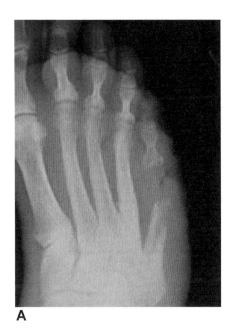 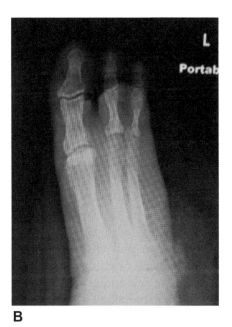

A   B

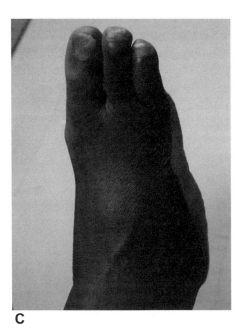

C

Figure 11-9: A: A preoperative X-ray of a lateral column amputation for osteomyelitis and long term clinical result. This preserves the function of the foot and is easily accommodated with shoe modifications. **B:** The postoperative X-ray of a lateral column amputation for osteomyelitis. **C:** The long term clinical photograph of a lateral column amputation for osteomyelitis.

Surgical Procedure:

The incisional approach for resection of the first and fifth rays is with a racquet incision that extends back proximally dorsomedially or dorsolaterally respectively a sufficient distance to resect the necessary segment of the metatarsal shaft (Fig. 11-10; Fig. 11-11). The incisional approach for a single central metatarsal is converging semielliptical incisions fashioned around the base of the toe involved that come to an apex both dorsally and plantarly (Fig. 11-12 A, B). The incision is perpendicular to the skin and is carried from skin to bone with no dissection by layers and no compression of the proximal skin edges with instrumentation. The involved digit is clamped with a traumatic clamp and the dorsal soft tissue is dissected off of the bone to the metatarsophalangeal joint where it is disarticulated and removed. The appropriate level of the bone resection is determined and it is resected with a power oscillating saw (Fig. 11-13; Fig. 11-14). In the case of osteomyelitis, that would be back to hard bleeding bone, and in polydactyly that would be the resection of the duplicated part of the metatarsal. With all of the bone cuts, there should be a bevel from dorsodistal to proximoplantar, and although some authorities advocate a particular angle, the exact angulation is not critical. In order to avoid sharp corners that could damage the skin with ambulation, the first metatarsal bevel should actually be from dorsal, distal, and medial to plantar, proximal, and lateral, and the fifth metatarsal bevel should be from dorsal, distal, and lateral to plantar, proximal, and medial. The bone edges can be further contoured with a rongeur in order to avoid any sharp edges. The surgical site is then irrigated with a high pressure lavage with two to four liters of fluid; if the amputation is for an infection, gram stain and culture and sensitivity from the deep tissue is taken at this time. There is no deep closure with absorbable suture for the previously stated reasons. Closure is with either 3-0 or 4-0 monofilament suture. In order to reduce tension on the wound and achieve deep closure to reduce dead space, several retention stitches are used and then the closure is completed with simple interrupted sutures between the retention stitches (Fig. 11-15; Fig. 11-16; Fig. 11-17). A compression dressing is then applied to the foot (Fig. 11-18).

Postoperative Management:

1. Immediate postoperative X-rays (Fig. 11-19; Fig. 11-20; Fig. 11-21).
2. Patient is placed non-weight bearing in posterior splint for minimum of three weeks.
3. Antibiotics are continued for two weeks if amputation is for infection.
4. Patient returns in one week for dressing change and to evaluate for purulence. If wound is purulent, remove the sutures, irrigate, and start on daily dressing changes.
5. Suture removal at three weeks if the wound did not become purulent.
6. Partial weight bearing at three weeks in a postoperative shoe is begun with the plan to progress to regular shoes by six weeks postoperatively. For single

lesser ray amputations no fillers, orthotics, or prosthetics should be needed. For first ray amputations, orthotic support is going to be needed to try and support the medial column. For a lateral column amputation, custom molded shoes are going to be needed to fit the foot.

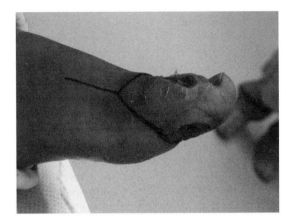

Figure 11-10: A clinical photograph of the racquet incision used for a first ray amputation.

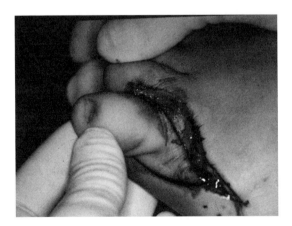

Figure 11-11: A clinical photograph of the racquet incision used for a fifth ray amputation.

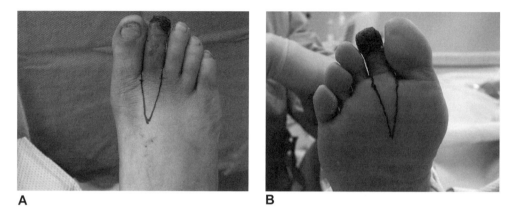

A   **B**

Figure 11-12: A: A clinical photograph of the dorsal part of a lesser ray amputation incision marked with a skin scribe. **B:** A clinical photograph of the plantar part of a lesser ray amputation incision marked with a skin scribe.

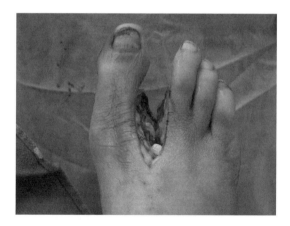

Figure 11-13: Resected second ray. The bone cut is made in the middle one third of the metatarsal to facilitate closure.

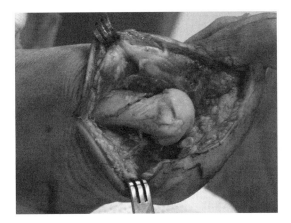

Figure 11-14: Clinical intraoperative photograph of first ray resection showing the first metatarsal marked with the angle of the resection to give the appropriate bevel to the bone cut.

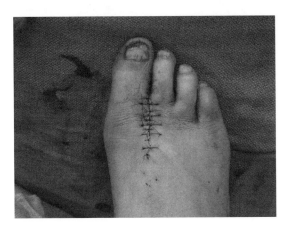

Figure 11-15: Clinical photograph of closure of a second ray resection that gives both a cosmetic and functional result.

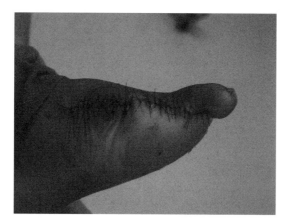

Figure 11-16: Clinical photograph of closure of a first ray resection that gives a good contour to the medial aspect of the foot in order to prevent shoegear irritation.

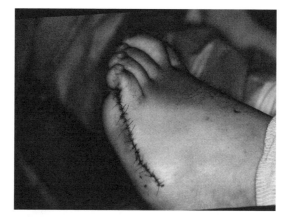

Figure 11-17: Clinical photograph of closure of a fifth ray resection that gives a good contour to the lateral aspect of the foot that is cosmetic and prevents shoegear irritation.

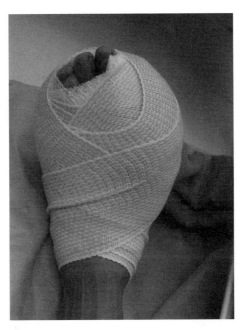

Figure 11-18: Clinical photograph illustrating a compression dressing utilizing fluffs and an ace wrap. The patient is then placed in a posterior splint and kept non-weight bearing.

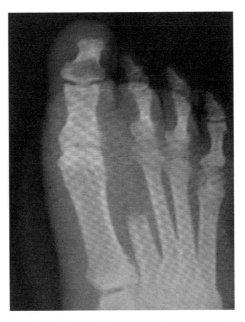

Figure 11-19: Postoperative X-ray of a second ray amputation. The bone cut is made in the middle one third of the metatarsal.

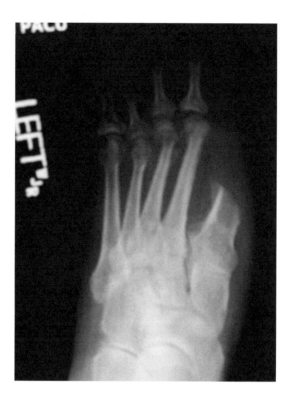

Figure 11-20: Postoperative X-ray of a first ray amputation illustrating the bevel of the cut from dorsal, distal, and medial to plantar, proximal, and lateral.

Complications:

1. Stump neuromas, wound dehiscence and further spread of infection are all possible as they are in digital amputations.

2. Transfer lesion to another metatarsal that can ultimately ulcerate, particularly in the neuropathic foot, requiring further surgical intervention.

3. First ray amputations can result in varus migration of the lesser digits with concomitant flexion contracture and irritation. Additionally, lateral weight transfer can result in stress fractures of the lesser metatarsals. An accommodative orthotic with filler to replace the first ray may prevent or minimize this complication.

4. Varus or valgus deformity of the foot if there is loss of the peroneus brevis or anterior tibial tendons respectively, which can be prevented or minimized by preserving or reattaching these structures.

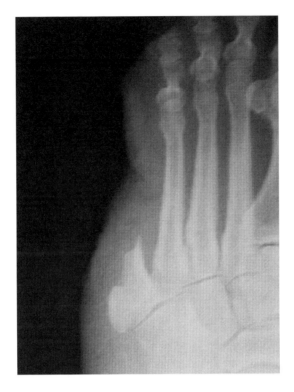

Figure 11-21: Postoperative X-ray of a fifth ray amputation illustrating the bevel of the cut from dorsal, distal, and lateral to plantar, proximal, and medial. If at all possible the base of the fifth mettarsal is preserved in order to maintain the attachment of the peroneus brevis.

Clinical pearls:

See digital amputations.

Transmetatarsal Amputation:

A transmetatarsal amputation (TMA) is the ablation of all five toes and all five metatarsal heads with the resection of the metatarsals being performed at various metatarsal lengths to treat a wide range of pathologies. It is a procedure that is advocated as a superior alternative to higher level amputations such as a transtibial amputation. The transmetatarsal amputation is used to preserve the residual limb length, to maintain function, and to reduce the energy expenditure of higher level amputations. Tantamount to the success of the procedure is the preservation of the extrinsic muscle insertions in order to prevent structural contractures from occurring. Specifically important is the preservation of the insertion of the peroneus brevis, peroneus longus, and the tibialis anterior tendons.

Indications:

1. Destruction of several toes and/or several metatarsal heads.

2. Two central rays need to be resected despite cause (an alternative to a TMA in this instance as discussed before would be the ablation of all of the lesser rays with the preservation of the first ray).

3. Two or more medial rays need to be removed.

4. Multiple ischemic digits.

5. Recurrent ulcerations of the digits or the metatarsal heads that are vascular or neuropathic in nature.

6. Failed digital amputations and ray resections.

7. Infection with wet gangrene and/or osteomyelitis of multiple digits and/or metatarsal heads.

8. Trauma to the forefoot that leaves it unsalvageable.

9. Congenital deformities – polydactyly and macrodactyly.

10. Tumors both benign and malignant.

Surgical Procedure:

Regardless of whether an equinus is present, the first step in a transmetatarsal amputation is to do an Achilles tenotomy through a stab incision. Different authorities differ on advocating a tendo-Achilles lengthening versus an Achilles tenotomy; the CSPM surgery department faculty prefers the tenotomy. This is done to try and prevent the development of an equinus and ultimately stump ulcers.

The dorsal incision for the transmetatarsal amputation is a slightly curving transverse incision approximately 1 cm distal to the level of the intended bone cuts. The incision is extended distally medially and laterally at approximately the midshaft point of the first and fifth metatarsals in the sagittal plane and then connected with a slightly curving transverse incision on the plantar aspect of the foot, thus creating a plantar flap (Fig. 11-22 A-C). The incisions are made skin to bone with no dissection by layers. The distal foot is grabbed with a traumatic clamp for manipulation. Dorsally the soft tissues are dissected off of the metatarsals giving enough exposure for the bone cuts. The bone cuts are made with either a power oscillating or sagittal saw, and done in a way to create a smooth metatarsal parabola. All of the bone cuts are done with a dorsal distal to plantar proximal bevel at no particular angle. Additionally, the first and fifth metatarsals need to be rounded at the medial and lateral sides of the foot: the bevel on the first is from dorsal, distal, and medial to plantar, proximal, and lateral, and the

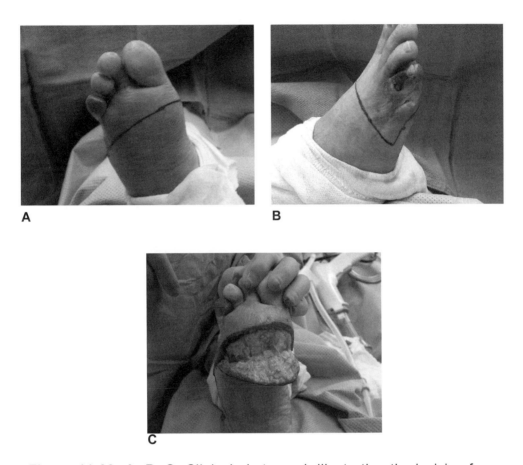

Figure 11-22: A, B, C: Clinical photograph illustrating the incision for a transmetatarsal amputation that creates a plantar flap.

bevel on the fifth is from dorsal, distal, and lateral to plantar, proximal, and medial. Once the bone cuts are complete, the dorsal distal foot is pulled up proximally and the soft tissue is dissected sharply off the metatarsals plantarly until the distal foot is disarticulated. This leaves a full thickness plantar flap. If there is an ulcer in the plantar flap, it can be excised with a "V" cut, and at closure it will create a "T" (Fig. 11-23 A, B). Any tendons in the flap are pulled distally, transected sharply, and allowed to retract proximally. The surgical site is inspected for any large lumens particularly looking for the dorsalis pedis artery, and they are ligated. Any small bleeders are

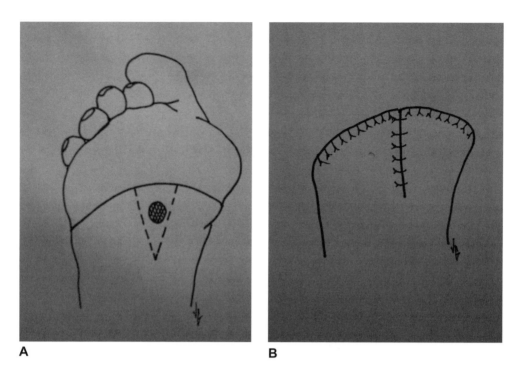

A   **B**

Figure 11-23: A: Drawing illustrates the utilization of a "V" cut in the plantar flap in order to excise an ulcer and allow primary closure. **B:** Drawing illustrates the primary closure of plantar flap with "V" cut to excise an ulcer in a transmetatarsal amputation.

cauterized. The surgical site is then irrigated with a high pressure lavage of at least 3 liters of fluid. The routine of the CSPM surgery department faculty is to use two 3 liter bags with the pulsating jet lavage. At this point outside gloves are removed, new drapes are put in place, and all previous instrumentation is no longer used. If the amputation was for an infection, the gram stain and culture and sensitivity specimens are collected at this time from the deep tissue. Any remodeling of the flap can be done at this time. If a drain is to be used it is put in place and must exit through a separate stab incision proximal to the amputation incision. The CSPM surgery department faculty does not usually use a drain. There are no deep or subcutaneous sutures used in closure, and the closure is completed with 3-0 or 4-0 monofilament suture. To reduce any wound tension and complete some deep closure to eliminate dead space, several retention stitches are used. The closure is completed with simple interrupted sutures in between the retention sutures (Fig. 11-24 A, B). A large and bulky compression dressing is applied and the foot is placed in a posterior splint.

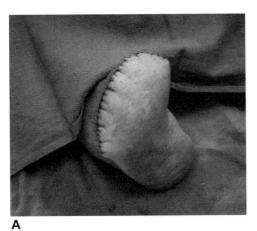 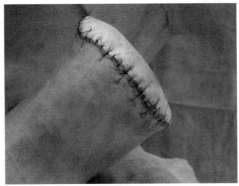

A   **B**

Figure 11-24: A, B: Clinical photograph showing the closure of a transmetatarsal amputation.

Postoperative Management:

1. Immediate postoperative X-rays (Fig. 11-25).

2. Patient will be non-weight bearing for three weeks or until sutures are removed.

3. Antibiotics are continued for two weeks if the amputation was for an infection.

4. Dressing change at one week to evaluate for purulence of the wound. If the wound is purulent, the sutures are removed, the wound is irrigated, and the patient started on daily dressing changes.

5. Suture removal occurs at three weeks if nothing untoward has occurred.

6. The patient is placed in a postoperative shoe at three weeks and made partial weight bearing.

7. At six weeks the patient is sent to a pedorthist to fashion a shoe filler that can go in the patient's regular shoes.

Complications:

1. Wound dehiscence and further spread of infection.

2. Equinus deformity of the foot resulting in stump ulceration.

3. Necrotic non-healing wound.

4. The need for an amputation at a higher level.

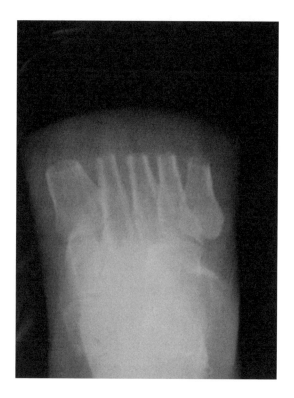

Figure 11-25: Postoperative X-ray of a transmetatarsal amputation.

Clinical Pearls:

1. The Achilles tenotomy will prevent any undue pressure on the distal stump and prevent the most significant problem of an equinus developing postoperatively.

2. Refer to the clinical pearls under digital amputations.

References:

Baumgartner R, Wetz HH. Forefoot Amputation. *Orthopaedics and Traumatology* 1:68-77, 1992.

Bowker JH, SanGiovanni TP. Minor and major lower limb amputation in persons with diabetes mellitus. The Diabetic Foot. 6th Ed. Bowker J, Pheifer M., Ed., Mosby, Inc., Philadelphia, Pa., 2001.

DeCotiis MA. Lisfranc and Chopart Amputations. *Clinics in Podiatric Medicine and Surgery* 22:385-393, 2005.

Dolce MD, Baruch K, Adamov DJ. The use of the distal Syme's procedure for treating onychopathy. *Clinics in Podiatric Medicine and Surgery* 21:689-697, 2004.

Early JS. Transmetatarsal and Midfoot Amputations. *Clinical Orthopaedics and Related Research* 361:85-90, 1999.

Freeman GJ, Mackie KM, Sare J, Walsh AKM, Pherwani AD. A Novel Approach to the Management of the Diabetic Foot: Metatarsal Excision in the Treatment of Osteomyelitis. *Eur J Vasc Endovasc Surg* 33:217-219, 2007.

Funk C, Young G. Subtotal Pedal amputations Biomechanical and Intraoperative Considerations. *JAPMA* 91:6-11, 2001.

Nguyen TH, Gordon IL, Whalen D, Wilson S. Transmetatarsal Amputation:Predictors of Healing. *The American Surgeon* 72:973-977, 2006.

Ohsawa S, Inamori Y, Fukuda K. Lower limb amputation for diabetic foot. *Arch Orthop Trauma Surg* 121:186-190, 2001.

Philbin TM, Berlet GC, Lee TH. Lower-Extremity Amputations in Association with Diabetes Mellitus. *Foot and Ankle Clinics* 11:791-804, 2006.

Pinzur MS, Gottschalk FA, Guedes de S. Pinto MA, Smith DG. Controversies in Lower-Extremity Amputation. *The Journal of Bone & Joint Surgery* 89A:1118-1127, 2007.

Pulla RJ, Kaminsky KM. Toe Amputations and Ray Resections. *Clinics in Podiatric Medicine and Surgery* 14:691-739, 1997.

Sage RA. Limb Salvage and Amputations. McGlamry's Comprehensive Textbook of Foot and Ankle Surgery 3rd Ed. Banks A, Downey M, Martin D, Miller S., Eds., Lippincott Williams & Wilkins, Philadelphia, Pa., 2001.

Smith DG, Assai M, Reiber GE, Vath C, LeMaster J, Wallace C. Minor environmental trauma and lower extremity amputation in high-risk patients with diabetes: incidence, pivotal events, etiology, and amputation level in a prospectively followed cohort. *Foot and Ankle International* 24:690-695, 2003.

Wagner FW. Lower-Extremity Amputations. The High Risk Foot in Diabetes. Frykberg R, Ed., Churchill Livingstone, New York, NY, 1991.

Wallace GF, Stapleton JJ. Transmetatarsal Amputations. *Clinics in Podiatric Medicine and Surgery* 22:365-384, 2005.

Wheelock FC, Rowbotham JL, Hoar CS. Amputations. Management of Diabetic Foot Problems Kozak G, Hoar C, Rowbotham J, Wheelock F, Gibbons G, Campbell D, Eds., WB Saunders, Philadelphia, Pa., 1984.

Congenital Deformities of the Forefoot   **12**

Albert E. Burns, DPM, FACFAS

Polydactyly

Introduction:

Polydactyly is the most common congenital deformity of the hand and the foot, and in the foot it accounts for 45 percent of all congenital deformities. It is defined as the presence of one or more supernumerary digits with or without accompanying metatarsals of the feet or metacarpals of the hand. The pattern of inheritance of simple polydactyly is autosomal dominant with incomplete penetrance. No gender predilection has been identified, and it involves the foot bilaterally in 25 to 50 percent of the reported cases. The reported incidence has ranged from 0.3-13.9 cases per 1,000 births with higher rates in blacks and Asians than whites.

Polydactyly is classified in accordance to its location and degree of duplication completeness. The most common classification is that of Temtamy and McKusick, who initially defined it as preaxial, referring to the tibial or radial side of a line bisecting the second ray or long finger, respectively, and postaxial, referring to the fibular and ulnar sides of the respective lines. This classification has come to be modified as *preaxial*, referring to the duplication of the hallux (Fig. 12-1); *postaxial,* referring to the duplication of the most lateral ray; and *central,* referring to duplication of the second, third, and fourth rays (Fig. 12-2). Since the condition occurs simultaneously in the hands and feet in one-third of the known cases, it is also referred to as crossed polydactyly. In crossed polydactyly, there is either preaxial or postaxial polydactyly of the hands and the opposite presentation in the feet. Mixed polydactyly is the presence of both preaxial and postaxial polydactyly of the same extremity.

Postaxial polydactyly accounts for 79 to 86 percent of all of the polydactyly seen in the hands and the feet, and so there has been additional sub-categorization of this entity. Temtamy and McKusick subcategorized it into either Type A or Type B. Type A is a fully developed extra digit articulating with either the fifth metatarsal or metacarpal (Fig. 12-3), and Type B is an accessory digit devoid of osseous components. The Venn-Watson classification of postaxial polydactyly describes five specific morphologic patterns based on the degree of metatarsal duplication. There is soft tissue duplication only, a wide metatarsal head (Fig. 12-4), a T-metatarsal, a Y-metatarsal (Fig. 12-5), and complete duplication of the fifth metatarsal.

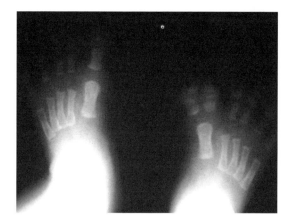

Figure 12-1: An X-ray of preaxial polydactyly showing duplication of the phalanges but within a common soft tissue envelop and no duplication of the metatarsal.

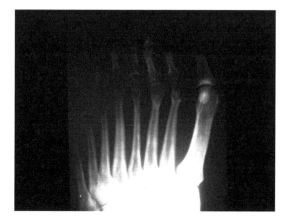

Figure 12-2: An X-ray of combined central and postaxial polydactyly with complete duplication of all of the involved metatarsals.

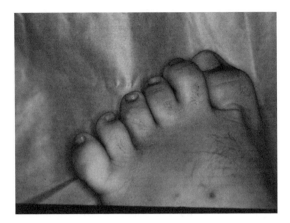

Figure 12-3: Clinical photograph of postaxial polydactyly with complete duplication into a fifth and sixth digits.

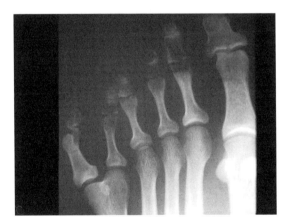

Figure 12-4: An X-ray of postaxial polydactyly with partial duplication of the fifth metatarsal in the form of a wide metatarsal head.

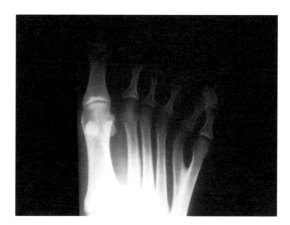

Figure 12-5: An X-ray of postaxial polydactyly with partial duplication of the fifth metatarsal in the form of a "Y" metatarsal.

Treatment:

The primary treatment for polydactyly is surgical removal. Shoe fitting and functional difficulties can be prognosticated, and removal of the extra digit or digits for psychological and cosmetic reasons is indicated. The most appropriate time for surgical intervention has varied opinions. It has been recommended that a rudimentary postaxial digit be tied off with ligature in the nursery. Other recommendations for removal have ranged from four months to 13 years. The decision of which digit to ablate, however, depends at least in part on the radiographic assessment of the development of the phalanges and metatarsals, so waiting until at least one year of age seems preferred. Additionally, since anesthesia is better tolerated after one year and adequate osseous development may not be complete until two to three years of age, it may be even more prudent to wait until then.

There are some general surgical tenets, which are used as guidelines for the surgical ablation of these supernumerary digits:

1. Remove the most peripheral digit – This would apply to preaxial and postaxial polydactyly and it facilitates the contouring of the foot.

2. Remove the most rudimentary digit – This rule can come into conflict with the first rule in preaxial and postaxial polydactyly and would take precedence over the first rule (Fig. 12-6). This may result in a gap between toes that will require another procedure such as a metatarsal osteotomy in order to properly contour the foot or to create an adequate cosmetic and functional result.

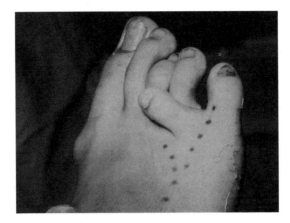

Figure 12-6: Clinical photograph of postaxial polydactyly where the most rudimentary digit is the fifth digit and is, therefore, the one that needs to be removed. This would require the addition of an osteotomy to the sixth metatarsal in order to bring the fourth and sixth digits into proper juxtaposition.

3. Ablate the duplicated part of the metatarsal.
4. Preserve and reattach tendons, ligaments, and capsules as needed to preserve function and reduce complications.
5. Resection through a physis will not cause growth disturbance.
6. Passing a smooth K-wire through the physis will not cause growth disturbance.

Surgical Procedures:

Preaxial Polydactyly – With partial duplication of the distal phalanx or of the distal and proximal phalanges within a common soft tissue envelope, it is the medial side that is usually ablated using a lenticular incision to remove the redundant osseous elements. Care must be taken to either preserve the attachment of the abductor hallucis tendon or to reattach it to the remaining phalanges. In complete duplication, the most medial digit is the one that is most often removed. This is accomplished with a racquet type incision, which allows for the removal of the redundant metatarsal. Unlike the guillotine type of incision utilized in gangrenous amputations, preaxial polydactyly requires more emphasis on restoring normal tendon and ligament relationships to correct this deformity. If the tibial hallux is removed, the abductor hallucis must be reattached to the remaining phalanx in addition to capsular repair in order to avoid the development of a hallux abductovalgus deformity. If the fibular hallux is to be removed, the incision is lenticular in the same fashion as for the central digits. In this situation, dissection would again be done in layers and the adductor hallucis reinserted into the remaining phalanx to avoid the development of a hallux varus deformity. Removing the fibular hallux would also leave a gap between the medial hallux and the digit of the second ray, and, therefore, require an osteotomy of the first metatarsal to move the hallux to an abutting position with the second digit. If an osteotomy is performed, it is fixed with a single K-wire. Deep closure is accomplished with 3-0 and/or 4-0 absorbable suture, and the skin closure is completed with 4-0 or 5-0 monofilament non-absorbable suture.

Central Ray Polydactyly - The most common duplication of the central rays involves the second digit, and the most common presentation is duplication of the distal phalanx or duplication of the distal and middle phalanges within a common soft tissue envelope. The most hypoplastic osseous elements are removed through a lenticular incision in a guillotine fashion. When there is complete duplication of central digit with either partial or complete duplication of the metatarsal a partial ray resection is performed. The purpose of central ray resections is to narrow the foot to normal width so that regular shoes may be worn. This is done through a lenticular incision and the metatarsal is resected somewhere in its middle third. Although it has been described to repair the deep transverse metatarsal ligament in order to close the gap created with the ray resection, it is really not necessary. Deep closure is accomplished with 3-0 and/or 4-0 absorbable suture, and the skin closure is complete with 4-0 or 5-0 monofilament non-absorbable suture.

Postaxial Polydactyly – Duplication of the fifth digit with some degree of duplication of the fifth metatarsal is the most frequent congenital disorder observed in the foot. If the duplication involves one or all of the phalanges within a common soft tissue envelope, the ablation is accomplished with the same technique described for the central digits, with the most peripheral phalanges usually being the ones to be removed (Fig. 12-7). With complete duplication of the digit into a fifth and sixth digit and variable duplication of the fifth metatarsal, the toe that has a radiographically dominant metatarsus should be retained. If the most peripheral or sixth digit is to be removed, it is done through a racquet type incision in a guillotine fashion (Fig. 12-8). There is no need to reattach tendons as there is in preaxial duplication. The duplicated metatarsal is removed with a power saw, taking care not to injure the articular surfaces of the fifth metatarsophalangeal joint (Fig. 12-9). If the fifth digit is to be removed, it is done through a lenticular incision as described for central ray ablation (Fig. 12-10). The redundant fifth metatarsal is removed with a power saw, protecting the sixth metatarsophalangeal joint. This will leave a gap between the fourth and sixth digits and require an osteotomy of the sixth metatarsal to move it medially and create abutment between the fourth and sixth digits (Fig.12-11 A, B). The level of the osteotomy will depend how wide the gap is, and the osteotomy is fixed with a K-wire that can cross the physis. Deep closure is accomplished with 3-0 and/or 4-0 absorbable suture, and skin closure is completed with 4-0 or 5-0 monofilament non-absorbable suture (Fig. 12-12).

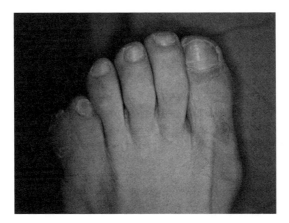

Figure 12-7: Clinical photograph of postaxial polydactyly with duplication of the phalanges within a common soft tissue envelope. The most peripheral or lateral phalanges would be the ones ablated.

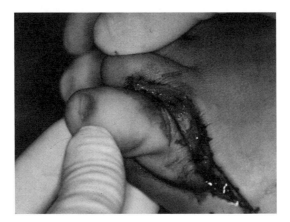

Figure 12-8: Intraoperative photograph showing the racquet incision to remove the sixth digit and the duplicated part of the fifth metatarsal.

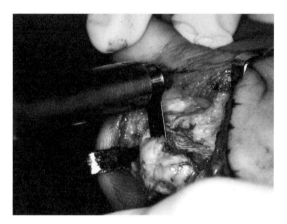

Figure 12-9: Intraoperative photograph illustrating the use of a power saw to remove the duplicated part of the metatarsal.

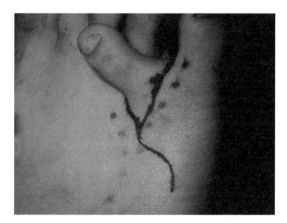

Figure 12-10: Intraoperative photograph illustrating a lenticular incision used to remove the fifth digit. The incision is modified slightly in a serpentine fashion proximally to allow easier access to the metatarsal for the osteotomy.

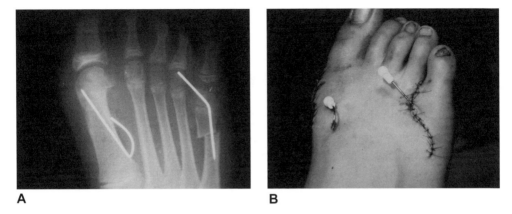

A   **B**

Figure 12-11: A: Postoperative X-ray showing ablation of the fifth digit and metatarsal osteotomy with fixation in order to abut the fourth and sixth digits. **B:** Postoperative clinical photograph illustrating ablation of the fifth digit in postaxial polydactyly and abutment of the fourth and sixth digits after osteotomy of the metatarsal.

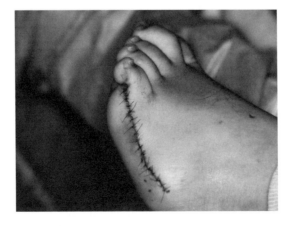

Figure 12-12: Clinical photograph showing closure of postaxial sixth digit ablation and creation of a normal contour to the foot.

Postoperative Management:

1. Immediate postoperative X-rays.

2. For medial and lateral peripheral ablations where there is no plantar incision, the patient can be ambulatory in a postoperative shoe. In central ray resections or where there are plantar incisions, the patient is made non-weight bearing in a posterior splint.

3. The patient returns to the office in one week for a dressing change to evaluate for infection.

4. Suture removal is at two to three weeks postoperatively.

5. After suture removal the patient can be progressed to weight bearing status unless an osteotomy was performed, then the weight bearing status will be determined by the radiographic evaluation of the healing of the osteotomy.

Inherent Complications:

1. Residual bone or soft tissue as a result of inadequate ablation.

2. Wound dehiscence due to excessive tension being placed on the ablation incision.

3. Hallux abductovalgus secondary to failure to reattach or inadequate tension of reattachment of abductor hallucis tendon.

4. Hallux varus secondary to failure to reattach adductor hallucis.

5. Development of plantar callosities due to malposition of osteotomies.

6. Pin track infection.

Clinical Pearls:

1. Preaxial dissection should be done in layers in order to facilitate reattachment of the tendons and ligaments.

2. Central and postaxial dissection should be done in a guillotine fashion since reattachment of tendons and ligaments are not necessary.

3. Reattachment of the deep transverse metatarsal ligament is not necessary in central ray ablations.

4. Flaps for amputations can be modified, so err to have too much flap rather than not enough, which would put excessive tension on the incision and compromise its vascularity.

5. Use a compression dressing in order to prevent hematoma and edema which may compromise your result.

6. Preserve the most normal digit.

7. There is no problem with either passing a pin across physis or bone resection through the physis.

Syndactyly

Introduction:

Syndactyly is a congenital or acquired deformity in which webbing persists between adjacent digits. It is a frequently encountered congenital anomaly that most often involves the second and third digit, and it may either be unilateral or bilateral with equal distribution between males and females. It is ten times more common in Caucasians than any other race and occurs in one of every 2,500 to 3,000 births. There are two classical ways in which it is classified: the Davis and German classification and the phenotypic classification.

The Davis and German classification:
Incomplete – webbing does not extend to the distal end of the toes
Complete – webbing extends to the distal end of the toes
Simple – a soft tissue connection alone exists
Complicated – the phalanges are abnormal in size, shape, number, or arrangement

Isolated syndactyly is divided into five phenotypic types that are all inherited as autosomal dominant disorders:

Type I Zygodactyly – Syndactyly of the third and fourth fingers and webbing between the second and third toes.

Type II Synpolydactyly–Syndactyly of the third and fourth fingers with polydactyly of the fourth finger and webbing of the fourth and fifth digits and polydactyly of the fifth digit.

Type III – Syndactyly of the fourth and fifth fingers and no involvement of the foot.

Type IV – Complete syndactyly of all the fingers and no foot involvement.

Type V – Syndactyly with metacarpal and metatarsal fusions.

Treatment:

Syndactyly of the foot is most often managed conservatively, because there is generally no functional implication and is more of a cosmetic problem. In the hand, the disability and functional loss is a primary indication for surgical intervention, but the lack of disability or functional loss in the foot and cosmesis that is not considered objectionable have led many to advocate that no treatment is necessary. Others suggest, however, that reconstruction of the toes may be indicated for cosmetic and psychological reasons. Conversely, synpolydactyly can cause a functional problem, resulting in shoe fitting problems and painful irritation due to a widened foot; surgical correction of this is well accepted. If surgical intervention is recommended, the surgeon typically waits until the child is at least eighteen months old; usually, the surgery is done between two and four years of age. Others have recommended surgical correction as early as six months of age.

Surgical Procedures:

Surgical desyndactylization of the toes is accomplished with flaps, grafts, or tissue expansion. Skin grafts have been used solely to cover the deficit created in separation of the toes or in conjunction with flaps when the flaps are incapable of covering the entire deficit. Full thickness skin grafts are recommended because split thickness grafts are more likely to contract. The graft is typically taken from the skin overlying the sinus tarsi. The disadvantages of donor site morbidity, pigmentation mismatch, and contracture and sloughing of the graft has resulted in surgeons avoiding their use. Tissue expansion is a substitute for skin grafting, but it requires staged operations and its long-term result is not clear.

To avoid skin grafts, various local flap techniques have been reported, and the two most prevalent are the dorsal rectangular flap and the dorsal or plantar pentagonal subcutaneous pedicled advancement flap. The use of the dorsal rectangular flap and simultaneous full-thickness skin graft has been the primary operative technique for syndactyly of the foot, but in order to avoid the use of the graft, a modification of the technique has included dorsal and plantar zigzag incisions, creating triangular flaps to cover the medial and lateral aspects of the desyndactylized toes. The apices of the triangular flaps extend to the midline of the phalanges with a flap angle of 45 to 60 degrees. All of the flaps are raised in a full-thickness fashion with minimal fat. Geometrically, this technique does not provide enough skin coverage without putting the flaps under tension and increasing the likelihood of vascular compromise, flap sloughing and contracture. A third alternative that has been advocated, therefore, is to use the rectangular flap to create the web and allow the remaining defects on the medial and lateral aspects of the effected toes to epithelialize spontaneously.

Another alternative to this, which allows primary closure with the initial surgical intervention, is the use of a dorsal or plantar pentagonal pedicled flap with the previously described dorsal and plantar triangular flaps (Fig. 12-13). The proximal pentagonal island flap is raised with the underlying subcutaneous tissue as a pedicle, allowing it to be used as a local advancement flap with a soft tissue pedicle. The deficit created by the pentagonal advancement flap is closed primarily, and the advancement flap itself is used to create the dorsal to plantar web. The remainder of the medial and lateral soft tissue deficit of the two effected toes is closed primarily with the dorsal and plantar triangular flaps.

In contrast to simple syndactyly, polysyndactyly can present with both a functional problem, causing issues with shoe fitting because of a widened forefoot, and a cosmetic problem. The fourth, fifth, and sixth digit are all contained within one soft tissue envelope. In most cases the problem is resolved by ablating the sixth digit and any duplication of the fifth metatarsal. There is more than enough skin flap coverage available with the removal of the osseous structures. Rarely there is partial webbing between the fourth and fifth digit and underdevelopment of the fifth digit. The previously described rectangular flap can be used to create a web between the fourth and sixth digit with medial and lateral rectangular flaps on the digits to cover the deficit created by the removal of the fifth digit. Again the redundant part of the fifth metatarsal would be removed and individual evaluation is needed to determine if an osteotomy is necessary in order to bring the fourth and sixth digit into proper juxtaposition to each other.

Postoperative Management:

1. A compression dressing is applied to any flaps or grafts.

2. If epithelialization is used, weekly dressing changes with a non-adherent dressing material is continued until coverage is complete.

3. If pins are used they are usually pulled at four weeks.

4. The child is allowed to be weight bearing, though some prefer to keep the patient non-weight bearing until the sutures and pins are removed.

5. Sutures are removed at two to three weeks.

6. After suture removal the child can progressed to activities of daily life unless an osteotomy was performed, then progression is based on radiographic evaluation of healing of the osteotomy.

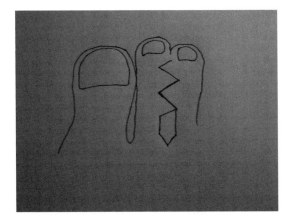

Figure 12-13: Drawing illustrating the use of a dorsal pentagonal pedicled flap with dorsal and plantar triangular flaps that allows primary closure in desyndactylization of adjacent digits.

Inherent Complications:

1. Creeping of the web resulting in a partial or even complete recurrence of the syndactyly.

2. Contracture resulting in structural or angulational deformity.

3. Hypertrophic scar formation or even the development of keloids.

4. Pigmentation and/or hairy mismatch if a skin graft is used.

5. Donor site morbidity if a skin graft is used.

6. Increased risk of infection if there are wounds left open or pin track infections when pins are used.

7. Flap and graft necrosis.

Clinical Pearls:

1. This is primarily a cosmetic problem that can result in both a worse cosmetic result and additional functional disability from surgical intervention, so parents should be completely counseled on the non-necessity of surgical correction.

2. As with any ablation, all of the previous pearls described should be followed.

3. Because of the high likelihood of contracture, the use of pins to maintain digital position is encouraged.

Macrodactyly

Introduction:

Macrodactyly is a rare congenital deformity of unknown origin that results in the enlargement of one or more digits of the hands and/or the feet. There is enlargement of the elements of the affected part including the bones, nerves, subcutaneous fat, nails and skin. The tendons and the blood vessels appear to be unaffected. The etiology of macrodactyly is unknown, but the most consistent pathological feature is the excessive accumulation of fibro-fatty tissue. Particularly there is an unusual increase in nerve size due to the infiltration with fatty tissue. In the foot, some combination of the first, second, or third toe involvement is almost invariable, with the second toe most commonly affected (Fig. 12-14). Increase in the length and breadth of the phalanges of the affected digit is an integral feature of macrodactyly, but metatarsal bone involvement is more variable (Fig. 12-15). Additionally, partial hypertrophy of the affected digit where only one side of the digit or just the distal end of the digit is involved can occur. There is never a presentation with midsection hypertrophy, and it involves males and females equally with no racial preference. There are two general

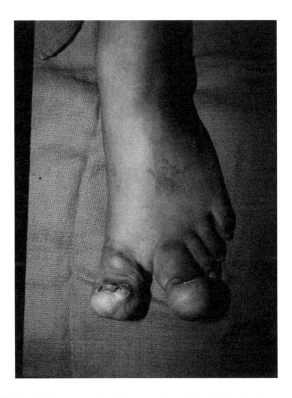

Figure 12-14: Clinical photograph of macrodactyly of the hallux and second digit.

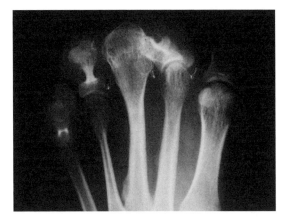

Figure 12-15: An X-ray of macrodactyly that affected the second, third and fourth digits with involvement of the metatarsal heads.

forms or classification of macrodactyly: static and progressive. In static macrodactyly or macrodactyly simplex congenita the enlargement is present at birth and the growth rate of the digit is proportional to the growth of the patient. In progressive macrodactyly or macrodystrophia lipomatosis progressiva, there is a disproportionately faster growth rate of the involved digit or digits until puberty. In progressive macrodactyly, there is the further complication of overgrowth of fatty tissue into the dorsum and plantar aspects of the foot.

Treatment:

Macrodactyly is primarily treated with surgery. The goal of surgery is to obtain a pain-free reasonably cosmetic plantigrade foot that fits into a regular shoe that is the same size as the contralateral foot. The deformities are managed by amputations of varying extent, combined with the removal of as much of the fibro-fatty tissue as possible. Digital amputation, ray resection, partial resection of phalanges together with soft tissue debulking, plastic shortening of the digit preserving the nail, and epiphysiodesis have all been recommended surgical approaches for macrodactyly. The choice of procedure, however, depends on both the classification of macrodactyly and the digit involved.

Three methods that simply don't have application in the foot are digital amputations, plastic shortening with preservation of the nail and epiphysiodesis. Digital amputation for the lesser toes is not only unappealing cosmetically, but it is not effective in addressing the enlargement of the forefoot. Ray resection results in the best cosmetic and functional outcomes in feet with involvement of the lesser toes. Because of the substantial contribution of the hallux and first metatarsal to weight bearing and gait, resection should be avoided altogether and treated with partial ablation and debulking procedures. Plastic reduction with preservation of the nail is a procedure that should be reserved for macrodactyly of the fingers. The procedure involves saving the nail and one-third of the dorsal side of the terminal phalanx and transposing it proximally, after an appropriate amount of the proximal phalanges are resected, and at the same time the necessary soft tissue debulking is accomplished. This will create a skin bulge, which is excised at a later date in a second operation. Vascular compromise is the primary concern in any macrodactyly surgery, and the increased dissection in this technique increases that risk for a cosmetic result that is not warranted in the foot. Epiphysiodesis can only shorten the toe and doesn't address the bulk. It is also not possible to calculate the timing of this procedure to have consistent length reduction.

Surgical Procedures:

Ray resection – A ray resection is indicated with either static or progressive macrodactyly when there is metatarsal involvement of the lesser digits. It would also be indicated in progressive macrodactyly of the lesser digits even without metatarsal involvement. It would also be considered as an alternative to a shortening and debulking procedure of the lesser digits in static macrodactyly. The incisional approach for an isolated ray resection of one of the internal digits is with converging semielliptical incisions fashioned around the base of the toe involved that come to an apex both dorsally and plantarly. The incisional approach for the fifth ray is with a racquet incision that extends back proximally dorsolaterally a sufficient distance to resect the necessary amount of the fifth metatarsal. The incision is perpendicular to the skin and is carried from skin to bone with no dissection by layers and no compression of the proximal skin edges with instruments. The bone is cut at some point in the middle one-third of the involved metatarsal and the ray is excised in toto. There is no exact angle of the bone cut but the internal metatarsals should have a bevel from dorsal distal to plantar proximal and the fifth metatarsal should be beveled from dorsal, distal and lateral to plantar, proximal, and medial. The bone edges can be further contoured with a rongeur in order to avoid any sharp edges. The surgical site is lavaged and deep closure is accomplished with 3-0 and/or 4-0 absorbable suture and skin closure is accomplished 4-0 or 5-0 monofilament suture. A compression dressing is applied to the foot. If multiple digits are involved then this would be an indication for a transmetatarsal amputation or an amputation of all the lesser digits with salvage of the hallux (Fig. 12-16 A, B, C).

Shortening and debulking procedure – Shortening and debulking procedures would be indicated in static macrodactyly of the lesser digits, when there is no metatarsal involvement. It would also be indicated in macrodactyly involving the first ray. This is a procedure that is done in stages. First the digit is reduced in length with ablation at the appropriate level (Fig. 12-17 A, B). This would usually involve disarticulation at the distal interphalangeal joint of the lesser digits or the interphalangeal joint of the hallux, or it would involve resection through the intermediate phalanx of the lesser digits or the proximal phalanx of the hallux. The level of the ablation would determine if any tendons need to be reattached as well as the need to arthrodese any remaining interphalangeal joint. After an interval of three months, the debulking of the soft tissue and possibly the reduction of the girth of the remaining bone can be completed in one or more stages (Fig. 12-18). The de-fatting is accomplished with lenticular incisions placed between the neurovascular elements, maximally removing 10 percent to 20 percent of the tissue. If additional soft tissue reduction is needed, it is done in a third stage on the other side of the digit five to six weeks later. During any of the soft tissue steps, the girth of the phalanges can be reduced with power instrumentation or bone forceps. Closure of this procedure is completed in the same manner as described for ray amputations.

Postoperative Management:

1. Immediate postoperative X-rays.
2. For ray resections or transmetatarsal amputations the patient is placed in a non-weight bearing posterior splint for three weeks.

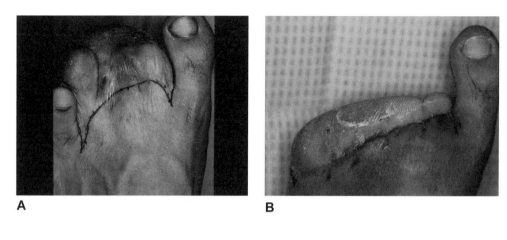

A

B

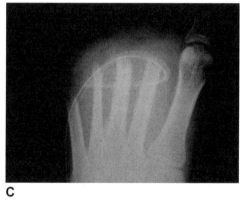

C

Figure 12-16: A: Preoperative clinical photograph of macrodactyly with metatarsal involvement of the second, third and fourth digits where a previous procedure had been performed in another country where the internal digits had been wired in a buckled position. **B:** Postoperative clinical photograph of a transmetatarsal amputation of macrodactyly of the internal digits with metatarsal involvement where the hallux has been preserved. **C:** Postoperative X-ray of a transmetatarsal amputation of macrodactyly of the internal digits with metatarsal involvement where the hallux has been preserved.

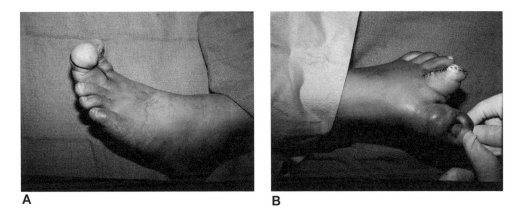

Figure 12-17: A: Preoperative clinical photograph of static macrodactyly of the hallux and second digit. **B:** Postoperative clinical photograph illustrating the first stage of correction with shortening of the second digit.

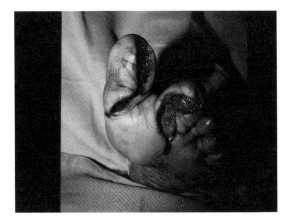

Figure 12-18: Intraoperative clinical photograph illustrating the debulking incisions for the reduction of the girth of both the hallux and second digit.

3. For the partial digital ablations and digital soft tissue debulking procedures, the patient can ambulate in a postoperative shoe.

4. The patient returns in one week for a dressing change and to evaluate for infection.

5. Suture removal at three weeks.

6. The patient will ambulate for the next one to three weeks in a postoperative shoe and then returns to normal shoe gear.

Complications:

1. Vascular compromise has a significant risk, since the vessels are not amongst the structures that are enlarged.

2. Subsequent regrowth of the fibro-fatty tissue due to inadequate de-fatting that results in further enlargement of the involved toe or of the bulk of the forefoot.

3. Toes that remain thick, heavy and non-cosmetic even after de-fatting.

4. Nerve entrapment or stump neuroma.

Clinical Pearls:

1. For single digit involvement, a ray resection is going to give the most functional, cosmetic, and predictable result, and it is the easiest to perform.

2. For multiple digit involvement that includes the hallux, a transmetatarsal amputation is the easiest to perform and gives the most predictable result without any of the complications associated with the reduction procedures.

3. For multiple digit involvement that does not include the hallux, salvaging the hallux and the first metatarsophalangeal joint will give the patient the most functional result.

4. For multiple digit involvement that does not involve the hallux but where there are degenerative changes of the first metatarsophalangeal joint, then preserving the hallux but fusing the first metatarsophalangeal joint will give the patient the most functional result.

5. If the size of the digit is so large as to dictate multiple debulking procedures, then ray resection is a better alternative.

Brachymetatarsia

Introduction:

Brachymetatarsia is defined as an abnormal shortening of a metatarsal or metatarsals. Quantitatively, it is considered brachymetatarsia when one metatarsal ends 5 mm or more proximal to the parabolic arc. It is due to a premature fusion or closure of the metatarsal physis. The exact etiology of the premature closure is unknown, but may be congenital, traumatic, iatrogenic, or environmental. It is associated with several disease processes, such as pseudohypoparathyroidism, pseudo-pseudohypoparathyroidism, poliomyelitis, malignancy, Down syndrome, Albright's hereditary osteodystrophy, diastrophic dysplasia, multiple epiphyseal dysplasia, myositis ossificans, and Turner syndrome. The first and fourth metatarsals are affected most commonly, and there is bilateral involvement in 72 percent of the congenital cases (Fig. 12-19). The incidence of brachymetatarsia is between 0.022 percent and 0.05 percent, and there is a female predominance of 25:1.

It does not appear at birth, and is rarely detectable until age five. The affected metatarsal is unable to bear weight, which results in transfer metatarsalgia and possible callus development under the adjacent metatarsals. The associated digit becomes displaced dorsally and is referred to as a "floating toe," which can be irritated by shoe gear. A skin cleft will develop under the involved metatarsophalangeal joint. Despite this most patients are asymptomatic and most often present with concerns of cosmetic appearance.

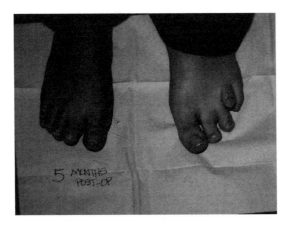

Figure 12-19: Clinical photograph of bilateral brachymetatarsia of the fourth ray. Postoperative correction of the right foot and preoperative condition of the left foot is illustrated.

Treatment:

Non-operative modalities should be used first in the treatment of brachymetatarsia. This would include callus debridement, metatarsal pads, orthotics and extra depth shoes. Controversy exists over whether cosmesis considerations justify surgical intervention. Although some investigators advocate surgical treatment only for painful deformity and transfer lesions, cosmesis is the most common indicator for surgical correction. Several procedures have been used to correct brachymetatarsia, including syndactylization, joint spacing implants, transpositional osteotomies, sliding osteotomies, osteotomies with bone grafting and callus distraction. Only two procedures should be considered to address this problem, however: a one stage lengthening with bone graft and callus distraction. One stage lengthening with bone graft needs a shorter period to bony union and has less morbidity, but it produces a proportionally smaller increase and more neurovascular complications than callus distraction. In evaluating a patient for the appropriate surgical approach, numerous variables must be assessed, including the number of rays affected, the amount of lengthening required, the possibility of combined adjacent metatarsal shortening and soft tissue contractures. It has been shown that the maximum amount of lengthening that can be achieved in one stage without causing neurovascular compromise is 15 mm, so a generally accepted guideline is to use the one stage interpositional bone graft technique when the lengthening required is less than 15 mm and to use the callus distraction technique when the lengthening required is 15 mm or greater. No matter which technique is used the maximum amount of length increase should not be more than 40 percent of the metatarsal length.

Surgical Procedures:

One stage interpositional bone graft lengthening – This procedure has been described as harvesting an autologous bone graft from the calcaneus, tibia, fibula, iliac crest, and from adjacent metatarsals when concomitant shortening of these metatarsals is part of the procedure. Using the adjacent metatarsals is recommended when possible, because it gives an appropriate size graft and eliminates creating a second donor surgical site. A dorsal longitudinal incision is made over the affected metatarsal and dissection by layers is completed. If there is significant skin contracture a Z-plasty incision may be used (Fig. 12-20). The periosteum is reflected sharply detaching the interosseous muscles to each side. It is not necessary to lengthen any of the soft tissue structures, if the planned length increase is less than 40 percent of the length of the metatarsal. An osteotomy with a power saw or corticotomy in the diaphyseal bone at approximately midshaft of the metatarsal is completed. A corticotomy is recommended to obviate any thermal necrosis of the bone from the saw. A 0.062 K-wire is passed distally through the metatarsal head, across the metatarsophalangeal joint, and through the toe crossing the interphalangeal joints. The wire is pulled out distally until it is flush with the resected metatarsal shaft. Passing the wire in this fashion will preclude subluxation of the toe when the lengthening is accomplished. In order to get maximum length and help avoid vascular spasm, the technique of gradually distracting the recipient site with a bone spreader over 20 to 30 minutes has been recommended. After the recipient site is completely prepared to accept the graft, the graft is harvested and transplanted immediately from the donor site to the recipient site (Fig. 12-21). The K-wire is retrograded through the graft into the base of the metatarsal or into tarsal bone and closure by layers is completed. If the graft was harvested from adjacent metatarsals, they are fixed with through and through wire, intramedullary K-wire, or crossed K-wires, and closure is accomplished (Fig. 12-22).

Callus distraction – The incisional approach and dissection is as it was described in the bone graft technique. The external fixator used is a unilateral device with 3 mm pins. For placement of the fixator it should be placed in the transverse plane for the peripheral metatarsals, at a 45 degree angle medially from the sagittal plane for the second metatarsal, and at a 45 degree angle laterally from the sagittal plane for third and fourth metatarsals (Fig. 12-23). Four pins are inserted into the metatarsal before the osteotomy or corticotomy is completed in order to have adequate stability (Fig. 12-24). Depending on the angle of placement of the device, the pins may need to be inserted percutaneously. After the first pin in inserted, the fixator is used as a guide to insert the remaining pins so that they are all parallel. An osteotomy or corticotomy is completed between the second and third pins, and an additional K-wire is passed across the metatarsophalangeal joint to prevent subluxation once the distraction starts (Fig. 12-25). Closure is completed in layers and a compression dressing is applied. Distraction is started at the seventh to tenth day postoperatively at a rate of 0.5-1.0 mm per day. This is done with a distraction of .25 mm every 12 or every six hours, which is a quarter turn of the fixator, until the desired length is achieved.

Postoperative Management:

1. Intraoperative X-rays or fluoroscopy is obtained to verify graft placement and alignment or device placement and alignment.

2. For the bone graft technique the patient is placed in a non-weight bearing posterior splint or below the knee cast. For the callus distraction technique, the patient is allowed to be weight bearing in a postoperative shoe.

3. The patient returns in one week for dressing change and evaluation for infection.

4. The patient returns at two to three weeks postoperatively for suture removal.

5. After suture removal the callus distraction technique requires twice a day pin cleansing with hydrogen peroxide. Any external K-wires also require twice a day pin cleansing.

6. K-wires in the bone graft technique are pulled at six to eight weeks. K-wires stabilizing the metatarsophalangeal joints are pulled after the total length increase is achieved.

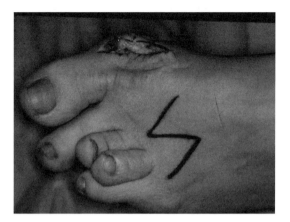

Figure 12-20: Clinical photograph of Z-plasty incision on the dorsum of the foot used to lengthen the contracture of the skin in a one-stage lengthening of the metatarsal or metatarsals.

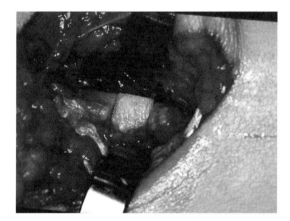

Figure 12-21: Intraoperative photograph of a graft harvested from adjacent metatarsals and fixed with an intramedullary K-wire.

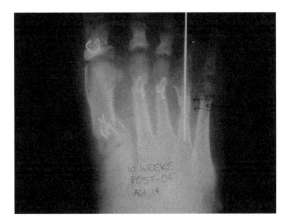

Figure 12-22: Postoperative X-ray illustrating concomitant lengthening of the brachymetatarsal and shortening of the adjacent metatarsals and utilization of bone graft from the adjacent metatarsals.

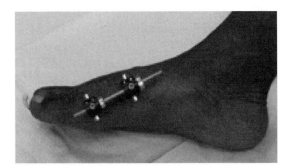

Figure 12-23: Postoperative clinical photograph of callus distraction of the first metatarsal with the external fixator applied in the transverse plane.

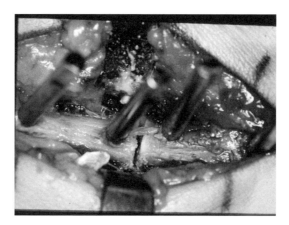

Figure 12-24: Intraoperative photograph illustrating the bone cut being placed between the second and third pins of the external fixation device.

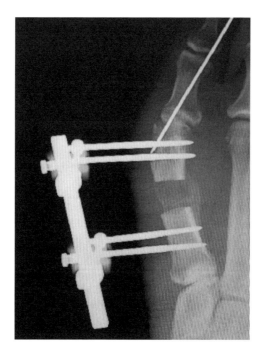

Figure 12-25: Postoperative X-ray of callus distraction technique of the first metatarsal illustrating healing bone and a K-wire passed across the metatarsophalangeal joint to prevent subluxation of that joint with the lengthening of metatarsal.

7. Serial radiographs are taken every two to three weeks to evaluate for bone graft incorporation or bone consolidation (Fig. 12-26 A, B).

8. The bone graft technique will require non-weight bearing for eight to 12 weeks.

9. With the callus distraction technique the device is left in place for twice the amount of time that it took to achieve the increased length of the metatarsal.

Complications:

1. Neurovascular compromise of the digit.

2. Subluxation of the metatarsophalangeal joint resulting in plantarflexion deformity of the digit.

3. Limitation of range of motion of the metatarsophalangeal joint.

4. Malunion with angulation of the metatarsal.

5. Donor site scar and pain.

6. Bone graft resorption or pseudarthrosis.

7. Pin track infections.

8. Fracturing of new bone.

9. Premature consolidation.

10. Delayed union or non-union.

11. Wire or pin breakage.

12. Hallux abductovalgus.

13. Inadequate length gain.

Clinical Pearls:

1. No matter how much lengthening is desired, a K-wire should be passed across the metatarsophalangeal joint in order to prevent subluxation.

2. External fixation may be used for any length increase, unlike the bone grafting technique, and the ability of the patient to be weight bearing with external fixation makes it the method of choice despite the concerns of dealing with the external apparatus.

3. Whenever a length of more than 40 percent increase in the length of the involved metatarsal is needed the procedure should be done in combination of shortening the other metatarsals.

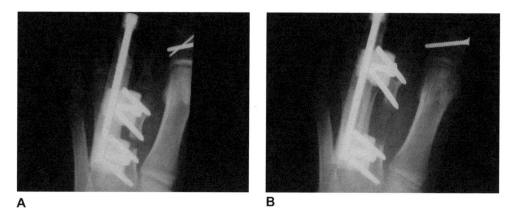

A   **B**

Figure 12-26: A: Early postoperative X-ray of callus distraction of the second metatarsal illustrating progressive lengthening and bone consolidation. **B:** Later postoperative X-ray of callus distraction of the second metatarsal illustrating further lengthening and bone consolidation.

Metatarsus Adductus

Introduction:

Metatarsus adductus is a positional or structural deformity where the metatarsals are medially deviated in the transverse plane in relation to the longitudinal axis of the lesser tarsus and the apex is at Lisfranc's joint. There has been inconsistency in the terminology used to describe this pathology in the past, but metatarsus adductus has become the accepted term for this isolated transverse plane deformity. Metatarsus adductus may also be one part of more complex multi-planar deformities such as metatarsus adductovarus, complex metatarsus adductus, talipes equinovarus, and cavoadductovarus. In metatarsus adductovarus or metatarsus varus, there is both a metatarsus adductus and a frontal plane varus of the metatarsus. Complex metatarsus adductus or skewfoot exists when an additional valgus deformity of the rearfoot occurs, creating a Z-foot where there is abduction of the lesser tarsus on the tarsus and adduction of the metatarsals on the lesser tarsus. Talipes equinovarus is the classic clubfoot where in addition to the metatarsus adductus, there is rearfoot varus and equinus. Cavoadductovarus is one of the manifestations of pes cavus where there is concomitant metatarsus adductus and rearfoot varus. The reported frequency is variable in the literature from 0.1 percent to 12 percent, and this is undoubtedly partially due to its association with other deformities such as those mentioned above and other lower extremity torsional abnormalities and even hip dysplasia. The identification of metatarsus adductus, therefore, mandates a complete musculoskeletal exam of the lower extremity. The etiology is still undetermined and examples of hereditary, intrauterine pressure and abnormal tendon insertions are replete in the literature. Part of the evaluation must, therefore, include a complete evaluation of muscle function.

Clinically, metatarsus adductus is commonly not recognized at birth and often not noted until one year of age, when the child starts to walk. The parents may describe how the child trips often, and the foot will appear "C" shaped with the convexity lateral and the concavity medially (Fig. 12-27). With the older child, the outer border of the foot can become callused and painful, there is medial breakdown of the shoes, and marked pronation of the foot as the child attempts to walk straight. Bisection of the heel and where that bisection passes in relation to the toes is used to determine the severity of the metatarsus adductus clinically. The adduction is also evaluated in terms of its flexibility or rigidity clinically as a way of prognosticating its amenability to conservative treatment. The clinical evaluation is done in conjunction with the radiographic evaluation. The metatarsus adductus angle is used specifically to quantitate the relationship of the metatarsals to the lesser tarsus. A metatarsus adductus angle of 15 degrees is considered normal for a rectus foot, and the severity of adduction is based on the deviance from this. A mild deformity is defined when the metatarsus adductus angle is 15 to 20 degrees, a moderate deformity when the angle is 21 to 25 degrees, and a severe deformity when the angle is greater than 25 degrees. Unfortunately, the lesser tarsus is radiographically silent in the infant and toddler, so it is not a measurable parameter. Two alternative methods of evaluating the deformity radiographically have been proposed. The first is to measure the angle formed by the lateral border of the calcaneus to the bisection of the second metatarsal (Fig. 12-28). This normally should be 15 plus or minus three degrees, but this actually measures forefoot adductus and not metatarsus adductus specifically, so the deformity could rest anywhere between the midtarsal joint and Lisfranc's joint. The second method is to determine the angle created by the bisection of the second metatarsal to the perpendicular to the line that connects the most proximal medial aspect of the first metatarsal to the most proximal lateral aspect of the fifth metatarsal (Fig. 12-29). The value of this angle should be 22 to 25 degrees at birth, 15 to 20 degrees in the toddler, and 15 degrees in the adult. Just as the evaluation for rearfoot deformity is done clinically, it should also be done radiographically. The anteroposterior talocalcaneal and cuboid abduction angles should be evaluated to determine if there is concomitant pronation of the rearfoot.

Treatment:

Mild foot deformities that are passively correctable generally do not need treatment, since they have a tendency to correct themselves spontaneously. Conservative treatment is through manipulation and serial casting. Reliable parents can be instructed in the technique of passive stretching and manipulation. The rearfoot is stabilized and simple continuous pulling on the forefoot will loosen it enough for

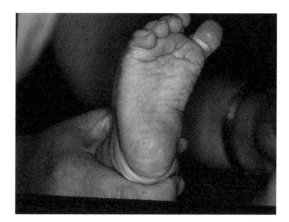

Figure 12-27: Clinical photograph illustrating the C-shaped deformity of the foot seen in metatarsus adductus.

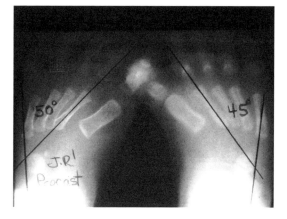

Figure 12-28: An X-ray illustrating a method of measuring the metatarsus adductus in an infant or a toddler using the angle created by the lateral border of the calcaneus to the bisection of the second metatarsal.

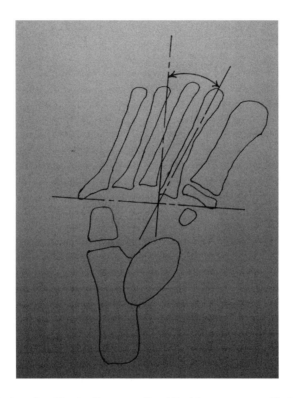

Figure 12-29: A drawing illustrating a method that is more specific to measuring the metatarsus adductus in the infant or toddler using the angle created by the bisection of the second metatarsal to the perpendicular to the line that connects the most proximal medial aspect of the first metatarsal to the most proximal lateral aspect of the fifth metatarsal.

manipulation. With one hand, the subtalar joint is stabilized and counterpressure is applied to the cuboid, and with the other hand, pressure is applied directly to the medial aspect of the first metatarsal head (Fig. 12-30). This would be done for 15 to 20 minutes a day for three to four weeks. Manipulation and serial plaster of paris casting has become the standard treatment in children with moderate and severe deformity. The manipulation is done as just described and a cast is applied to maintain the correction on a weekly basis in infants less than three months old and biweekly in children over three months of age (Fig. 12-31).

Surgical correction of metatarsus adductus is only advocated in the pediatric patient after two years of and following unsuccessful results with conservative treatment modalities. The Heyman, Herndon and Strong procedure, which is a complete tarsometatarsal soft tissue release, was the standard procedure, but high

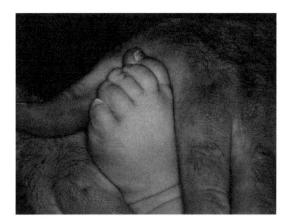

Figure 12-30: Clinical photograph illustrating the manipulation technique for treatment of metatarsus adductus.

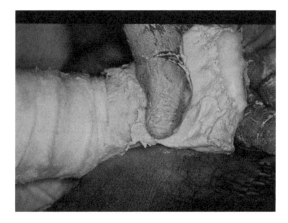

Figure 12-31: Clinical photograph illustrating application of the serial plaster cast technique for the treatment of metatarsus adductus.

failure rates and consistent postoperative fibrotic and stiff feet has resulted in not recommending this procedure. Instead, it has led to recommending continuation of conservative modalities until the child is four to five years old and then performing an osseous procedure. The model for the osseous procedures is metatarsal base osteotomies described by Berman and Gartland. Numerous modifications of this procedure in fashioning the osteotomies to provide greater stability and lend itself to ASIF fixation have been described. The technique described by Lepird has become the most accepted way of performing the procedure. Alternatively, a closing wedge osteotomy of the cuboid and third cuneiform and an opening wedge osteotomy of the medial and intermediate cuneiform that is used for the treatment of severe forefoot adductus could be used for severe metatarsus adductus.

Surgical Procedure:

Lepird procedure – Three dorsal longitudinal incisions are used for access to the five metatarsal bases. Each incision is approximately 3 to 4 cm in length with one dorsomedial over the base of the first metatarsal, one between the bases of the second and third metatarsals, and one between the bases of the fourth and fifth metatarsals. Dissection is by layers, and the bases of the metatarsals are exposed subperiosteally. Lepird originally described the procedure with oblique closing wedge osteotomies of the first and fifth metatarsals and oblique through and through osteotomies of the lesser metatarsals directed from dorsal proximal to plantar distal (Fig. 12-32). The osteotomy on the first metatarsal should be at least 6 mm distal to the proximal physis. The amount of bone removed from the first and fifth metatarsal would be based on the amount of correction desired. A described modification to the Lepird procedure is to employ the same type of osteotomy on the fifth metatarsal as the internal metatarsals. The problem with the oblique closing wedge osteotomy of the first metatarsal is that it does not provide sagittal plane stability and predetermines how much correction is to be achieved disallowing any adjustment intraoperatively. A further modification, therefore, is to perform the same osteotomy on the first as the rest of the metatarsals. This is the osteotomy described by Mau that goes from dorsal distal to plantar proximal and is approximately parallel to the weight bearing surface. This osteotomy has superior intrinsic stability because of the dorsal shelf that resists dorsal displacement forces, and it provides good bone apposition for fixation (Fig. 12-33 A, B). It is also simple to perform. The osteotomies have been described as being only partially completed, applying the fixation without compression, finishing the osteotomies and rotating the distal segments and then compressing the fixation. Pragmatically, this is not necessary and complicates the procedure. What further simplifies the technique is the use of the small 3.0 mm cannulated screws. The osteotomies are completed, the pins for all five screws are inserted, the forefoot is rotated to the desired position, and the screws are inserted securing the first and fifth metatarsals initially. Closure is by layers and a compression dressing is applied.

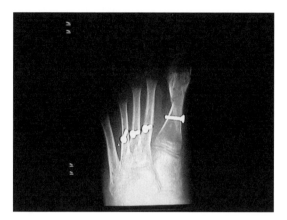

Figure 12-32: Postoperative X-ray illustrating the Lepird procedure where an oblique closing base wedge osteotomy of the first metatarsal was used.

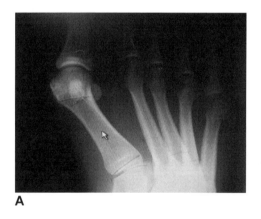

A

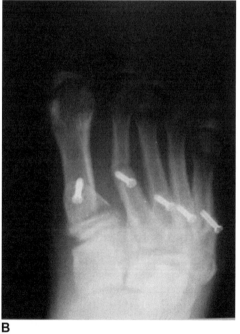

B

Figure 12-33: A: Preoperative X-ray of a metatarsus adductus foot where the Lepird procedure was used. **B:** Postoperative X-ray illustrating the Lepird procedure for correction of metatarsus adductus where the Mau osteotomy was used on all of the metatarsals.

Postoperative Management:

1. Intraoperative X-rays or fluoroscopy is used to verify correction and position of all osteotomies.

2. A below the knee non-weight bearing cast or posterior splint is used for six to eight weeks.

3. The patient returns at one week for dressing change and evaluation for infection.

4. The patient returns at two to three weeks for suture removal.

5. Serial radiographs are taken every two to three weeks to evaluate for osteotomy healing.

6. With radiographic evidence of healing osteotomies the patient is progressed to partial weight bearing in a postoperative shoe for two to three weeks and then progressed to full weight bearing in their regular shoes.

Complications:

1. Damage to the physis of the first metatarsal.

2. Shortening of a metatarsal resulting in a lack of weight bearing that could result in a floating toe and transfer metatarsalgia.

3. Elevation of a metatarsal either by performance of the osteotomy or premature weight bearing and the sequelae associated with lack of weight bearing.

4. Hallux varus or hallux valgus if the soft tissue structures are not adequately evaluated and addressed.

5. Undercorrection resulting in continued irritation and symptomatology and rearfoot compensation.

6. Overcorrection resulting in a structurally abducted foot and medial column collapse.

7. Delayed union or non-union of one or more osteotomy site.

8. Stiff and fibrotic foot.

Clinical Pearls:

1. Intraoperatively, a gross but effective method of assuring proper alignment is to look at the lateral border of the foot and verify that it is a straight line.

2. Take the time intraoperatively to make sure that the cannulated screw pins are all inserted plumb to the respective osteotomies.

3. Use Intraoperative fluoroscopy to not only verify the apposition of the osteotomies but that a normal metatarsal parabola exists.

References:

Agnew PS. Metatarsus adductus and allied disorders. <u>McGlamry's Comprehensive Textbook of Foot and Ankle Surgery</u>. Banks AS et al, Ed., Lippincott Williams & Wilkins, Philadelphia, Pa., 2001.

Akin, S. An unusual and nonclassified central polydactyly of the foot. *Annals of Plastic Surgery* 53:86-88, 2004.

Baek GH, Chung MS. The treatment of congenital brachymetatarsia by one-stage lengthening. *J Bone Joint Surg (Br)* 80-B:1040-1044, 1998.

Barsky AJ. Macrodactyly. *J Bone Joint Surg (Am)* 49-A:1255-1266, 1967.

Berman A, Gartland JJ. Metatarsal osteotomy for the correction of adduction of the fore part of the foot in children. *J Bone Joint Surg (Am)* 53-A:498-506, 1971.

Burns AE. Revised tarsectomy for correction of relapsed clubfoot. *J Foot Surg* 23:275-278, 1984.

Chang CH, Kumar SJ, Riddle EC, Glutting J. Macrodactyly of the foot. *J Bone Joint Surg (Am)* 84-A:1189-1194, 2002.

Christensen JC, Leff FB, Lepow GM, Schwartz RI, colon PA, Arminio ST, Nixon P, Segel D, Leff S. Congenital polydactyly and polymetatarsalia: classification, genetics, and surgical correction. *J Foot Surg* 20:151-158, 1981.

Coppolelli BG, Ready JE, Awbrey BJ, Smith LS. Polydactyly of the foot in adults: literature review and unusual case presentation with diagnostic and treatment recommendations. *J Foot Surg* 30:12-18, 1991.

Dennyson WG, Bear JN, Bhoola KD. Macrodactyly in the foot. *J Bone Joint Surg (Br)* 59-B: 355-359, 1977.

DeValentine SJ. Miscellaneous Congenital Deformities. <u>Foot and Ankle Disorders in Children</u>. DeValentine SJ, Ed., Churchill Livingstone, New York, NY, 1992.

Fagan JP. Metatarsus Adductus. <u>Foot and Ankle Disorders in Children</u>. DeValentine SJ Ed. Churchill Livingstone, New York, NY, 1992.

Giorgini RJ, Rostkowski T, Japour C. Desyndactylization of the first and second toes using full-thickness autologous skin graft from the ankle. *J Am Pod Med Assn* 96:513-517, 2006.

Glover JP, Hyer CF, Berlet GC, Lee TH. Early results of the Mau osteotomy for correction of moderate to severe hallux valgus: A review of 24 cases. *J Foot & Ankle Surg* 47:237-242, 2008.

Goforth WP, Overbeek TD. Brachymetatarsia of the third and fourth metatarsals. *J Am Pod Med Assn* 91:373-378, 2001.

Gordon E, Luhmann SJ, Dobbs MB, Szymanski DA, Rich MM, Anderson DJ, Schoenecker PL. Combined midfoot osteotomy for severe fore foot adductus. *J Pediatr Orthop* 23:74-78, 2003.

Haber LL, Adams HB, Thompson GH, Duncan LS, DiDomenico LA, McCluskey WP. Unique Case of Polydactyly and a new classification system. *Pediatr Orthop* 27:326-328, 2007.

Hayashi A, Yanai A, Komuro Y, Nishida M. A new surgical technique for polysyndactyly of the toes without skin graft. *Plastic and Reconstructive Surg* 114(2):433-438, 2004.

Heyman CH, Herndon CH, Strong JM. Mobilization of the tarsometatarsal and intermetatarsal joints for the correction of resistant adduction of the fore part of the foot in congenital club-foot or congenital metatarsus varus. *J Bone Joint Surg (Am)* 40-A:299-310, 1958.

Itoh Y, Arai K. A new operation for syndactyly and polysyndactyly of the foot without skin grafts. *Br J Plastic Surg* 48(5): 306-311, 1995.

Kawabata H, Ariga K, Shibata T, Matsui Y. Open treatment of syndactyly of the foot. *Scand J Plast Reconstr Surg Hand Surg* 37:150-154, 2003.

Kim HT, Lee SH, Yoo CI, Kang JH, Sub JT. The management of brachymetatarsia. *J Bone Joint Surg (Br)* 85-B:683-690, 2003.

Kim JS, Black GH, Chung MS, Yoon PW. Multiple congenital brachymetatarsia. *J Bone Joint Surg (Br)* 86-B:1013-1015, 2004.

Kotwal PP, Farooque M. Macrodactyly. *J Bone Joint Surg (Br)* 80:651-653, 1998.

Lagoutaris ED, DiDomenico LA, Haber LL. Early surgical repair of macrodactyly. *J Am Pod Med Assn* 94:499-501, 2004.

Lee HS, Park SS, Yoon JO, Kin JS, Youm YS. Classification of Postaxial polydactyly of the foot. *Foot & Ankle Intl* 27:356-362, 2006.

Lim YJ, Teoh LC, Lee EH. Reconstruction of syndactyly and polysyndactyly of the toes with a dorsal pentagonal island flap: a technique that allows primary skin closure without the use of skin grafting. *J Foot & Ankle Surg* 46:86-92, 2007.

Manifis T. Surgery of metatarsus adductus. Curtin Health Science/Dept Podiatry Encyclopedia 1-15, 2007.

Marcinko DE, Hetico HR. Structural metatarsus adductus deformity, surgical case report. *J Foot Surg* 31:607-610, 1992.

Martin DE. Callus distraction. McGlamry's Forefoot Surgery Banks AS, et al Ed. Lippincott Williams & Wilkins, Philadelphia, Pa., 2004.

Masada K, Fujita S, Fuji T, Ohno H. Complications following metatarsal lengthening by callus distraction for brachymetatarsia. *J Pediatr Orthop* 19:394-397, 1999.

Masada K, Tsuyuguchi Y, Kawabata H, Ono K. Treatment of preaxial polydactyly of the foot. *Plast & Reconstr Surg* 79:251-258, 1987.

Morley SE, Smith PJ. Polydactyly of the feet in children: suggestions for surgical management. *Br J Plast Surg* 54:34-38, 2001.

Peabody CW, Muro F. Congenital metatarsus varus. Presented at the Annual Meeting of the American Orthopaedic Association, June 17, 1932.

Ponseti IV, Becker JH. Congenital metatarsus adductus: The results of treatment. *J Bone Joint Surg (Am)* 48-A:702-711, 1966.

Schimizzi A, Brage M. Brachymetatarsia. *Foot & Ankle Clinics* 9:555-570, 2004.

Shim JS, Park SJ. Treatment of brachymetatarsia by distraction osteogenesis. *J Pediatr Orthop* 26:250-254, 2006.

Togashi S, Nakayama Y, Hata J, Endo T. A new surgical method for treating lateral ray polydactyly with brachydactyly of the foot: lengthening the reconstructed fifth toe. *J Plast Reconstr & Aesth Surg* 59:752-758, 2006.

Toriyama K, Kamei Y, Morishita T, Matsuoka K, Torii S. Z-plasty of dorsal and plantar flaps for hallux varus with preaxial polydactyly of the foot. *Plast & Reconstr Surg* 117:112-115, 2006.

Tsuge K. Treatment of Macrodactyly. *Plast & Reconstr Surg* 39:590-599, 1967.

Turra S, Gigante C, Bisinella G. Polydactyly of the foot. *J Ped Ortho* 16:216-220, 2007.

Uda H, Sugawara Y, Niu A, Sarukawa S. Treatment of lateral ray polydactyly of the foot: focusing on the selection of the toe to be excised. *Plast & Reconstr Surg* 109:1581-1591, 2002.

Wagreich CR. Congenital Deformities. McGlamry's Comprehensive Textbook of Foot and Ankle Surgery. Banks A, et al, Ed. Lippincott Williams & Wilkins, Philadelphia, Pa., 2001.

Wan SC. Metatarsus adductus and skewfoot deformity. *Clinics in Podiatric Med & Surg* 23:23-40, 2006.

Watanabe H, Fujita S, Oka I. Polydactyly of the foot: an analysis of 265 cases and a morphological classification. *Plast & Reconstr Surg* 89:856-877, 1992.

Yamada N, Yasuda Y, Hashimoto, Iwashiro H, Uchinuma E. Use of internal callus distraction in the treatment of congenital brachymetatarsia. *Br J Plast Surg* 58:1014-1019, 2005.

Yu GV, John B, Freireich R. Surgical management of metatarsus adductus deformity. *Clinics in Podiatric Med & Surg* 4:207-232, 1987.

Index

Page numbers followed by an *f* denote figures.